Vivas and Communication Skills in
SURGERY

Commissioning Editor: Laurence Hunter
Project Development Manager: Siân Jarman
Project Manager: Nancy Arnott
Designer: Erik Bigland
Illustrator: Amanda Williams

Vivas and Communication Skills in SURGERY

Kathryn McCarthy MRCS(Eng) MRCS(Ed)
Research Fellow, Barts and The London NHS Trust, London, UK

Matthew Hacking FRCA
Consultant Anaesthetist, Royal Marsden Hospital, London, UK

Ragheed Al Mufti MB BCh BAO MSc MD FRCS(Eng)
FRCSEd(Gen)
Consultant Surgeon, Barts and The London NHS Trust,
London, UK

Jonathan Hewitt MSc MRCP
Research Fellow, NHS Research and Development,
Eastern Region, UK

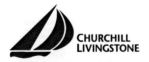
CHURCHILL
LIVINGSTONE

EDINBURGH   LONDON   NEW YORK   OXFORD   PHILADELPHIA
ST LOUIS   SYDNEY   TORONTO 2004

CHURCHILL LIVINGSTONE
An imprint of Elsevier Science Limited

First published 2004

ISBN 0-443-07342-2

British Library Cataloguing in Publication Data
A catalogue record for this book is available from the British Library

Library of Congress Cataloging in Publication Data
A catalog record for this book is available from the Library of Congress

Notice
Medical knowledge is constantly changing. Standard safety precautions must be
followed, but as new research and clinical experience broaden our knowledge,
changes in treatment and drug therapy may become necessary or appropriate.
Readers are advised to check the most current product information provided by
the manufacturer of each drug to be administered to verify the recommended
dose, the method and duration of administration, and contraindications. It is
the responsibility of the practitioner, relying on experience and knowledge of
the patient, to determine dosages and the best treatment for each individual
patient. Neither the Publisher nor the authors assumes any liability for any
injury and/or damage to persons or property arising from this publication.
The Publisher

The
publisher's
policy is to use
**paper manufactured
from sustainable forests**

Transferred to Digital Printing in 2009

This book has been written to aid any candidate preparing to sit a surgical viva, including undergraduate surgical finals, the MRCS examination and even as a brush-up to surgical registrars prior to the exit exam. It includes a broad range of topics from basic science through to clinically relevant scenarios and also incorporates some of the wider surgical issues such as epidemiology.

The viva component of the MRCS examination is traditionally the most feared and elusive part of the exam. Until recently, it constituted the final hurdle in a long, slow process. The viva component is now examined before the final clinical skills and communication skills bay. This may dampen the 'grande finale' effect of the viva, as the clinical stage traditionally has higher success rates; however, there will be no change in the level of knowledge required to pass the viva.

The Royal Colleges of Surgeons have provided a syllabus for the exam through a comprehensive list of core and system modules. There are ten in all. This certainly provides more structure to the exam than the previous haphazard reading of random chapters in a list of books. It is hard, however, as a candidate to imagine that, even if you managed to read up on the entire syllabus, it would equip you to deal with the onslaught of an oral exam.

It is our experience that some areas of the syllabus are 'exam favourites' and are more commonly asked than others. We have compiled a list of topics with commonly asked questions in viva style. Answers provided have been reviewed by college examiners and give the candidate some idea of how to deal with viva questions and what is required in order to pass the exam.

Unfortunately, half the battle is technique. As the exam looms nearer, many horror stories fly amongst candidates of previously asked nightmare questions or grossly unfair viva topics leading to exam failure. The best advice we can give is that if you fail the exam, you have failed it on your own merits. The examiner is rarely 'out to fail you'. They are meant to begin with simple questions and then test you to the limits of your knowledge. If you work hard and ensure you have a good understanding of the basic topics, you will not be caught out. Keep your answers simple and logically structured and you won't fail the exam.

The aim of this book is to provide some idea about the structure of this exam. We hope that it will help you improve your performance on the day.

London 2004

K.M.
M.H.
R.A.M.
J.H.

The authors would like to acknowledge the following individuals for their input to this text:

Dr Robert Whitaker MD MChir FRCS
Assistant Clinical Anatomist, University of Cambridge. MRCS examiner for RCS England and Edinburgh. Former Consultant Paediatric Urologist, Addenbrooke's Hospital, Cambridge

Mr Richard Novell MChir FRCS
Consultant Colorectal Surgeon, Luton and Dunstable Hospital. MRCS examiner for RCS England

Dr Simon Harrod FRCA
Consultant Anaesthetist, Barts and The London Queen Mary School of Medicine and Dentistry

Dr Liam Smeeth MRCGP MSc PhD
MRC Clinical Lecturer, London School of Hygiene and Tropical Medicine

Mr Mark Latimer MA MRCS(Eng) MRCS(Ed)
Specialist Registrar in Orthopaedic surgery, Eastern Region

Mr Adel Rateme FRCS(Ed) (illustrations)
Senior Specialist Registrar in General Surgery, Barts and The London Queen Mary School of Medicine and Dentistry

Dr Simon Clarke FRCA
Consultant Anaesthetist, University College Hospital

Dr Jonathon Cousins FRCA
Consultant Anaesthetist Hammersmith Hospital

Dr Paul Flynn BSc MRCP FRCA
Specialist registrar in Anaesthetics, University College Hospital

In addition, the authors wish to thank:

Philip Kelly and Naveen Cavale

Full details about the MRCS examination, including the new intercollegiate examination, can be found on the UK College websites: *www.rcseng.ac.uk, www.rcsed.ac.uk* and *www.rcpsglasg.ac.uk.*

The intercollegiate MRCS examination is divided into three parts. Parts 1 and 2 are MCQ papers on applied basic sciences and clinical problem solving. Part 3 is the viva and clinical skills examination and communication skills examination. This book deals with the viva and communication skills elements of Part 3.

In order to enter the MRCS viva examination you must first have obtained a pass in both MCQ papers. Requirements for the exam also include completion of 20 months of basic surgical training, completion of the ATLS course and Basic Surgical Skills course and an up-to-date, neatly filled in log book.

The MRCS viva examination comprises six 10-minute oral vivas grouped into three 20-minute slots. The slots are as follows;

- Applied surgical anatomy, operative surgery
- Clinical pathology, principles of surgery
- Applied physiology, critical care

The vivas are always paired in this manner, i.e. applied surgical anatomy is always examined in the same 20-minute slot as operative surgery. However, due to logistics on the day, you may find that the first viva you enter is in fact applied physiology and critical care. You will be taken to each viva site by an examination assistant and given full instructions. A bell is rung to indicate the end of each 20-minute viva. You should then return promptly to the assembly point, where you will be taken to the next part of the viva.

The clinical skills part of the exam is also accompanied by a communication skills section. It is not designed to test medical knowledge; however, you are expected to be accurate and examiners are allowed to fail you if you give wrong information.

There are three sections to the communications skills, as follows:

- Section 1 – giving information to a patient/relative (actor)
- Section 2 – ability to take a history and present relevant information to a hospital consultant (the examiner)
- Section 3 – ability to gather relevant information from a set of notes and communicate via a letter to the GP. This is a written test.

If any of the viva, clinical skills or communication skills section are failed, it is possible to retake them separately at a later date. If you fail the viva section alone, you would have to resit it at the next available sitting. You must pass the viva section before you can proceed to the final clinical skills examination for the MRCS. You will have to pass the communication skills section separately before being awarded the MRCS exam.

GENERAL TIPS

It is advisable to be as punctual as possible. You won't give your best performance if you are running late and have no idea where you are supposed to be. It is stressful enough without making things worse for yourself; after all, you may well be shown straight into the communication skills section.

It is always a good idea to make an effort with your appearance. Don't worry about 'overdressing' for the occasion. Almost all the men will turn up in suits. The women have a little more leeway; however, it is still advisable for them to dress smartly. It is not recommended that you bring in any sort of bag into the actual viva setting; there is usually a waiting area where you can ask another petrified candidate if they can keep an eye on it for you. Men should ensure that ties do not fall into the cadavers during the anatomy viva; the same applies to those with long hair.

The best approach to take on the day is a confident and honest one. It is a long day for the examiners and it is easier for them to give you marks if you take the time to answer the question in a logical manner, speaking clearly. This is best achieved by pausing for a short while after the question has been asked and not blurting out the first thing that comes to mind, unless you are absolutely sure it is correct. Honesty is definitely the best policy. You have been trained through a lifetime of MCQs to make logical guesses; however, in an oral exam you will instil more confidence in the examiner if you honestly admit when you don't know something, as opposed to making the answer up. If you are wrong, you will be deemed to be unsafe and they will be obliged to fail you. If you state that you don't know the answer to the question, the examiner will have no choice but to move on to a different topic which you may know extremely well and, chances are, they may forget the whole incident.

Examiners have been strictly warned not to say 'good' or 'well done'. This may give you a falsely positive impression. Therefore don't look for any sort of recognition about your performance. It is generally thought that the more questions you get asked, the better you are doing. Once you have answered a question, you may be swiftly moved on to a new topic. Go with the flow and just hope that you are racking up the points. The general rule of the day is to begin with what the examiners consider to be an easy question and then take you to the limits of your knowledge. The initial question, therefore, is more or less pass/fail. If you think the questions are very difficult, then you are either doing extremely well, or you have not quite reached the standard required to pass the exam. If you have done the right amount of work it may be possible for you to lead the viva. This is the best way of turning the situation to your advantage. You don't have to be arrogant or aggressive, just keep on the ball and try to lead the discussion in the direction you would like it to go in. Try finishing your answer with a topic you are familiar with, which can then lead on to further discussion. The examiner will get very bored and infuriated if he/she has to drag the answers out of you.

Examiners are now limited to a list of topics that they can ask you. Gone are the days when they can ask you their little 'pet favourite' questions. Believe it or not, they are all trying to pass you. They can't pass you if they think that you are unsafe.

APPLIED SURGICAL ANATOMY/OPERATIVE SURGERY

This section lasts 10 minutes for each part, separated by a bell. There will be three people sitting behind the desk as you approach. One will be the clinical anatomist who will start off the first 10-minute viva; the second one will be a surgeon who will take your log book off you and will browse through it during the anatomy part of the exam. The third person will also be a surgeon who will observe the 20-minute exam and give his/her opinion on marking once you have left.

The clinical anatomist may lead you to a cadaver which usually comprises a whole body that has been dissected. You may be given a stick to point with, so watch out for shakiness. Once you have been asked several questions such as 'Show me where the ureter is?' or 'Where is the vagus nerve in the neck?' you may then be led back to the desk where you will see a selection of bones. Common exam bones include the skull, the hand (carpal bones), the radius, the femur and the clavicle; however, be prepared for anything from an atypical rib to a lumbar vertebra. It is considered to be an outright fail if you cannot side or articulate obvious bones such as the tibia and femur. In Edinburgh, you are not likely to come across any cadavers. Instead you may be handed plastic specimens, such as the bronchopulmonary segments, rather than being shown a cadaver. Often there are plastic specimens, for example skulls, lying on the desk and you may well not be asked about them at all. It is a good idea to visit a dissection room before the exam as it may have been a long time since you last saw a cadaver. It is all very well learning the anatomy off by heart from a book, but there is no substitute for looking comfortable with the cadaver on the day. That also includes the way you handle the specimen. All these aspects give the examiner some idea of the extent of your revision. Obviously the anatomy demonstrators have an advantage; however, it doesn't take a huge amount of effort to develop similar confidence with cadavers.

Occasionally you may come across a volunteer sitting on a couch in a dressing gown, waiting to be examined. As part of the anatomy viva you may be shown to the model and asked to demonstrate some surface anatomy such as, 'Show me the spinal root of the accessory nerve?' or 'Show me the surface markings of the pleura?' It upsets the examiner greatly if you make a meal of introducing yourself to the 'patient'. They are there for the purposes of the anatomical demonstration only. It is good enough to simply be polite and say 'hello' and swiftly move on to what you have been asked to do.

For the operative surgery viva the surgeon will usually ask you something from your log book. If you have performed an operation yourself, you will be expected to have a reasonable knowledge about it. Alternatively, you may be asked something like 'I see you have some experience in cardiothoracic surgery, tell me how you would manage an aortic dissection'. It pays to go through your log book carefully before the exam so that you won't get caught out.

CLINICAL PATHOLOGY/PRINCIPLES OF SURGERY

This part of the viva is usually quite straightforward. You will begin with pathology while the other surgeon peruses your log book. You may well be given a case scenario leading to various topics such as methods of histological diagnosis.

Pathologists are also hot on definitions, so learn them well as it may be all you get asked. In the second viva, you will be asked on general topics that you should be familiar with, regardless of whether or not it appears in your log book, i.e. retention of urine.

APPLIED PHYSIOLOGY/CRITICAL CARE

This part of the exam is said to have the highest fail rate. The examiners are usually physiologists and ITU consultants. Alternatively, there may be a surgeon who examines for physiology. There is no escaping proper revision of your basic medical sciences at this point. It will become quite obvious to the examiner if you have not put the hours in. As long as you demonstrate a good level of understanding of the basic concepts, you should be able to pass this part of the exam. The examiners are not deliberately trying to catch you out.

You may be handed a blank piece of paper and asked to draw the venous waveforms encountered as you insert a Swann–Ganz catheter or a graph demonstrating oxygen dissociation. Do a few practice runs beforehand – particularly graphs, as it suddenly becomes difficult to label the x and y axes when you are under pressure.

MARKING SCHEME

Each viva is marked out of 5.

    1 = outright fail
    2 = bare fail
    3 = pass
    4 = good pass
    5 = outstanding.

There are six vivas in all, therefore you will get a mark out of 30. It is currently understood that the pass mark is effectively 17. You are in fact expected to pass (obtain a '3') in all sections. However, there is some leeway for the examiners to allow a '2' in one section. If you were to get two '2's' then you would need a '4' in another section in order to pass. You will be failed, however, if you are awarded two 2's in the same section, i.e. anatomy and operative surgery, or if you get more than two '2's'. Similarly, it is frowned upon to perform badly in anatomy and you may be failed on the basis of that alone.

The average mark awarded for a good candidate is 3. In order to be awarded a '4', you will need a good working knowledge of all that's asked and confidently be able to answer more in-depth questions. To obtain a '5', your level of knowledge and ability to answer questions must be excellent. Before awarding a '5', the examiner may see how you perform in the second of the two vivas to get an overall impression of the breadth of your knowledge. Most good candidates should have a high standard in all sections. It is unlikely that you will be awarded a '5' in one viva and a '2' in the accompanying viva.

READING LIST

The Royal College of Surgeons provides a reading list that covers the MCQ papers, the viva and the clinical skills section. The following books may also be useful in preparing for the viva examination:

Abrahams PH, Marks SC, Hutchings R. McMinns' Colour Atlas of Human Anatomy. 5th edn. Mosby, 2002.
Burnand KG, Young AE. The New Aird's Companion in Surgical Studies. 2nd edn. Churchill Livingstone, 1998.
Despopoulos A, Silbernagl S. Color Atlas of Physiology. 5th edn. Thieme, 2003.
Lumley JSP. Surface Anatomy. 3rd edn. Churchill Livingstone, 2002.
Sinnatamby CS. Last's Anatomy. 10th edn. Churchill Livingstone, 1999.
Underwood JCE. General and Systematic Pathology. 3rd edn. Churchill Livingstone, 2000.
Whitaker RH, Borley N. Instant Anatomy. 2nd edn. Blackwell Science, 2000.

APPLIED SURGICAL ANATOMY

SURFACE ANATOMY CHEST WALL

Q. Where would you palpate the apex of the heart?

A. The apex of the heart may be palpated at the left fifth intercostal space, in the mid-clavicular line.

Q. If you auscultated the heart in this area what would you hear?

A. It should be possible to hear the mitral valve closing at the apex of the heart.

Q. What are the surface markings of the heart?

A. The heart may be traced from the third rib at the right sternal edge to the second rib at the left sternal edge. From here, the heart may be traced to the apex at the mid-clavicular line, fifth intercostal space. The inferior border of the heart can then be traced horizontally across the midline to the right sternal edge at the level of the sixth rib. The heart may then be followed back to the third rib at the right sternal edge. (Remember 3–2–5½–6.)

Q. What are the surface markings of the right pleura?

A. The right pleura extends approximately 3 cm above the middle of the medial third of the clavicle. From here it travels anteriorly to meet the left pleura at the sternum. They travel together until the fourth rib when they begin to diverge. The right pleura is still parasternal at the sixth rib; however, it then travels to the mid-clavicular line at the level of the eighth rib. From there, it travels to the mid-axillary line at the tenth costal cartilage and travels along the 12th rib. (Remember 4–6–8–10–12 (even numbers).)

Q. How does this differ on the left side?

A. On the left the pleura has to make way for the heart. As a result, the left pleura comes away from the sternum at the sixth costal cartilage instead of at the eighth. Otherwise, the surface markings are the same on both sides.

Q. How do the surface markings of the lungs correspond to this?

A. The lungs correspond to the markings of the pleura except inferiorly. Here they extend two rib spaces above the pleural markings, below the sixth rib.

Q. What are the surface markings of the lung fissures?

A. The surface markings of the lung fissures include:

- Oblique fissure (both sides) – coincides with a line from the third thoracic spine to the sixth costochondral junction
- Horizontal fissure (right lung only) – follows a line from the oblique fissure in the mid-axillary line to the fourth costal cartilage on the right-hand side.

Q. Where does the trachea divide?

A. The trachea divides at the level of the sternal angle.

Q. What are the surface markings of the female breast?

A. The female breast lies on the pectoralis major, serratus anterior and external oblique. It extends from the second to the sixth rib. Medially it extends to the lateral border of the sternum and laterally it reaches the anterior wall of the axilla.

In males, the nipple lies at the level of the fourth intercostal cartilage at the mid-clavicular line.

Q. What types of thoracotomy incisions do you know?

A.
- Midline sternotomy – this approach is used for most cardiac operations
- Left anterolateral thoracotomy – at the level of the fifth rib, useful in operations involving the mitral valve
- Left posterolateral thoracotomy – through the fourth rib when trying to access the hilum of the lung and the seventh/eighth rib when trying to access the posterior mediastinum or oesophagogastric region.

SURFACE ANATOMY ABDOMEN

Q. What is the surface marking of the gallbladder?

A. The surface marking of the gallbladder is at the level of the right ninth costal cartilage at the mid-clavicular line.

Q. Where does the abdominal aorta bifurcate?

A. The abdominal aorta bifurcates at the level of the umbilicus or the fourth lumbar vertebra.

Q. Where is the transpyloric plane?

A. The transpyloric plane is a plane horizontal to a line connecting the jugular notch and the pubic symphysis. It is approximately halfway between the xiphisternum and umbilicus.

Q. What structures may be found at this level?

A. The plane passes through:

- Fundus of the gallbladder
- Lower border of L1 vertebra
- Spinal cord ends
- Pylorus
- Neck of pancreas
- Attachment of the transverse mesocolon
- Superior mesenteric artery branching off the aorta
- Portal vein formed from the superior mesenteric vein and splenic vein
- Hilum of both kidneys

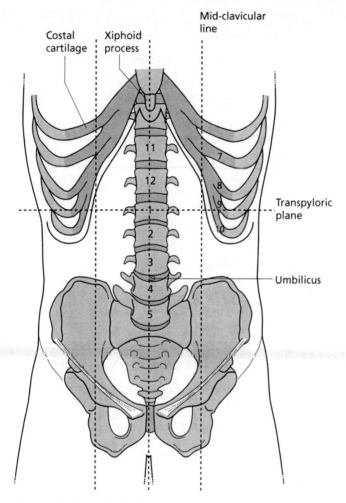

Fig. 1 The transpyloric plane

- Second part of the duodenum
- Hilum of the spleen
- Duodenojejunal junction.

Q. What dermatome surrounds the umbilicus?

A. The umbilicus is at the level of the L4 vertebra and its dermatome is T10.

SURFACE ANATOMY | LONG SAPHENOUS VEIN

Q. What is the course of the long saphenous vein in the lower leg?

A. The long saphenous vein passes anterior to the medial malleolus. From here, it obliquely crosses the lower end of the medial surface of the tibia. It then runs up the medial surface of the tibia towards the knee. At the knee, the long saphenous vein lies one hand's breadth behind the medial aspect of the patella and from there it travels along the medial aspect of the thigh to the saphenous opening in the cribriform fascia. Here it joins up with the femoral vein which travels into the pelvis.

Q. Do you know of any veins that drain into the long saphenous vein at the level of the saphenous opening?

A. Commonly, there are four veins that drain into the long saphenous vein:

- Superior epigastric
- Superficial external pudendal
- Deep external pudendal
- Superficial circumflex iliac.

SURFACE ANATOMY | ACCESSORY NERVE

Q. What is the surface marking of the spinal root of the accessory nerve in the posterior triangle?

A. The spinal root of the accessory nerve may be found emerging one third of the way down the posterior surface of the sternocleidomastoid muscle and travelling downwards beneath the anterior surface of the trapezius, two thirds of the way down.

Q. What does the accessory nerve supply?

A. The cranial root of the accessory nerve joins the vagus and the spinal root supplies the trapezius and sternocleidomastoid muscles.

Q. What occurs if the spinal root of the accessory nerve is damaged in this area?

A. If the spinal root of the accessory nerve is damaged before it enters the sternocleidomastoid, the patient will be unable to turn his/her face to the opposite side. If the nerve is damaged in the posterior triangle, however, the trapezius will be paralysed and so the patient will be unable to shrug their shoulder on the affected side.

Q. Where are the groups of lymph nodes in the neck situated?

A. There are essentially two rings and two chains of lymph nodes in the neck. The two rings are superficial and deep. The deep ring is situated around the nasopharynx and includes:

- Palatine tonsil
- Oropharynx
- Nasopharynx.

The superficial ring includes:

- Occipital
- Retro-auricular
- Superficial parotid
- Deep parotid
- Submental
- Submandibular nodes.

The deep cervical lymph chain follows the internal jugular vein and includes:

- Digastric nodes
- Carotid triangle nodes
- Omohyoid group
- Nodes in the posterior triangle.

The superficial lymph chain follows the external and anterior jugular veins.

EMBRYOLOGY   DEVELOPMENT OF THE HEART

It is unlikely that you will be asked questions on this topic; however, it is a good idea to have some knowledge of it, although because it is a difficult topic you won't be expected to have a detailed knowledge.

Q. How does the primitive heart develop from the yolk sac?

A. The primitive heart begins as angioblasts on the wall of the yolk sac which develop into blood vessels. A single heart tube is produced by two blood vessels that join together. The heart tube then develops a muscular wall and becomes pulsatile. It grows in a cephalo–caudal direction and divides into four parts called:

- Bulb
- Ventricle
- Atrium
- Sinus venosus.

It is surrounded by a cavity that later develops into the pericardium.

Due to the rapid growth of the heart tube, folding occurs within the pericardium. This results in the bulb and ventricle lying anterior to the atrium and sinus venosus.

Q. How does the aorta develop?

A. The aorta and pulmonary trunk both develop from the bifurcation of the truncus arteriosus. The truncus arteriosus develops from the upper region of the bulb.

Q. What develops from the lower part of the bulb?

A. The lower part of the bulb develops into the smooth outflow area of the right ventricle. The left ventricle is primarily derived from the ventricle of the original single heart tube.

Q. Where is the foramen ovale situated?

A. The foramen ovale is situated within the septum dividing the right and left atria. It is formed from a gap beneath the septum secundum which leads to the secondary foramen (*ostium secundum*) in the septum primum.

Q. What is its significance?

A. The foramen ovale allows blood to pass from the right to the left atrium as a crucial part of the fetal circulation.

Q. What happens to the foramen ovale after birth?

A. The foramen ovale generally closes at birth with the onset of respiration. This results from an increase in left atrial pressure which forces the septum primum and secundum to oppose and then fuse.

Occasionally, complete fusion does not occur and a passage remains at the site of the foramen ovale. It is not usually physiologically significant. However, it may be possible to demonstrate it during cardiac angiography.

Q. What is the significance of the pectinate muscles?

A. The pectinate muscles constitute the 'rough' area of the wall of the right atrium. It represents the embryonic remains of the original atria.

Q. What congenital abnormalities of the heart do you know about?

A. Common congenital cardiac abnormalities may be classified into:

- Atrial septal defects – these include abnormalities of the septum primum or secundum
- Ventricular septal defects – mostly affecting the upper fibrous area of the septum
- Fallot's tetralogy – pulmonary stenosis, ventricular septal defect, right ventricular hypertrophy and an overriding aorta.

Other common congenital cardiac abnormalities include patent ductus arteriosus, coarctation of the aorta and, more rarely, transposition of the great vessels.

EMBRYOLOGY FETAL CIRCULATION

Q. How is blood oxygenated in the fetal circulation?

A. Blood is oxygenated via the placenta which acts as the 'lung' of the fetal circulation.

Q. How does this oxygenated blood travel from the placenta to the fetus?

A. Oxygenated blood travels via the left umbilical vein into the porta hepatis of the fetus. In adult life, the remnant of this structure is called the ligamentum teres. From here it passes into the ductus venosus, partially bypassing the liver, and then into the inferior vena cava.

Q. What is the name of this structure in adult life?

A. The ductus venosus thromboses and becomes fibrous in adult life. It is then known as the ligamentum venosum.

Q. Where does oxygenated blood go once it's in the right atrium?

A. Once in the right atrium, oxygenated blood then travels through the foramen ovale, within the interatrial septum, to the left atrium. This way the lungs are completely bypassed. From the left atrium blood travels into the left ventricle, aorta and then to the head via the carotid arteries and the upper limbs via the subclavian arteries.

Q. How does venous blood return to the placenta for reoxygenation?

A. Venous blood from the head returns via the brachiocephalic veins to the superior vena cava. It enters the right atrium and flows into the right ventricle without mixing with the oxygenated blood travelling to the left atrium. From the right ventricle it passes into the pulmonary trunk. It then passes into the ductus arteriosus due to the high vascular resistance within the pulmonary vasculature and the low resistance within the fetal aorta and placental vessels.

The ductus arteriosus connects the left pulmonary artery to the aorta just distal to the origin of the left subclavian artery. From here the venous blood mixes with the oxygenated blood that hasn't reached the carotids. Most of the fetal oxygenated blood, therefore, is used to supply the head.

Once in the aorta, the venous blood travels back to the placenta via two umbilical arteries which are branches of the common iliac arteries.

Q. What is the name given to the ductus arteriosus in adult life?

A. It is called the ligamentum arteriosum.

Q. What is a patent ductus arteriosus?

A. A patent ductus arteriosus (PDA) is where the ductus arteriosus remains open after birth. At birth, there is a dramatic increase in aortic pressure as the blood ceases to flow through the placenta. There is also a dramatic fall in pulmonary artery pressure with the expansion of the lungs and hence blood flow reverses within the ductus arteriosus. It is thought that this reversal of blood flow causes the ductus to be exposed to much higher levels of oxygen within the blood and, in response, the muscular walls constrict and the ductus closes. This usually occurs within 12 hours of birth. Other theories attribute the failure to close to the vasodilatory effects of prostaglandins which may be overcome by administering indomethacin.

If the ductus arteriosus remains patent, a shunt may develop from the left to the right side of the heart. If the shunt becomes large, blood is pumped from the high-pressure left side of the heart to the low-pressure right side. The right side can become overloaded as a result and the PDA may need to be ligated.

EMBRYOLOGY DEVELOPMENT OF THE GUT

Questions on this topic are similarly not likely to be asked. However, I came across one candidate who was asked on this topic and he had missed it out of his revision because it was unlikely to come up.

Q. Can you describe what happens to the gut at 4 weeks?

A. At 4 weeks, the embryological gut exists as a single tube from the mouth to the cloaca. It is suspended in the dorsal mesentery which is attached to the posterior abdominal wall. The dorsal mesentery attaches to the anterior surface of the aorta in order to allow branches of the aorta to supply the length of the gut.

Q. What are the names of these branches and the areas that they supply?

A. The branches are called:

- Coeliac artery (trunk) – supplies the foregut including lower oesophagus, stomach, duodenum, liver, pancreas and spleen
- Superior mesenteric artery – from the duodenum (distal to the bile duct) to the distal transverse colon
- Inferior mesenteric artery – distal transverse colon to the anal canal.

Q. What happens to the gut at the sixth week?

A. By the sixth week, the gut is growing at such a rate, the size of the abdominal cavity is unable to keep up. As a result, it herniates out through the umbilicus until approximately 4 weeks later when the abdomen has grown big enough to allow it to return.

Q. Which part of the gut usually herniates?

A. It is usually the midgut that herniates. It remains attached to the abdomen by the vitellointestinal duct.

Q. What happens to the vitellointestinal duct after birth?

A. In postnatal life, the remnant of the vitellointestinal duct may persist and is known as Meckel's diverticulum. It is 2 inches long, is situated along the antimesenteric border and is characteristically found two feet proximal to the iliocaecal junction. It is more commonly found in men.

Q. What is the name given to the condition where the herniated gut contents fail to return to the abdomen?

A. Exomphalos.

EMBRYOLOGY   PHARYNGEAL ARCHES AND POUCHES

Q. What are the pharyngeal pouches?

A. The pharyngeal pouches are otherwise known as branchial pouches. They are pouches which develop from the lining of the pharynx between the pharyngeal arches.

Q. What are the pharyngeal arches?

A. Pharyngeal arches are derived embryologically from mesodermal structures that grow ventrally from the lining of the pharynx. They fuse in the midline to form six arches.

Each arch contains cartilage, muscle, an artery and a cranial nerve to supply all that develops within it.

Q. What are the names of the arches and their contents?

A. The names of the pharyngeal arches include:

First arch (mandibular)

- Meckel's cartilage
- Mandible
- Mucous membrane (anterior two thirds of the tongue)
- Muscles of mastication
- Mandibular nerve
- Maxillary artery.

Second arch (hyoid)

- Muscles of facial expression
- Stapes, styloid process, stylohyoid ligament, lesser horn and superior part of body of hyoid bone
- Facial nerve.

Third arch

- Greater horn and inferior part of hyoid bone
- Stylopharyngeus muscle
- Glossopharyngeal nerve.

Fourth and sixth arches

- Thyroid, cricoid, epiglottic, arytenoids cartilage
- Intrinsic muscles of the larynx and pharynx
- Laryngeal and pharyngeal branches of the vagus nerve.

Fifth arch

- Disappears.

Q. What is a branchial cyst?

A. A branchial cyst is the persistence of the ectoderm of the cervical sinus. This sinus forms as the pharyngeal clefts fuse. Usually the ectoderm that forms the cervical sinus disappears. Clinically it presents as a lump in the anterior triangle of the neck present from birth.

UPPER LIMB | SHOULDER JOINT

Q. What type of joint is the shoulder joint?

A. The shoulder is a ball and socket synovial joint which is made up of the head of the humerus and the glenoid cavity.

Q. Can you tell me any other ball and socket joints that you know of?

A. Yes, the hip joint. Also the sternoclavicular joint and the talocalcaneonavicular joints both act as ball and socket joints.

Q. What features are specific to the shoulder ball and socket joint?

A. The head of the humerus is approximately four times the size of the glenoid cavity, which is also quite shallow. The joint capsule is also lax inferiorly allowing for a wide range of movement.

Q. You mentioned that the humeral head is four times the size of the glenoid. What makes the shoulder joint stable?

A. Yes, the disproportionate size of the humerus with the glenoid cavity and the laxity of the capsule make the shoulder joint inherently unstable; however, there are several features that contribute to the joint's stability. Firstly, the labrum of the glenoid is made of fibro-cartilage and deepens the glenoid cavity. Secondly, there is support from the glenohumeral and coracohumeral ligaments, which reinforce the capsule. The capsule is also strengthened by the insertion of the rotator cuff muscles.

Q. What is the rotator cuff made up of?

A. The rotator cuff comprises the subscapularis, supraspinatus, infraspinatus and teres minor. They fuse with the superior and lateral side of the capsule and attach onto the humerus.

Q. What types of shoulder dislocation do you know about?

A. The most common dislocation of the shoulder is downwards and anteriorly. It is also possible to dislocate the shoulder posteriorly, although it is less common.

Q. Why is this?

A. This is because the shoulder is least supported at the inferior joint margin and after being forced out of joint inferiorly, the arm then hangs by the side of the body pushing the humeral head in front of the glenoid.

Q. What muscles are involved in abduction of the shoulder joint?

A. Firstly, the supraspinatus initiates the movement of abduction. Then, the deltoid acts by further and more powerfully abducting the arm. The scapula must then rotate, bringing the glenoid upwards. This is performed by the trapezius and serratus anterior. Then lateral rotation of the humerus occurs via the infraspinatus and teres minor.

UPPER LIMB AXILLA

Q. Describe the boundaries of the axilla.

A. The axilla is bounded anteriorly by the pectoralis major, pectoralis minor, sub-clavius and the clavipectoral fascia. This makes up the anterior axillary fold. The posterior axillary fold is made up of the subscapularis and teres major. Medially the serratus anterior is covered by axillary fascia. The lateral margin is the bicipital groove. The axilla extends to the level of the fourth rib.

Q. What are the contents of the axilla?

A. The axilla contains the axillary artery which is a continuation of the subclavian artery, the axillary vein, the brachial plexus and the axillary lymph nodes.

Q. At what point does the subclavian artery become the axillary artery?

A. The axillary artery is formed when the subclavian artery passes over the outer border of the first rib and enters the axilla. It becomes the brachial artery at the lower border of the teres major.

Q. What groups of lymph nodes are present in the axilla?

A. There are approximately 25–30 lymph nodes in total present in the axilla. There are thought to be five groups of nodes in the axilla. These are called the anterior, posterior, lateral, central and apical. All groups are thought to drain into the apical group before draining into either the thoracic duct or the subclavian vein.

Q. Where does the breast drain to?

A. The breast drains primarily to the axilla. Commonly the anterior groups are affected first and these lie along the distal border of the pectoralis minor. The medial breast also drains along the internal mammary vessels. Occasionally there may be drainage along the intercostal vessels, and lymphatic channels exist from one breast to the other; therefore, drainage is possible across the chest wall. Rarely there may be direct drainage to the supra-clavicular nodes; these shouldn't be missed out on a breast examination.

Q. What do you know about 'sentinel node localization' in breast surgery?

A. Sentinel node biopsy is a new technique that is being developed in breast surgery. It stems from the need to accurately stage the axilla in order to give useful information about the prognosis of the disease. If we were to perform an axillary clearance on every person who had breast cancer then we would see a lot of morbidity as a result. For some small tumours it is possible to perform an axillary sample where we remove approximately four lymph glands blindly from the axilla in order to gain information about possible nodal involvement. This is associated with much less morbidity.

Sentinel node localization provides us with a way of obtaining more reliable information about which node the tumour drains to first. It is performed using methylene blue dye which is injected around the tumour site at operation and preoperative infiltration of the area using radioisotope colloid injection. On inspection of the axilla at operation, the sentinel node should demonstrate a blue discoloration, and this may be confirmed as 'hot' by counts detected using a Geiger counter.

This technique allows us to identify the 'sentinel node' with a high degree of certainty. The node can then be assessed histologically for the presence of metastases. It may also be possible to use this technique to guide an axillary sampling procedure.

Q. You mentioned that there is morbidity associated with axillary dissections. What do you mean by this?

A. As I mentioned before, it is often important to perform an axillary procedure in order to gain useful information about the prognosis of the breast cancer. It is also useful in minimizing uncontrollable axillary recurrence.

Common problems encountered following an axillary dissection include wound infection and poor wound healing. Seromas are also a common occurrence; however, it is debatable whether this is actually a complication or natural sequelae. A stiff shoulder is also a common complaint postoperatively. Nerve injury may occur intraoperatively. The most commonly affected nerve is the intercostobrachial nerve (T2) which carries sensory fibres to the upper medial aspect of the arm. Patients affected complain of numbness and tingling in this distribution. Other nerves at risk include the long thoracic nerve of Bell and the thoracodorsal nerve. Injury to these would result in a winged scapula and a paralysed latissimus dorsi respectively.

Also, a small proportion of patients develop lymphoedema in the affected arm. This is more common in patients who undergo axillary clearance as opposed to a sample. It is also far more likely to occur if surgery to the axilla is combined with radiotherapy. It is usually managed effectively by symptomatic treatment with arm sleeves, use of antibiotics when necessary and regular follow-up with the breast-care nurses.

UPPER LIMB BRACHIAL PLEXUS LESIONS

Q. Where is the brachial plexus?

A. The brachial plexus supplies the upper limb and is formed in the root of the neck. It emerges between the scalene muscles, passes through the posterior triangle of the neck and behind the clavicle before innervating the upper limb.

Q. What are the root values of the brachial plexus?

A. The roots of the brachial plexus are made up from the anterior rami of C5–T1 originating from the cervical spinal cord.

Q. What comprises a spinal nerve?

A. A spinal nerve is made up of anterior and posterior nerve roots which leave the spinal cord and join together to form a spinal nerve. They are also accompanied by sympathetic fibres to their final destination and provide vasomotor, sudomotor and pilomotor function to the skin. C1 is the only spinal nerve that doesn't supply skin and there are 31 pairs of spinal nerves in total. After leaving the intervertebral foramen the spinal nerve then divides into anterior and posterior rami. The anterior rami then become plexuses such as the brachial or lumbar plexus. The posterior rami supplies the erector spinae, transversospinalis and the levator costae muscles of the thorax.

Q. What type of fibres do the anterior and posterior roots contain?

A. The anterior roots provide motor supply and the posterior roots provide sensory innervation.

Q. What are the first three branches from the roots of the brachial plexus?

A. The first branch is called the dorsal scapular nerve (C5). This nerve primarily supplies the rhomboids and also gives a branch to the levator scapulae. The second branch is the nerve to the subclavius (C5, 6). The third is the long thoracic nerve of Bell (C5, 6, 7) which supplies the serratus anterior (see Tip).

Q. What clinical sign might you see when the long thoracic nerve is injured?

A. A winged scapula.

Q. What types of brachial plexus injuries do you know of?

A. Brachial plexus injuries may be partial or complete. Complete avulsion of the brachial plexus is an extremely rare injury often sustained during high-speed motorcycle accidents. Partial brachial plexus injuries may be divided into those that affect the upper roots, known as Erb's paralysis (C5, 6) and those affecting the lower roots known as Klumpke's paralysis (C8, T1).

Q. How would you differentiate these injuries?

A. Complete avulsion of the brachial plexus would result in the affected limb hanging by the side. It would be completely immobile, numb, and may have an associated Horner's syndrome if the nearby sympathetic fibres to the pupil are affected (T1). It may be possible to detect the level of injury by testing muscle groups in the upper limb. For example, if the serratus anterior and rhomboids are working, then the level of injury will be below the roots.

Erb's paralysis is the commonest injury of the brachial plexus. It is caused by downward traction on the upper limb during childbirth. It affects roots C5 and 6 and results in paralysis of abduction and lateral rotation of the arm. The muscles affected include the supraspinatus, deltoid, infraspinatus, teres minor and the supinators (biceps and supinator). The arm hangs by the side of the body, is medially rotated and pronated. Also there is loss of sensation affecting the lateral arm including the lateral forearm and thumb.

Klumpke's paralysis involves damage to the lower roots C8 and T1. It may be caused by a childbirth injury when the child is delivered breech and the arm is pulled forcibly upwards. It may also be caused by a cervical rib. This condition results in 'claw hand' due to paralysis of the intrinsic muscles of the hand. It also causes loss of sensation of the medial forearm and the ulnar one and a half digits.

✔ TIP

It is a good idea to learn all the branches of the various parts of the brachial plexus. It may seem very laborious; however, it is best not to be caught out and will impress the examiner if you have taken the time to learn them all.

Branches of the roots (3)
- Dorsal scapular nerve
- Nerve to subclavius
- Long thoracic nerve of Bell.

Branch of the upper trunk (1)
- Suprascapular nerve.

Branches of the lateral cord (3)
- Lateral pectoral nerve
- Musculocutaneous nerve
- Lateral head of the median nerve.

✔ **TIP–cont'd**

Branches of the medial cord (5)
- Medial pectoral nerve
- Medial head of median nerve
- Medial cutaneous nerve of the arm
- Medial cutaneous nerve of the forearm
- Ulnar nerve.

Branches of the posterior cord (5)
- Upper subscapular nerve
- Thoracodorsal nerve
- Lower subscapular nerve
- Axillary nerve
- Radial nerve.

UPPER LIMB   CUBITAL FOSSA/ELBOW

Q. Where is the cubital fossa?

A. It is a triangular space in the elbow at the level of the humeral epicondyles. It is bounded by the pronator teres and the brachioradialis.

Q. What does it contain?

A. It contains the median nerve, brachial artery, tendon of the biceps, radial nerve and its posterior interosseous branch.

Q. What is the position of the brachial artery in relation to the median nerve at this level?

A. It lies lateral to the median nerve.

Q. What are the branches of the median nerve above the level of the elbow joint?

A. The only branches of the median nerve above the elbow include a vascular branch to the brachial artery and occasionally a branch to the pronator teres.

Q. What is the course of the posterior interosseous nerve in the cubital fossa?

A. The posterior interosseous nerve is a branch of the radial nerve and comes off in the cubital fossa. From there it supplies the extensor carpi radialis brevis and supinator. It then leaves the cubital fossa between the two heads of the supinator muscle to supply the forearm extensors.

Q. What are the branches of the ulnar nerve in the arm?

A. The ulnar nerve has no branches in the arm. Its first branch is to the elbow joint which comes off in the groove of the medial epicondyle of the humerus.

Q. What type of joint is the elbow?

A. It is a synovial hinge joint involving the lower end of the humerus and the radius and ulna. Flexion and extension are the only movements possible at this joint.

Q. How are pronation and supination possible in the forearm, given this limitation of movement at the elbow?

A. Pronation and supination occur at the superior and inferior radioulnar joints. In pronation, the head of the radius rotates in the fibro-osseous ring which is made up of the annular ligament and the radial notch of the ulnar. The capsule of the elbow does not attach to the radius; instead it attaches to the annular ligament allowing the radius to move freely within it.

Q. What muscles are responsible for these movements?

A. The pronator quadratus and pronator teres are responsible for pronation. The biceps and supinator are responsible for supination. Supination is the more powerful movement, maximally so when the elbow is flexed.

Q. Do you know of any lymph nodes around the elbow?

A. The supratrochlear nodes are situated around the medial epicondyle of the humerus. They drain the medial forearm and hand, and pass to the lateral axillary lymph nodes.

Q. What do you know about the 'carrying angle' of the elbow?

A. The carrying angle is the angle of the ulna in relation to the humerus when fully extended. It is approximately 170°. It means that when the arms hang by the side of the body, the elbow fits into the waist. It is more obvious in women.

Q. What are the risks associated with supracondylar fractures in children?

A. Supracondylar fractures in children tend to be a result of a fall onto an out-stretched hand. The elbow is hyper-extended and the result is a posterior displacement of the distal humerus and elbow joint beyond the fracture site. It is associated with neurovascular injuries. Nerve injury may affect the brachial, ulnar or median nerves. The brachial artery may be injured by the extreme anterior displacement of the proximal fragment of the humerus or may be lacerated on sharp fracture-site fragments. It is therefore important to diagnose the condition early to prevent irreversible ischaemia.

Other relevant complications include compartment syndrome which may occur on its own or may develop after reduction and immobilization. If this isn't diagnosed early and treated, Volkmann's ischaemic contracture may develop.

In the long term, if the child's fracture malunites they may develop a cubitus valgus or varus deformity where there is excessive angulation at the elbow. They may also suffer with elbow stiffness for a considerable amount of time after treatment.

UPPER LIMB   ANATOMICAL SNUFFBOX

Q. What do you understand by the term 'anatomical snuffbox'?

A. The anatomical snuffbox is a depression that occurs on the radial side of the wrist when the thumb is fully extended.

Q. Can you tell me what its boundaries are?

A. The ulnar border of the snuffbox is the extensor pollicis longus. The radial border is made up of the extensor pollicis brevis and abductor pollicis longus tendons. The floor of the snuffbox is made up of the base of the thumb metacarpal, trapezium, scaphoid and radial styloid.

Q. What are the contents of the anatomical snuffbox?

A. Essentially the main content of the snuffbox is the radial artery which lies on the floor beneath the tendons. Also cutaneous branches of the radial nerve cross superficial to the tendons. The cephalic vein is formed from the radial side of the dorsal venous network in the roof of the snuffbox and travels from here along the radial side of the forearm towards the antecubital fossa.

Q. What is the significance of tenderness in the anatomical snuffbox?

A. Anatomical snuffbox tenderness is a clinical sign of a possible scaphoid injury.

Q. What do you know about the management of scaphoid injuries?

A. The scaphoid is a carpal bone which articulates with the lunate, trapezium at the base of the thumb metacarpal and the wrist joint. It is the most commonly fractured carpal bone. It is usually injured by a high-impact fall onto an outstretched hand. It may be difficult to diagnose radiologically; therefore emphasis is placed on clinical findings such as anatomical snuffbox tenderness and swelling. Treatment involves either a ventura splint or a full scaphoid cast immobilization, depending on the degree of clinical suspicion. Repeat scaphoid radiographs should then be repeated in 10 days' time if the fracture was difficult to diagnose at presentation. It must be remembered that you should be guided by your clinical suspicion at this time and should continue with cast immobilization until you are happy that the injury has healed.

If it is quite obvious that there is a clear fracture present, open reduction and internal fixation using a Herbert screw may be attempted.

Q. What is the problem associated with fracture of the scaphoid?

A. The scaphoid receives its blood supply from the distal end; therefore fractures through the waist of the scaphoid may lead to avascular necrosis of the proximal fragment. If a fracture goes unnoticed the end result may be accelerated osteoarthritis and a reduced level of function in the wrist. It may also be complicated by reflex sympathetic dystrophy in the longer term.

Q. Do you know of any other bones where avascular necrosis can occur?

A. The head of the femur and talus are both subject to avascular necrosis.

UPPER LIMB   CARPAL TUNNEL

Q. What are the boundaries of the carpal tunnel?

A. The carpal tunnel is a canal which lies between the flexor retinaculum and the carpal bones in the hand.

Q. What are the attachments of the flexor retinaculum?

A. The flexor retinaculum forms the roof of the carpal tunnel in the hand. It is a fibrous band that originates from the pisiform and hook of hamate and attaches to the tubercle of the scaphoid and the ridge of the trapezium.

Q. Can you tell me what important structures pass through the carpal tunnel?

A. The median nerve and all the long flexor tendons of the thumb and fingers.

Q. What about the ulnar nerve?

A. No, the ulnar nerve lies with the ulnar artery and these both lie superficial to the flexor retinaculum.

Q. Tell me what you know about flexor sheaths.

A. A common flexor sheath covers all superficial and deep flexor tendons.

Q. Does this sheath completely cover the flexor tendons?

A. No, the covering is deficient on the radial side. This enables the tendons to have an arterial blood supply.

Q. What are the symptoms of carpal tunnel syndrome?

A. Carpal tunnel syndrome results in median nerve compression and may be idiopathic or caused by pregnancy, diabetes, arthritis and acromegaly. Symptoms include abnormal sensation over the radial three and a half digits and wasting of the thenar muscles. The tingling is characteristically at night and may be reproduced by percussion over the median nerve. This is called Tinel's test.

Q. How would you distinguish a high median nerve lesion in the forearm as opposed to carpal tunnel compression?

A. In the case of carpal tunnel syndrome, sensation over the thenar eminence is intact as the palmar cutaneous branch of the median nerve which comes off before the carpal tunnel supplies this patch of skin. In high lesions, this sensation will be lost.

UPPER LIMB HAND

Q. What is the function of the flexor retinaculum?

A. It prevents 'bowstringing' of the flexor tendons.

Q. To what is it attached?

A. On the radial side – to the scaphoid tubercle and the trapezium; on the ulnar side – to the hook of hamate and pisiform.

Q. What structures pass through the carpal tunnel?

A. These include:

- Flexor digitorum superficialis
- Flexor digitorum profundus
- Flexor pollicis longus
- Median nerve
- Flexor carpi radialis.

Q. Which structures are at risk when performing a carpal tunnel decompression?

A. 1. Palmar cutaneous branch – this branch of the median nerve takes a variable course superficial to the flexor retinaculum and supplies sensation to the skin overlying the thenar eminence.
2. Recurrent motor branch – usually distal and radial to the operative field, this branch of the median nerve is less often damaged but the consequences are more significant. It supplies the muscles of the thenar eminence.
3. Superficial palmar arch – this terminal branch of the ulnar artery crosses the palm at the level of the distal border of the abducted thumb.

Q. Where do the digital flexor tendons insert?

A. Flexor digitorum profundus inserts at the base of the distal phalanx, flexor digitorum superficialis at both sides of the midsection of the middle phalanx.

Q. Where and how do these two tendons cross?

A. Flexor digitorum superficialis bifurcates into two slips at the base of the first phalanx. Flexor digitorum profundus (FDP) passes between these two slips. The slips briefly reunite deep to FDP before splitting once more to insert either side of the midshaft of the middle phalanx.

Q. What prevents these tendons from 'bowstringing' as the fingers are flexed?

A. Thickenings of the fibrous flexor sheath are firmly attached to bone to form pulleys. A pulley may be incised without loss of function in treating a trigger finger.

Q. What factors predict restoration of function following repair to a divided flexor tendon?

A.
1. Site of injury
2. Nature of injury (clean cut/crush)
3. Timing of repair
4. Surgical planning and technique
5. Postoperative hand therapy.

Q. The extensor tendons are in six discrete compartments overlying the distal radius and ulnar; how are these compartments arranged?

A.
I   Abductor pollicis longus/extensor pollicis brevis (note abductor pollicis brevis is muscle of thenar eminence)

II   Extensor carpi radialis

III Extensor pollicis longus (direction of action modified by 'pulley' of Lister's tubercle)

IV Extensor digitorum

V   Extensor digiti minimi

VI Extensor carpi ulnaris.

Q. Where may surgically important hand infections occur?

A.
- Nail – acute or chronic paronychia may require surgery. Abscesses of the paronychium (skinfold on the lateral border of the nail) or of the skinflap superficial to the proximal nail may be treated by simple incision and drainage. If there is pus under the nail or the nail is involved in chronic infection, then all or part of the nail may be removed.
- Pulp – a felon or pulp abscess is often exquisitely painful. The pulp is divided into numerous small compartments by strong fibrous septa. A midline longitudinal palmar incision or accurate lateral incision cutting the fibrous septa may be used.
- Web space – often originating in the palmar calluses of horny handed labourers, these track dorsally. Adequate drainage usually requires palmar and dorsal incisions. The web itself should not be incised.
- Deep fascial spaces – abscesses of the thenar or midpalmar spaces are usually secondary to inadequately treated tenosynovitis. Systemic sepsis often complicates any further delay in drainage.
- Tenosynovitis – aggressive early antibiotics may prevent spread. If pus is present it must be drained. Long-term functional deficits are common.

Clinical signs include:

- tenderness over the involved sheath
- fixed flexion of the digit
- pain on attempted passive extension
- swelling of the digit.

Closed irrigation, if adequately performed, probably causes fewer long-term problems than open drainage.

- Radial and ulnar bursae – the radial bursa contains flexor pollicis longus whilst the ulnar bursa contains flexor digitorum profundus and flexor digitorum superficialis. These bursae often communicate. Early closed irrigation is the treatment of choice.
- Septic arthritis – metacarpophalangeal joint sepsis is often caused by the collision of fist with tooth. A low threshold should be maintained for exploring knuckle injuries sustained in this way. Interphalangeal joint infection acquired haematogenously or through local trauma should be washed out immediately and vigorously.

 TIP

Hand injuries are extremely common. Delays or mistakes in the management of hand injuries often have irreversible (and thus costly) functional implications. In exams and real life, hand injuries requiring treatment are easily missed. If in doubt, it is always safer to seek an orthopaedic opinion.

UPPER LIMB CLAVICLE

Q. What is the function of the clavicle?

A. It forms a cantilever between the axial skeleton and the appendicular skeleton of the upper limb. It also affords protection to structures of the root of the neck.

Q. How does it ossify?

A. Initially by intramembranous ossification in condensed mesenchyme. Later, longitudinal growth occurs by growth of terminal cartilage and subsequent endochondral ossification. It is the first bone to ossify (5–6 weeks' gestation) and the last to fuse (25 years).

Q. What are the articulations of the clavicle?

A. Medially it articulates with the manubrium and first costal cartilage. The sternoclavicular joint (SCJ) is a complex atypical synovial joint. The articular surfaces are fibro-cartilage and the joint contains an articular disc.

Laterally it articulates with the acromion. The acromioclavicular joint (ACJ) is a simple atypical synovial joint which often has a small disc.

Q. Are fractures or dislocations of the clavicle more common?

A. Fractures are extremely common (5% of all fractures).

Dislocations are relatively uncommon due to the strong ligaments that reinforce the sternoclavicluar and acromioclavicular joints.

Q. What are these ligaments called?

A. • Sternoclavicular joint – costoclavicular, interclavicular, anterior and posterior sternoclavicular ligaments
• Acromioclavicular joint – acromioclavicular and coracoclavicular ligaments (trapezoid and conoid parts).

Q. What is the usual mechanism for acromioclavicular joint dislocation?

A. Downwards excursion of the clavicle is blocked by the thoracic cage. Thus a downwards blow on the acromion disrupts first the acromioclavicular then the coracoclavicular ligaments.

If the coracoclavicular ligaments are intact, treatment is with a broad arm sling. If these are ruptured some surgeons would advocate temporary coracoclavicular screw fixation.

Q. What is the usual mechanism of sternoclavicular joint dislocation?

A. The sternoclavicular joint is relatively unstable in compression; thus a lateral blow to the shoulder may cause the medial clavicle to dislocate in front of or behind the sternum.

Q. Which direction of sternoclavicular joint dislocation is more hazardous?

A. Posterior dislocations may injure the great vessels, trachea, oesophagus, heart or pleura.

Q. How are sternoclavicular dislocations treated?

A. Posterior dislocations are usually stable following closed reduction.

Anterior dislocations are usually unstable. Conservative management results in a visible bulge; resection of the medial clavicle carries risks and leaves a scar.

Q. Which part of the clavicle usually breaks?

A. Medial 5%, middle 85%, lateral 10%.

Q. What are the implications of the site of fracture?

A. Medial fractures are associated with high-energy trauma and carry a higher risk of injury to underlying structures.

Lateral fractures more commonly result in non-union and the outer end is pulled up by the deltoid.

Q. How are clavicle fractures treated?

A. The commonest treatment is a broad arm sling for 6–8 weeks. This leads to a non-union rate of 0.1–0.5%.

Operative treatment carries a risk of injury to underlying structures and leads to a non-union rate of 4–5%.

Q. Why operate then?

A. • Open fracture/tented skin
• Polytrauma/floating shoulder
• Neurovascular injury.

UPPER LIMB HUMERUS

Q. What sort of joint is the shoulder joint?

A. The glenohumeral joint is a typical synovial multi-axial ball and socket joint.

Q. What factors enhance the mobility of the shoulder?

A. 1. Large humeral head in shallow glenoid fossa
2. Capsular laxity (glenohumeral joint may be distracted 2–3 cm in 'relaxed' patient)
3. Scapulothoracic excursion.

Q. What factors enhance the stability of the joint?

A. The stability of the joint is enhanced by:

The rotator cuff

• Anterior – subscapularis
• Superior – supraspinatus
• Posterior – supraspinatus, infraspinatus and teres minor

and the glenoid labrum.

Q. In what position is the shoulder least stable?

A. Abduction, extension and external rotation (American 'taking the oath' position). Glenohumeral dislocation is the commonest joint dislocation (38%); 98% of all glenohumeral dislocations are anterior and inferior.

Q. What complications may accompany dislocation?

A. Complications include:

• Bankart lesion (fracture to the anterior glenoid labrum)
• Hill–Sachs lesion (intra-articular fracture to the humeral head)
• Rotator cuff tear
• Neurovascular injury (especially the axillary nerve).

Q. Where is the humerus commonly fractured?

A. The elderly commonly fracture the surgical neck of the humerus when falling onto an outstretched hand. They may also fracture the greater tuberosity at the same time. A fracture through the shaft in this age group is usually due to a metastasis.

Younger patients usually sustain a spiral fracture to the shaft of the humerus. They may also sustain an oblique or transverse fracture through the shaft or occasionally may break the proximal humerus in multiple places.

Adolescents may suffer a fracture separation of the upper humeral epiphysis causing the shaft to move away from the humeral head in the joint.

Q. Which nerves are at risk in humeral fractures?

A. There are several nerves at risk in fractures of the humerus.

Axillary nerve

Seen in humeral neck fractures (also glenohumeral dislocation).

Radial nerve

- Humeral shaft fractures (nerve lies against the bone in spiral groove)
- Supracondylar fracture.

Median nerve

Supracondylar fracture.

Ulnar nerve

- Medial epicondylar fracture
- 'Tardy ulnar palsy' 2° to progressive cubitus valgus following lateral condylar fracture.

Q. Why classify anything in medicine?

A. 1. To guide treatment
2. To predict prognosis
3. To allow objective comparison of outcomes in clinical research.

Q. How may distal humeral fractures be classified?

A. • Supracondylar (65% of all paediatric elbow fractures, high risk of neurovascular injury)
- Transcondylar (less common and less stable than supracondylar fractures, thus lower threshold to fixation)
- Intercondylar ('T'-, 'Y'- or 'V'-shaped fractures)
- Condylar (25% of paediatric elbow fractures)
- Epicondylar.

Q. What radiographic clues may imply an unseen elbow injury?

A. The appearance of pathological fat pads implies a tense effusion. Treat as an undisplaced radial head or supracondylar fracture until proven otherwise.

A visible posterior fat pad is always pathological; an anterior fat pad may be seen flush to the bone but is pathological if displaced from the bone.

A third of the capitulum should be seen in front of a line drawn down the front of the humerus (see supracondylar fractures). The capitulum should always be aligned with the radius.

 TIP

In exams and real life, elbow injuries requiring treatment are easily missed. If in doubt, it is always safer to seek an orthopaedic opinion.

LOWER LIMB   FASCIA LATA

Q. Where is the fascia lata?

A. The fascia lata is a layer of fascia that surrounds the thigh.

Q. Does it completely enclose the thigh?

A. Yes, it completely encloses the thigh in a stocking-like fashion and overlaps at the top to form the saphenous opening.

Q. What is the tensor fasciae latae?

A. It is a muscle of the thigh which arises from the iliac crest between the tubercle and the anterior superior iliac spine and inserts into the iliotibial tract.

Q. What is its function?

A. It tenses the iliotibial tract and is assisted by the gluteus maximus in locking the extended knee. It also helps to stabilize the pelvis during walking.

Q. Where does the iliotibial tract insert?

A. The iliotibial tract is a thickening of the fascia lata on the lateral aspect of the thigh and inserts into the smooth circular facet on the lateral condyle of the tibia, anterior to the line of the knee joint.

Q. What muscle also inserts into it?

A. Three quarters of the gluteus maximus inserts into it.

Q. How does the iliotibial tract stabilize the extended knee?

A. The iliotibial tract is able to maintain the knee in a hyper-extended position because it passes anterior to the knee joint when straight. This enables the quadriceps to relax and the patella to be mobile and hence the knee is able to comfortably 'lock' in the hyper-extended position.

Q. What is the nerve supply of the tensor fascia lata?

A. The superior gluteal nerve (L4, 5, S1).

LOWER LIMB PATELLA

Q. How many articular facets does the patella have?

A. It has three: the lateral, medial and most medial. (At this point you may be handed a patella and asked to 'side it'. It is worth remembering that the patella lies comfortably on the broader, lateral facet. Therefore you can work out which side it is from.)

The narrowest facet is the medial which is subdivided into two articular facets.

Q. What does each facet articulate with?

A. The most medial facet articulates with the medial condyle of the femur and the lateral facet articulates with the lateral femoral condyle.

Q. What type of bone is the patella?

A. The patella is a sesamoid bone.

Q. Within which tendon is it enclosed?

A. The quadriceps tendon.

Q. Do you know of any congenital abnormalities of the patella?

A. Yes, the patella develops from several centres of ossification that fuse to form one bone. If this fusion doesn't occur a bipartite patella may result.

Q. How would you differentiate a bipartite patella from a fracture on X-ray?

A. Generally, the edges of a bipartite patella would be smooth and rounded off. A newly fractured patella would have sharper edges; however, these may be difficult to distinguish when the fracture is a bit older. It would also be sensible to X-ray the other side; if fractured, only the side in question would demonstrate the abnormality.

Q. What deficit would you expect to find in a knee if a patella was badly fractured and needed to be avulsed?

A. Immediately after the operation the knee would be stiff and painful. It may take extensive physiotherapy to assist extension of the knee; however, it is quite possible that the knee returns to the full range of movement despite the loss.

Q. How stable is the patella?

A. The patella is very mobile. Inserting into it superiorly is the quadriceps tendon and medially the vastus medialis.

Q. In what direction do they pull the patella?

A. The general direction of pull by the quadriceps tendon is lateral; however, the vastus medialis counterbalances this by pulling medially.

Q. Lateral dislocation of the patella is quite a common condition. Who gets it?

A. Lateral dislocation of the patella is common in tall, thin adolescent girls. This is because they tend to have a knock-knee deformity (*genu valgum*) and the lateral condyle of the femur is unable to prevent the patella from sliding over it.

Q. What else prevents the patella from dislocating laterally?

A. Usually the lateral condyle of the femur is bony or prominent enough to prevent dislocation. Also, the medial patellar retinacular fibres provide some tension on the patella as do the lower fibres of the vastus medialis inserting low down on the medial surface of the patella.

Q. Does the patella have a cartilage layer?

A. Yes, the posterior surface of the patella is covered with hyaline cartilage.

LOWER LIMB   HIP

You may be handed a femur in this section and asked to 'side it'. Don't be caught out – it is easy to get confused and you will have a long way to come back if you get the first question wrong. The femur has a long shaft with a rounded head at the top end and two condyles at the lower end. Look at the rounded head; it has a greater and lesser trochanter on its lateral aspect. The lesser trochanter should be facing medially and the greater one facing laterally. The neck of the femur should incline upwards and medially. It is angled at approximately 125° to the shaft of the femur. The anterior surface of the femur is smooth and convex; however, the posterior surface has a palpable ridge called the linea aspera that gives muscular attachment. If you are still unable to accurately side it, look at the condyles – the lateral condyle projects forward more than the medial in order to prevent lateral dislocation of the patella. The medial condyle also has the prominent adductor tubercle above the medial condyle that is readily palpable.

Q. Show me where the capsule of the joint attaches.

A. The capsule of the hip joint is attached to the acetabulum and the transverse acetabular ligament. From here, it passes anteriorly over the neck of the femur to the intertrochanteric line. Posteriorly, it only reaches halfway down the neck of the femur.

Q. What ligaments support the capsule?

A. Three ligaments support the capsule:

- Iliofemoral
- Pubofemoral
- Ishiofemoral.

The iliofemoral is the strongest.

Q. What are its attachments?

A. The iliofemoral ligament arises from the anterior inferior iliac spine and inserts 'Y-shaped' into the trochanteric line.

Q. What type of joint is the hip joint?

A. The hip joint is a ball and socket synovial joint. It allows a wide range of movement.

Q. What is its blood supply?

A. In a child, a branch from the obturator artery reaches the head of the femur through the ligament of the head of the femur. At approximately 10 years of age, the blood supply of the head and neck is taken over by the medial circumflex femoral artery and the trochanteric anastomosis. Nutrient arteries also pass through the retinacular fibres of the capsule to supply the head of the femur.

Q. How stable is the hip joint?

A. The hip joint is stable due to the tightly fitting labrum of the acetabulum and its reinforcing ligaments. It is also supported by the gluteal muscles. It is least stable in the flexed, adducted position; however, it is so stable that a dislocation is usually associated with a forceful injury and an acetabular fracture.

Q. What surgical approaches to the hip do you know of?

A. There are several surgical approaches to the hip. These include:

- Anterior approach – between the tensor fascia lata and sartorius, then dividing the rectus femoris and the anterior third of the gluteus medius.
- Lateral approach – this involves splitting through the fibres of the tensor fascia lata, gluteus medius and minimis or detaching them from the greater trochanter.
- Posterior approach – this involves splitting through the fibres of the gluteus maximus and detaching the piriformis, obturator internus and gemelli from the femur.

Q. Which nerves may be at risk?

A. The superior gluteal nerve is at risk during the lateral approach and the sciatic nerve is at risk during the posterior approach.

LOWER LIMB | KNEE

Q. What sort of joint is the knee joint?

A. It is a complex compound synovial joint. It is the largest joint in the body.

- Compound – it involves both the bicondylar tibio-femoral and sellar patello-femoral joints
- Complex – it contains menisci.

Q. What movements occur at the knee joint?

A. Flexion/extension and rotation.

Q. What are the attachments of the capsule?

A. The articular margins of the tibia, femur and patella *except supero-anteriorly*.

The capsule is deficient above the patella; thus the joint is continuous with a large supra-patellar bursa or pouch.

Q. Is this clinically significant?

A. Fluid from this pouch must be excluded before a small effusion can be detected.

Pus in this pouch will also enter the joint, a surgical emergency (this is not the case for an infectious pre-patellar bursitis).

Q. Is the capsule reinforced?

A. Medially by the intrinsic part of the medial collateral ligament; posteriorly by the popliteal ligament.

Q. What other ligaments stabilize the knee?

A. The anterior cruciate ligament, posterior cruciate ligament and the extrinsic part of the medial collateral ligament.

Q. What soft tissue structures of the knee are most commonly damaged in sports injuries?

A. The medial collateral ligament, anterior cruciate ligament and the medial meniscus.

Q. How are injuries to these structures treated?

A. Medial collateral ligament

Clinical examination – sprain without laxity treat with physiotherapy; sprain with laxity treat with a cast brace.

Anterior cruciate ligament

Clinical examination and/or arthroscopy – partial tear treat with physiotherapy; complete tear treat by debriding remnant and physiotherapy.

The majority of patients with a complete anterior cruciate ligament rupture achieve adequate dynamic stabilization of the knee through physiotherapy. The rest should be considered for surgical replacement.

Meniscus

Clinical examination and/or arthroscopy – peripheral (vascularized) tear treat with repair; central (avascular) tear treat by debriding.

LOWER LIMB FOOT AND ANKLE

It is quite likely that you may be handed a bone or two in this section. For example, you may be handed a tibia and calcaneus (articulated with the rest of the foot) and asked to articulate them. It is worth knowing then that the lower end of the tibia has a medial malleolus; therefore, first work out which way up the tibia goes, then position the medial malleolus medially and the ankle joint should be correctly articulated.

Alternatively, you may be handed a fibula and asked to 'side it'. The fibula is a notoriously difficult bone to 'side'. It is long and slender and can be difficult to orientate each end. The proximal end is quite square shaped and the lower end is flatter with a notch in it called the malleolar fossa. A trick a colleague taught me is to hold the fibula upright between your thumb and index finger. If it fits snugly in the left thumb, it is the left fibula and similarly if it fits the right thumb comfortably, it's the right fibula (i.e. the notch is posterior).

Q. What type of joint is the ankle joint?

A. It is a hinged synovial joint.

Q. What movements does it allow?

A. It allows dorsi flexion/extension and plantar flexion of the foot.

Q. Where does inversion and eversion of the foot occur?

A. Inversion and eversion occur at the subtalar and midtarsal joints.

Q. And which muscles are responsible for these movements?

A. The tibialis anterior and tibialis posterior are attached to the medial aspect of the foot and hence bring about inversion. The peroneus longus, brevis and tertius are attached to the lateral aspect of the foot and so evert the foot.

Q. What bones make up the medial longitudinal arch of the foot?

A. The medial longitudinal arch is made up of:

- Calcaneus
- Talus
- Navicular
- Three cuneiform bones
- Three metatarsal bones.

Q. How is this arch maintained?

A. The arch is made up of the above bones; however, it gains most of its stability from its muscular attachments. Mostly the flexor hallucis longus and the flexor digitorum longus maintain the arch with some help from the plantar aponeurosis.

Q. What are the phases the foot must go through in order to walk?

A. The four phases of walking include:

- Heel strike
- Stance phase

- Push-off phase
- Swing.

Q. You may be handed a cadaveric foot and asked where the flexor retinaculum is.

A. The flexor retinaculum is a thickening of fascia that connects the medial malleolus to the calcaneus.

Q. What passes underneath the flexor retinaculum?

A. Underneath the flexor retinaculum lie the tendons of the deep calf muscles on their way to the sole of the foot. These include:

- Flexor digitorum longus
- Flexor hallucis longus
- Tibialis posterior.

Q. In what order do they pass beneath the medial malleolus?

A. They pass as follows from medial to lateral:

- Tibialis posterior
- Flexor digitorum longus
- Flexor hallucis longus.

I usually remember this with the mnemonic Tom, Dick and Harry.

Q. What nerve supplies these muscles?

A. The tibial nerve (S1, 2).

Q. What does the superficial peroneal nerve supply?

A. The superficial peroneal nerve is a branch of the common peroneal. It supplies sensation to most of the dorsum of the foot except the skin of the first cleft which is supplied by the deep peroneal nerve. It also supplies sensation to the distal, lateral third of the leg.

Q. If this nerve was injured, would you expect to see a foot drop?

A. No, I would expect to see a sensory loss affecting the distal third of the lateral leg and the dorsum of the foot apart from the first cleft. If a foot drop was present, I would suspect an injury had occurred to the deep peroneal nerve which supplies the leg extensors.

LOWER LIMB FEMUR

Q. What is the position of the femoral neck in relation to its shaft?

A. The neck is anteverted to 10–15° and angled at approximately 125°. This is widest at birth and lessens with age (less so for females).

Q. Where does the psoas major attach to the femur?

A. To the middle surface of the lesser trochanter with the iliacus.

Q. What is its action on the hip?

A. It flexes the hip.

Q. What is the blood supply to the femoral head?

A. This includes:

- Retinacular vessels – these are derived from the greater trochanteric anastomosis (from branches of the lateral and medial circumflex arteries, branches of the profunda femoris)
- Nutrient arteries (from the profunda femoris)
- Artery of the head (accompanies the ligamentum teres), derived from the acetabular artery (a branch of the internal iliac artery). It has limited significance in adults.

Q. How does your knowledge of this vascular anatomy guide the treatment of fractures of the neck of the femur?

A. The goal of hip fracture surgery is to preserve the head of the femur if it has a reasonable chance of survival. Displaced intracapsular fractures are likely to disrupt the blood supply and thus precipitate avascular necrosis. For these fractures, attempts to save the head often fail and thus in most cases the head should be abandoned and replaced.

Thus the common fracture patterns are usually treated as follows:

- Extracapsular – internal fixation (e.g. dynamic hip screw)
- Undisplaced intracapsular – internal fixation (e.g. cannulated screws)
- Displaced intracapsular – hemiarthroplasty (e.g. Austin—Moore).

Q. What features would you look for on an X-ray to diagnose a fractured neck of the femur?

A. I would look for:

- An obvious fracture line
- Alignment of the trabecular lines
- Presence of any abnormal bone shadows
- Length of the femoral neck (shortened in impacted fractures).

Q. Do you know of any classifications for femoral neck fractures?

A. Garden's classification is based on an anteroposterior radiograph and includes:

- Stage I – partial fracture (incomplete/impacted, trabeculae malaligned)
- Stage II – complete fracture but no displacement (trabeculae aligned)
- Stage III – complete fracture with some displacement (retinacular fibres still attached, therefore trabeculae appear malaligned on X-ray)
- Stage IV – complete fracture with total displacement (trabeculae appear normally aligned on X-ray as the head is free to lie in the correct position in the acetabulum).

Q. When is a fracture of the neck of the femur an emergency?

A. The benefit of preserving the head of the femur is much greater in young patients. Thus biologically young patients with displaced intracapsular fractures are often rushed to theatre for emergency open reduction and fixation. There is no evidence to support this practice. There is a wealth of evidence to demonstrate that a wait of up to 48 hours will not prejudice the outcome of hip fracture surgery. After 48 hours the mortality doubles.

Q. What are the possible complications of femoral neck fractures?

A. Complications include:

- Avascular necrosis – high risk in displaced fractures due to disruption of the blood supply. Eventually femoral head collapse may occur causing pain and loss of function.
- Non-union – high risk in displaced fractures.
- Osteoarthritis – may develop prematurely causing pain and loss of function.
- Non-specific – deep vein thrombosis, pulmonary embolism, chest infection, pressure sores.

Q. What is a positive Trendelenburg's sign?

A. The contralateral pelvis does not rise when weight is taken on the affected side.

Q. What are the causes of this sign?

A. • Weak abductors (gluteus medius and minimus)
- Short femoral neck
- Medial migration of the femoral head
- Neuropathy
- Pain.

THORAX | DIAPHRAGM

Q. How does the diaphragm develop embryologically?

A. The diaphragm develops from:

- Septum transversum (central tendon)
- Pleuro-peritoneal mesodermal membranes
- Dorsal oesophageal mesentery
- Cervical myotomes (muscular input into the septum transversum, before its descent).

Q. Where would a congenital diaphragmatic hernia commonly arise?

A. The commonest congenital diaphragmatic hernia is known as Bochdalek's foramen which is the failure of the development of the pleuro-peritoneal membrane. It occurs posteriorly and is more common on the left-hand side.

Q. What other types of hernia do you know about?

A. Acquired diaphragmatic hernias are far more common than congenital ones. For example, a hiatus hernia is extremely prevalent within the population. This is where the gastro-oesophageal junction slides through the oesophageal opening of the diaphragm. It is known as a sliding hiatus hernia and is associated with reflux oesophagitis and Barrett's oesophagus. A less common type of hiatus hernia is known as the 'rolling' or para-oesophageal hernia. Here, the gastro-oesophageal junction remains in position and an area of stomach and peritoneum nearby slides upwards along the oesophagus and into the thorax.

Q. What is the blood supply of the diaphragm?

A. The diaphragm derives most of its blood supply from the lower five intercostal arteries and the subcostal arteries. There are also contributions from the inferior phrenic arteries (branches of the aorta) and from the pericardiophrenic and musculophrenic arteries which are branches of the internal thoracic artery.

Q. What is the nerve supply of the diaphragm?

A. The diaphragm has a motor supply only – the phrenic nerve: C3, 4, 5.

Q. At what level does the aorta pass through the diaphragm? What other structures pass with it?

A. The aorta passes through the diaphragm at the level of T12. With it passes the azygous vein and the thoracic duct.

✱ TEACHING NOTE

It is worth learning the diaphragmatic openings off by heart:

- T8 – inferior vena caval opening and right phrenic nerve
- T10 – oesophageal opening and right and left vagi and oesophageal branches of the left gastric artery and lymphatics
- T12 – aortic opening and azygous vein and thoracic duct.

Q. Where does the left phrenic nerve pass through the diaphragm?

A. The left phrenic nerve passes on its own through the muscular part of the left dome of the diaphragm.

✱ TEACHING NOTE

It is worth learning all the other structures that pass through the diaphragm:
- Hemiazygous vein – passes with the aorta through T12
- Greater, lesser and least splanchnic nerves – pass through each crus
- Sympathetic trunk – passes behind the medial arcuate ligament
- Superior epigastric vessels – pass between the xiphisternum and costal fibres of the diaphragm
- Subcostal neurovascular bundle – passes behind the lateral arcuate ligament.

THORAX   MUSCLES OF RESPIRATION

Q. How does the diaphragm contribute to respiration?

A. The diaphragm aids inspiration via contraction resulting in an increase in lung volume.

Q. What other muscles contribute to inspiration?

A. Other muscles contributing to inspiration include:

- The scalenus muscles
- Pectoralis major and minor
- Latissimus dorsi (inspiration and expiration)
- Serratus anterior
- Sternocleidomastoids
- The external intercostal muscles.

During quiet inspiration, it is mainly the movements of the diaphragm and the external intercostals that are responsible for the majority of the work. The diaphragm contracts and hence the lung bases expand. This is accompanied by a bucket handle movement of the ribs to increase the transverse diameter of the thorax. The contraction of the diaphragm causes the inferior vena cava to be opened wider in order to help venous return. It also results in an increase in intra-abdominal pressure.

Q. What muscles assist with expiration?

A. Expiration mostly occurs passively due to the elastic recoil of the diaphragm. It may also be aided by the internal intercostal muscles. In some circumstances, such as chronic obstructive airway disease (COAD), the muscles of the abdominal wall and reverse actions of the scalenus, pectoralis and latissimus dorsi aid with forced expiration.

Q. What is the difference between the movement of the upper and lower ribs during inspiration?

A. The contraction of the external intercostal muscles during inspiration results in the elevation of the second to the seventh ribs. This causes an increase in the anteroposterior diameter of the thorax by pushing the sternum forwards. In the lower ribs, this contraction results in an increase in the transverse diameter of the thorax by the bucket handle movements of the ribs.

THORAX   HEART

Q. What are the contents of the mediastinum?

A. The mediastinum is situated within the centre of the thorax between the lungs. It contains the heart and its great vessels, the trachea, oesophagus, thoracic duct, several lymph nodes, the phrenic and vagus nerves and the thymus.

Q. Where is the plane of Louis and what is its significance?

A. The plane of Louis relates to a plane that divides the mediastinum. It passes horizontally through the manubriosternal joint which is at the level of the second costal cartilage towards the lower border of vertebra T4. It divides the mediastinum into the superior and inferior mediastinum. The superior mediastinum lies above this line and the inferior lies below it. The inferior is subdivided into the anterior, middle and posterior mediastinum according to its relationship to the pericardium.

At the level of the plane of Louis:

- The trachea bifurcates
- The aorta arches over
- The azygous vein enters the superior vena cava
- The thoracic duct crosses the left side of the oesophagus.

Lying within the plane is the ligamentum arteriosum and the left recurrent laryngeal nerve below it.

Q. What are the courses of the phrenic and vagus nerves in the thorax?

A. Essentially the main difference between the two nerves is that the phrenic nerve passes in front of the lung root and the vagus nerve passes behind it.

The phrenic nerve arises from C4, travels over the anterior scalenus muscle and behind the subclavian vein. The right phrenic nerve travels lateral to the right brachiocephalic vein, the superior vena cava, the right atrium and the inferior vena cava. It then passes through the diaphragm through the same opening as the inferior vena cava. The left phrenic nerve is lateral to the left common carotid, subclavian artery and the superior intercostal vein. It then travels over the pericardium of the left ventricle and leaves the diaphragm on its own through the muscular region, lateral to the pericardium.

The right and left vagi travel alongside the trachea. The left vagus crosses the arch of the aorta and gives off a branch at this point known as the left recurrent laryngeal nerve. This nerve hooks around the ligamentum arteriosum and travels back up to the neck in the tracheo-oesophageal groove. The left vagus nerve then passes behind the lung root and gives off branches to the pulmonary and oesophageal plexuses. The right vagus also has a right recurrent laryngeal branch, however, this is given off much higher in the neck and hooks around the subclavian artery before travelling back up to the neck.

Q. Where is the base of the heart?

A. The base of the heart is otherwise known as the posterior surface. It is made up of the left atrium and four pulmonary veins.

Q. What is the blood supply to the heart?

A. The heart is supplied by coronary arteries which are branches of the ascending aorta. The right coronary artery leaves the aorta in the anterior aortic sinus, passes into the atrio-ventricular groove and runs posteriorly at the inferior border of the heart. It tends to anastomose with the circumflex branch of the left coronary artery. It is responsible for branches to the sino-atrial node and atrio-ventricular node in two thirds of cases.

The left coronary artery leaves the aorta in the left posterior aortic sinus. It gives off the anterior descending branch (LAD) which travels along the interventricular groove to anastomose with the posterior branch from the right coronary artery. The left coronary artery then becomes the circumflex artery which travels to the posterior aspect of the heart giving off branches before anastomosing with the right.

The veins of the heart do not follow the arteries. Most of the venous blood drains into the coronary sinus via the great, middle, small and anterior cardiac veins. The coronary sinus lies in the posterior atrio-ventricular groove and drains into the posterior aspect of the right atrium. There are also several venae cordis minimae which are small veins in the walls of the four chambers that drain directly into each of the chambers.

Q. What are the branches of the thoracic aorta?

A. The thoracic aorta begins at the lower border of T4 and finishes at T12 where the aorta leaves the thorax by passing through the diaphragm, between the crura.

The branches include:

- Nine pairs of posterior intercostal arteries
- Subcostal arteries
- Bronchial arteries
- Oesophageal arteries
- Pericardial arteries
- Branch to the phrenic nerve.

✱ TEACHING NOTE

In the London exam, it is likely that you will be led to a cadaver, handed a pointer and brought to the heart. The examiner will then ask you various questions such as the ones above. It is assumed, therefore, that you will actually be able to point out the various anatomical structures such as the right and left vagus nerves with their recurrent laryngeals branching off. If you don't manage to identify the structure in question, the examiner will move on to another area that you may be able to correctly identify before asking you questions about it.

THORAX OESOPHAGUS

The examiner may begin this area by asking you to identify the oesophagus within the cadaver.

Q. What type of muscle is the oesophagus made up of?

A. The oesophagus is a muscular tube made up of an outer longitudinal layer and an inner circular one. The upper half is mainly skeletal muscle and the lower part mainly smooth muscle.

Q. What type of epithelium lines the muscularis mucosa?

A. The surface epithelium of the oesophagus is mainly stratified squamous epithelium. This becomes columnar at the level of the gastro-oesophageal junction. It doesn't always occur strictly at this level; however, if it occurs above 3 cm from the junction, it is thought to be abnormal and is called Barrett's oesophagus.

Q. What is the significance of Barrett's oesophagus?

A. Barrett's oesophagus is a pre-malignant condition. It is due to the presence of columnar epithelium within the lower oesophagus above normal limits and is thought to occur by metaplasia. Metaplasia is the transformation of one differentiated cell type into another and the stimulus for this change is reflux of gastric contents into the lower oesophagus.

The condition may require regular endoscopic surveillance to detect the development of squamous cell carcinoma.

Q. What usually prevents this condition from occurring?

A. There is no lower oesophageal sphincter as such that prevents the reflux of gastric contents; however, there is a natural area of high pressure at the lower end of the oesophagus that acts as a sphincter.

Q. What is the blood supply of the oesophagus?

A. The oesophagus may be divided into upper, middle and lower. The upper oesophagus is supplied by the inferior thyroid arteries, the middle oesophagus by aortic branches and the lower oesophagus by branches from the left gastric artery.

The venous drainage from the upper oesophagus is to the brachiocephalic veins, the middle third to the azygous system and the lower third drains to the left gastric vein and then into the portal vein.

Q. What is the clinical condition known as where anastomoses form between the portal and systemic venous systems?

A. Oesophageal varices.

THORAX LUNGS

You may be led to the lung roots and asked the following questions.

Q. Can you name these structures within the right and left lung roots?

A. In the left lung root, the pulmonary artery lies superiorly and the left bronchus lies inferiorly. There is also a pulmonary vein lying in front of and below the left bronchus.

In the right lung root the bronchus to the right upper lobe has already branched off; therefore, the upper lobe bronchus and its pulmonary artery lie superiorly in the lung root. Inferiorly is the main bronchus and pulmonary artery. There are also two pulmonary veins which lie in front of and below the main bronchus as in the left lung root.

Q. Are there any other structures to be found in the lung root?

A. Yes, each lung root also contains lymph nodes, nerves and some bronchial vessels. (It is reasonable to conclude when asked 'What structures pass through it?' that a nerve/artery/vein/lymphatics may be the right answer.)

Q. Where does the trachea begin and end?

A. The trachea begins at C6 and bifurcates into two main bronchi at the upper border of T5.

Q. What type of cartilage is the trachea made out of?

A. The tracheal rings are incomplete rings of hyaline cartilage whose function is to stay open in order to maintain a patent airway. There is a high content of elastic fibres in order that recoil may occur during respiration.

Q. What is the surface epithelium of the trachea?

A. The surface epithelium is typical pseudostratified columnar ciliated respiratory epithelium. It is characterized by goblet cells and mucous glands.

Q. Does this epithelium also line the epiglottis?

A. No, the epiglottis is lined with stratified squamous epithelium.

Q. Where does this change in epithelium take place?

A. It occurs along the upper part of the posterior aspect of the epiglottis.

Q. Does this mean that the vocal cords are lined with respiratory epithelium?

A. No, the vocal cords are lined with stratified squamous epithelium.

Q. How many bronchopulmonary segments does each lung contain?

A. There are ten bronchopulmonary segments in each lung.

Q. Can you name them?

	Right lung	Left lung
Upper lobe	Apical	Apico-posterior
	Posterior	Anterior
	Anterior	
Middle lobe	Medial	Superior lingular
	Lateral	Inferior lingular
Lower lobe	Apical	Apical
	Medial basal	Medial basal
	Anterior basal	Anterior basal
	Lateral basal	Lateral basal
	Posterior basal	Posterior basal

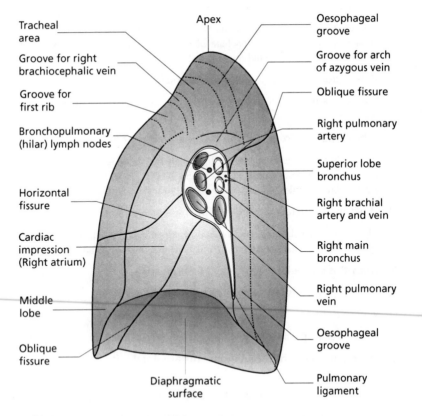

Tracheal area

Groove for right brachiocephalic vein

Groove for first rib

Bronchopulmonary (hilar) lymph nodes

Horizontal fissure

Cardiac impression (Right atrium)

Middle lobe

Oblique fissure

Apex

Diaphragmatic surface

Oesophageal groove

Groove for arch of azygous vein

Oblique fissure

Right pulmonary artery

Superior lobe bronchus

Right brachial artery and vein

Right main bronchus

Right pulmonary vein

Oesophageal groove

Pulmonary ligament

(A)

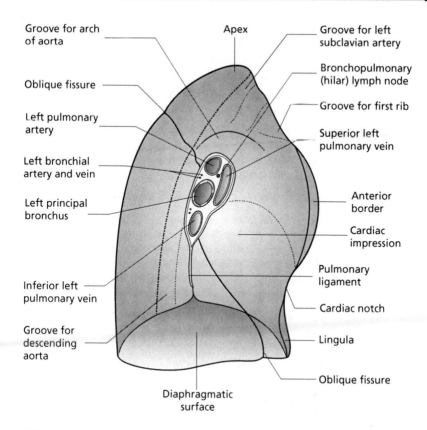

(B)

Fig. 2   The medial (mediastinal) surfaces of (A) the right lung and (B) the left lung

THORAX   STERNUM/RIB CAGE

In this section, it is highly likely that you will be presented with a bone and asked about it.

Q. You may be handed the vertebral column (articulated) and then a rib and asked to articulate the rib on the spine.

A. In this scenario, it is a good idea to have familiarized yourself with the ribs and the thoracic spine prior to the exam. If you haven't, you should know that a typical rib has a head, neck, shaft and tubercle that faces posteriorly from the lateral margin of the neck. In order to orientate the rib, you should know that the shaft of the rib slopes down and back up until the angle and then twists forward. The upper surface is blunt and the lower surface has a sharp, well demarcated costal groove. This should enable you to work out which way up the rib lies. Then, you should feel the two articular facets on the head of the rib. You should know that the lower facet articulates with its own vertebra and the upper facet articulates with the vertebra above. It is worth mentioning at this point that both joints are synovial.

It is also worth knowing that the tubercle of the rib has two facets and it is the medial facet that articulates with the transverse process of its own vertebra.

Having correctly articulated at these two areas, it will then be possible for you to correctly demonstrate how the rib moves with respiration. If you have been handed one of the higher ribs, this will be an 'up and down' movement, whereas a lower rib will move like a bucket handle.

Q. Where is the costal groove and what is its significance?

A. The costal groove is present at the lower edge of the rib. The external intercostal muscle attaches to the lower, outermost edge; the internal intercostal attaches within the intercostal groove; and the transversus thoracis attaches to the innermost surface. The intercostal neurovascular bundles lie deep within the costal grooves between the internal intercostal muscle and the transversus thoracis. It lies in the order *vein–artery–nerve (VAN)* from up to down.

The clinical significance of the costal groove is that when attempting pleural aspiration, it is advisable to aim the needle above any rib as opposed to below it in order to avoid penetrating this neurovascular bundle.

Q. What type of joint does the sternum make with the costal cartilages?

A. Atypical synovial joints except for the first.

Q. Is that true of all costal cartilages articulating with the sternum?

A. No, the first costal cartilage articulates with the manubrio-sternum by a primary cartilaginous joint.

Of note here is that the clavicle is the first to articulate with the manubrium and does so via an atypical synovial joint.

Q. What is the difference between a primary cartilaginous and a synovial joint?

A. Cartilaginous joints may be primary or secondary. A primary cartilaginous joint, as in the first costal cartilage, is where bone attaches to hyaline cartilage. It is characteristically a rigid joint.

Typical synovial joints involve two ends of bone meeting, with hyaline cartilage covering each bone end and the whole thing being surrounded by a joint capsule. The joint capsule encloses a joint cavity that is lined with synovial epithelium. The joint is characteristically mobile.

✳ TEACHING NOTE

It is worth learning off by heart all the different types of joints encountered in the body so that you don't get caught out.

Definitions of joints

Fibrous	Bone – connective tissue – bone
	Little movement i.e. skull sutures
Primary cartilaginous	Bone – hyaline cartilage
	Little movement i.e. first rib to manubrium
Secondary cartilaginous	Bone (hyaline cartilage) – fibro-cartilage – (hyaline cartilage) bone
	Small amount of movement i.e. midline (pubis, intervertebral discs)
Typical synovial	Bone (hyaline cartilage) – synovial cavity and joint capsule – (hyaline cartilage) bone
	Good range of movement – most joints
Atypical synovial	Bone (fibro-cartilage) – capsule – (fibro-cartilage) bone
	Good range of movement i.e. TMJ, costosternal

Examples to learn

- Clavicle – manubrium: atypical synovial
- First costal cartilage – manubrium: primary cartilaginous
- Second costal cartilage – sternum: atypical synovial
- Manubrium – sternum: secondary cartilaginous
- All costal cartilages – 12 ribs: primary cartilaginous
- All epiphyses: primary cartilaginous
- Bones of skull: fibrous
- Lower tibia-fibular syndesmosis: fibrous
- Pubic symphysis: secondary cartilaginous
- Intervertebral discs: secondary cartilaginous
- All limb joints: typical synovial
- Sternoclavicular joint: atypical synovial
- Temporomandibular joint: atypical synovial.

ABDOMEN RECTUS SHEATH

Q. What muscles make up the anterior abdominal wall?

A. The anterior abdominal wall is made up of:

- External oblique
- Internal oblique
- Transversus abdominis.

The rectus abdominis muscle is also situated in the midline at the point where all the above muscles meet.

Q. What are the functions of the anterior abdominal wall?

A. The anterior abdominal wall:

- Protects the intestines
- Aids with forceful expiration
- Compresses the abdomen when necessary i.e. defecation, parturition.

Q. What is the blood supply of the anterior abdominal wall?

A. The anterior abdominal wall is supplied by:

- Intercostal vessels
- Superior and inferior epigastric arteries
- Lumbar arteries
- Deep circumflex iliac arteries.

Q. In which layer do the vessels travel?

A. The vessels travel between the internal oblique and transversus abdominis.

Q. What is the rectus sheath and what does it contain?

A. The rectus sheath is a midline structure made up of all the aponeuroses of the anterior abdominal wall. The external oblique aponeurosis fuses to form its anterior layer; the transversus aponeurosis fuses to form the posterior layer. Between the costal margin and the umbilicus, the internal oblique aponeurosis splits around the rectus abdominis to contribute to the anterior and posterior layers. Halfway between the umbilicus and pubic symphysis, all three aponeurotic layers fuse anteriorly to the rectus abdominis. At this level the posterior layer has a free edge known as the *arcuate line*. It is here that the inferior epigastric artery enters the rectus sheath to supply the rectus abdominis.

The contents of the sheath include:

- Rectus abdominis
- Pyramidalis
- Lower six thoracic nerves
- Superior and inferior epigastric arteries and veins.

Q. Where does the inferior epigastric artery originate?

A. It is a branch of the external iliac artery just proximal to the inguinal ligament.

Q. Where is the linea alba?

A. The linea alba runs between the two rectus abdominis muscles in the midline of the anterior abdominal wall. It is a strong, dense aponeurosis made up from the anterior and posterior layers of the rectus sheath. It is attached to the xiphoid process and to the pubic symphysis. It is narrow at the level of the pubic symphysis and widens out nearer the xiphisternum. It is characterized by three tendinous intersections. These occur at the level of:

- Xiphisternum
- Umbilicus
- Midway between the xiphisternum and the umbilicus.

They give the muscle a characteristic bulging appearance when contracted.

ABDOMEN   INGUINAL CANAL

Q. What is the most common type of inguinal hernia?

A. A direct inguinal hernia is the most common. It tends to occur in men over 30 years of age and is due to a weakness in the transversalis fascia or conjoint tendon of the posterior wall of the inguinal canal.

Q. What is the difference between this and an indirect inguinal hernia?

A. Indirect inguinal hernias tend to be due to a congenital abnormality and so are seen frequently in young children but also in adults. The hernia occurs due to the presence of a patent processus vaginalis. As a result, the hernial sac passes through the inguinal canal and downwards to the scrotum.

Q. How can you distinguish between the two?

A. Clinically it should be possible to differentiate between the two hernias by occluding the deep inguinal ring. If occlusion of the deep ring controls the hernia then it is an indirect hernia, if it bulges out next to your fingers then it is a direct hernia.

Anatomically, it is classified as an indirect hernia if it lies lateral to the inferior epigastric artery which lies at the medial edge of the deep inguinal ring. It is a direct hernia if it passes medially to this.

Q. What are the boundaries of the inguinal canal?

A. The boundaries are as follows:

- Floor – in-rolled edge of the inguinal ligament
- Roof – in-rolled edges of the internal oblique and transversus abdominis (which become the *conjoint tendon*)
- Anterior border – aponeurosis of the external oblique and laterally some fibres of the internal oblique
- Posterior border – transversalis fascia with conjoint tendon medially.

Q. What are the contents of the inguinal canal?

A. The inguinal canal contains:

- Spermatic cord
- Ilioinguinal nerve
- Round ligament (females).

Q. What does the ilioinguinal nerve supply?

A. It supplies:

- Upper medial thigh
- Anterior third of the scrotum/labium major
- Conjoint tendon
- Root of penis.

Q. How would you differentiate clinically between an inguinal and a femoral hernia?

A. They can be differentiated clinically by their relationship to the pubic tubercle. An inguinal hernia lies above and medial to it, and a femoral hernia lies below and lateral.

ABDOMEN   PERITONEUM

Q. What is the name of the ligament that connects the liver to the anterior abdominal wall above the umbilicus?

A. The falciform ligament.

Q. Is that the same as the ligamentum teres?

A. No, the ligamentum teres lies in the inferior margin of the falciform ligament and attaches inferiorly to the notch.

Q. What is its significance?

A. It was the left umbilical vein embryologically.

Q. Where would you find the remnants of the umbilical arteries?

A. The remnants of the umbilical arteries are contained within the medial umbilical folds on the posterior surface of the lower anterior abdominal wall.

Q. What is the difference between the visceral and parietal peritoneum?

A. The parietal peritoneum lines the abdominal cavity from the diaphragm to the pelvis; it is supplied by somatic nerves. It becomes the visceral peritoneum in the areas where it leaves the abdominal wall to cover viscera i.e. the mesentery of the small intestine. This is supplied by autonomic nerves.

Q. What are the boundaries of the lesser sac?

A. The lesser sac is situated posterior to the stomach. Its boundaries include:

- Anterior wall – posterior layer of the lesser omentum, peritoneum covering the posterior stomach and posterior layer of the greater omentum
- Posterior wall – the greater omentum, anterior surface of the transverse colon and transverse mesocolon.

Above the transverse mesocolon, the posterior wall is made up of peritoneum that covers the pancreas, upper left kidney and left suprarenal gland.

Q. What are the names of the peritoneal ligaments that connect the stomach to the spleen and left kidney?

A. They are known as the gastrosplenic and lienorenal ligaments.

Q. What do each of these ligaments contain?

A. The gastrosplenic ligament contains the short gastric and left gastroepiploic vessels. The lienorenal ligament contains the splenic vessels and the tail of the pancreas.

Q. Does the sigmoid colon have its own mesentery?

A. Yes, it is called the sigmoid mesocolon. Its shape is an inverted 'V' at the site of the bifurcation of the common iliac artery, on the left side of the pelvic brim.

ABDOMEN DUODENUM

You may be asked to point out the duodenum in a cadaver.

Q. How many parts make up the duodenum?

A. The duodenum is divided up into four parts: first, second, third and fourth.

Q. At what level do they lie?

A. The first part lies at L1, the second part at L2, the third at L3 and the fourth at L2.

Q. What is important about the second part of the duodenum?

A. Within the second part of the duodenum is the major duodenal papilla. This is where the ampulla of Vater opens into the duodenum.

Q. What is the ampulla of Vater made up of?

A. It is made up of the bile duct and the major pancreatic duct.

Q. During endoscopy, how far does the duodenal papilla usually lie from the pylorus?

A. 10 cm.

Q. What structures relate to the third part of the duodenum?

A. The third part of the duodenum lies over the right psoas muscle. Anterior to the psoas and hence posterior to the duodenum lie the right gonadal vessels and ureter. The third part of the duodenum then passes across the inferior vena cava and aorta to reach the left side where it meets the left psoas muscle. It is crossed anteriorly by the superior mesenteric vessels and the inferior mesenteric artery commences beneath it. The pancreas lies on the superior aspect of the third part of the duodenum.

Q. What is the blood supply of the duodenum?

A. The superior and inferior pancreaticoduodenal arteries supply most of the duodenum. There is also some contribution from the hepatic, gastroduodenal, right gastric and right gastroepiploic arteries.

Q. What is different about the mucosa in the first part of the duodenum?

A. The duodenal mucosa is thrown into multiple folds called valvulae conniventes which are characteristically seen throughout the entire small intestine. The initial part of the duodenum, however, is smooth and has a characteristic appearance on imaging. It tends to appear shorter than it actually is on an anteroposterior (AP) radiograph due to the fact that it travels upwards and backwards.

ABDOMEN GALLBLADDER

The examiner may point to the gallbladder within a cadaver and ask you what it is. If you don't know what it is, you will be expected to make some intelligent suggestions. For example, the examiner will have pointed to the right upper quadrant of the abdomen. That limits your options as to what it may or may not be. It is acceptable to gently handle the cadaver in order to gain more information. For example, if you have an idea that it is the gallbladder, you may lift up the right lobe of the liver gently in order to expose the gallbladder. If you are feeling confident, then you may use a pointer to point out the *fundus*, *body* and *neck* of the gallbladder running into the cystic duct.

Q. What arteries supply the gallbladder?

A. The gallbladder usually derives its blood supply from the cystic artery which is usually a branch of the right branch of the hepatic artery. Occasionally the cystic artery may arise from the left branch of the hepatic artery or even from the common hepatic artery itself.

Q. Is it the same for the venous drainage?

A. No, the venous drainage of the gallbladder is via several small veins draining directly into the liver through the gallbladder bed. They generally don't accompany the cystic artery.

Q. What are the boundaries of the foramen of Winslow?

A. The foramen of Winslow is the entrance to the lesser sac. The anterior boundary is made up of a free edge of lesser omentum containing the portal vein posteriorly with the bile duct and hepatic artery anteriorly. Posteriorly is the inferior vena cava covered with parietal peritoneum from the posterior abdominal wall. The upper boundary is the caudate process of the liver and the lower boundary is the first part of the duodenum.

Q. How is the portal vein formed?

A. The portal vein is formed by the superior mesenteric vein and the splenic vein behind the neck of the pancreas.

Q. What areas of porto-systemic anastamoses do you know of?

A. There are five in total:

- Lower oesophagus – the middle part drains systemically to the azygous vein and the lower part drains to the portal system via the left gastric vein.
- Upper anal canal – the upper veins drain via the superior rectal to the inferior mesenteric vein (portal system) and the lower drains into the internal iliac vein (systemic system).
- Bare area of liver.
- Peri-umbilical region – the veins above and below the umbilicus drain systemically to the lateral thoracic and to the great saphenous veins respectively (systemic system). Around the umbilicus, a few veins accompany the ligamentum teres and drain into the portal vein.
- Retroperitoneum – anastomoses may occur where the ascending and descending colon are in contact with the posterior abdominal wall. The colon drains via the superior and inferior mesenteric veins to the portal system and the posterior abdominal wall drains systemically.

Q. When do they become clinically significant?

A. They become clinically significant when portal hypertension prevents normal portal venous drainage, resulting in the development of a collateral circulation. It can lead to potentially life-threatening clinical conditions such as oesophageal varices.

Q. What surface markings would you use in order to perform a needle biopsy of the liver?

A. First, I would confirm the indications for the procedure and then I would obtain informed consent. I would position the needle through the right eighth/ninth intercostal space in the mid-axillary line. I would go in above the rib so as to avoid the intercostal vessels. At this level I would hope that my needle would be below the level of the lung. I would only insert the needle up to the 6 cm mark in order to avoid damage to the inferior vena cava.

Q. What are the complications of this procedure?

A. The complications include:

- Damage to the intercostal muscles/intercostal vessels
- Pneumothorax
- Liver injury/haemorrhage (clotting must be checked preoperatively)
- Damage to the inferior vena cava.

ABDOMEN PANCREAS

Q. How would you recognize the pancreas in the abdomen?

A. The pancreas is a long, thin glandular structure lying transversely in the upper abdominal cavity. It has a large head lying on the right-hand side, it crosses the midline and has a thinner tail on the left-hand side of the abdomen.

Q. What is the blood supply of the pancreas?

A. The pancreas derives most of its blood supply from the splenic artery which is a branch of the coeliac trunk. It runs along the superior aspect of the pancreas on its way to the spleen and gives off a large branch midway known as the *arteria pancreatica magna*. There are also some contributions from the superior and inferior pancreaticoduodenal arteries.

Q. What forms underneath the neck of the pancreas?

A. The commencement of the portal vein from the superior mesenteric and splenic veins lies beneath the neck of the pancreas.

Q. What is the function of the pancreas?

A. The pancreas is an exocrine and endocrine gland. As an exocrine gland it is responsible for the secretion of enzymes that can be released into the duodenum via the pancreatic duct to help digest food. As an endocrine gland, it produces hormones into the circulation, such as insulin and glucagon, which are responsible for the control of carbohydrate metabolism.

Q. How does the pancreas develop embryologically?

A. The embryological development of the pancreas occurs via a dorsal and ventral bud at the junction between the foregut and the midgut. The rotation of the foregut results in the retroperitoneal placement of the developing pancreas. The two buds fuse in order to form the developed pancreas. Once developed, the pancreas is made up of a tail, body, neck, uncinate process and head.

Q. Do you know of any embryological abnormalities that may occur?

A. The commonest embryological abnormality of the pancreas is where the ventral bud fails to rotate and fuse with the dorsal bud. As a result, the pancreas is formed in a continuous ring around the second part of the duodenum. In this scenario, there may be two pancreatic ducts joining the duodenum.

ABDOMEN POSTERIOR ABDOMINAL WALL

Q. What is the root value of the lumbar plexus?

A. The lumbar plexus originates from the anterior rami of L1, 2, 3 and 4.

Q. What are the main branches that come off it?

A. The main branches include:

- Ilioinguinal and iliohypogastric (L1)
- Genitofemoral nerve (L1, 2)
- Lateral cutaneous nerve of the thigh (L2, 3)
- Femoral nerve (L2, 3, 4: posterior division)
- Obturator nerve (L2, 3, 4: anterior division).

Q. What is the relationship of these branches to the psoas muscle?

A. The lumbar plexus lies within the substance of the psoas muscle. The genitofemoral nerve emerges from the anterior aspect of the muscle; the ilioinguinal, iliohypogastric, lateral femoral cutaneous and femoral nerves all emerge from its lateral edge. The obturator and lumbosacral trunk emerge from its medial edge.

Q. What are the attachments of the psoas muscle?

A. The psoas originates from the transverse processes of the five lumbar vertebrae, the sides of the bodies and their intervertebral discs. It attaches as a tendon to the lesser trochanter of the femur.

Q. What is its action?

A. It is a powerful flexor of the hip. It also laterally flexes the vertebral column and aids in flexion of the trunk.

Q. How would a psoas abscess present?

A. A psoas abscess may present with systemic systems such as fever, anorexia and malaise. Clinically, pus may track down the sheath that encloses the psoas and result in a tender, hot swelling in the groin or upper thigh.

Q. Where else may it produce a hot, tender swelling?

A. If untreated, it may travel along the femoral vessels and present as a swelling in the popliteal fossa.

Q. What are the branches of the abdominal aorta?

A. The branches of the abdominal aorta include:

- Inferior phrenic arteries
- Coeliac trunk
- Superior mesenteric artery
- Inferior mesenteric artery
- Suprarenal arteries
- Renal arteries
- Testicular/ovarian arteries
- Four lumbar branches on each side.

It bifurcates into the two common iliac vessels and the median sacral artery at L4.

PELVIS RECTUM

Q. Where does the rectum begin and end?

A. The rectum begins at the level of S3. It is a continuation of the sigmoid colon. It ends as the anal canal in front of the tip of the coccyx.

Q. Does the rectum have a mesentery?

A. No, it doesn't; however, there is a fascial layer covering the rectum known as the mesorectum. It is thought to contain lymphoid tissue and is removed by some colorectal surgeons when performing an anterior resection for colorectal carcinoma.

Q. Is the rectum covered with peritoneum?

A. Yes. The upper third is covered along its front and sides, and the middle third is covered anteriorly only. The lower third is not covered in peritoneum at all.

Q. What nerves may be damaged when performing an anterior resection for a colorectal carcinoma?

A. An anterior resection involves the removal of the rectum through an abdominal approach. It is possible to remove the rectum also through a two-stage abdominal and peroneal approach if the tumour is positioned in the lower rectum.

The nerves that may be injured include the sympathetics that accompany the inferior mesenteric and superior rectal arteries and the parasympathetics from the pelvic splanchnic nerves. Damage to these nerves would lead to erectile dysfunction and impotence.

Q. What is the blood supply of the rectum?

A. The rectum is supplied by the superior rectal artery which is a continuation of the inferior mesenteric artery. It bifurcates at the level of S3 into branches that supply most of the length of the rectum. There are also some contributions from the middle rectal artery which is a branch of the internal iliac artery and the inferior rectal which is a branch of the internal pudendal artery.

Q. What can be felt on rectal examination?

A. It is possible to palpate:

- Coccyx and sacrum
- Ischial spines
- Prostate (males)
- Cervix, uterosacral ligaments and occasionally the ovaries (females).

PELVIS UROGENITAL REGION

Q. What are the contents of the perineal space?

A. The deep perineal space lies above the perineal membrane. It contains:

- Membranous urethra
- Sphincter urethrae
- Deep transverse perineal muscles
- Internal pudendal vessels
- Bulbo urethral glands
- Dorsal nerve of the penis.

Q. Is the urethral sphincter present in women?

A. No.

Q. What structure immediately surrounds the urethra in the male?

A. The corpus spongiosum leading to the glans penis.

Q. Is this connected to the corpus cavernosum?

A. No, they are completely separate structures.

Q. What are the contents of the spermatic cord?

A. The cord contains:

- Vas deferens
- Testicular artery, artery to the ductus and cremasteric artery
- Pampiniform venous plexus
- Lymphatics
- Genital branch of the genitofemoral nerve and sympathetic branches that accompany arteries
- Processus vaginalis.

Q. What layers do you pass through when operating on the testis?

A. The layers are as follows:

- Skin
- Subcutaneous tissue (no fat) containing dartos muscle
- External spermatic fascia
- Cremaster muscle and fascia
- Internal spermatic fascia
- Tunica vaginalis
- Tunica albuginea.

Q. From what does the internal spermatic fascia arise?

A. The internal spermatic fascia is a continuation of the transversalis fascia as it passes through the deep inguinal ring.

Q. Where does the epididymis lie in relation to the testis?

A. The epididymis is attached to the posterior–lateral surface of the testis.

Q. How does semen produced in the testes end up in the urethra prior to ejaculation?

A. Sperm is produced by seminiferous tubules in the testes. From here it travels to the epididymis and into the vas deferens. The vas passes within the spermatic cord and through the inguinal canal. It enters the abdomen through the deep inguinal ring and crosses over the ureter posteriorly to enter the posterior aspect of the bladder. Here it joins with the seminal vesicles which provide seminal fluid and together they form the ejaculatory duct. The ejaculatory duct opens into the verumonatum within the prostatic urethra. From here, the ejaculatory fluid is propelled into the penile urethra by the bulbospongiosus muscle and is prevented from passing backwards by the external urethral sphincter.

Q. Is the semen stored in the seminal vesicles prior to ejaculation?

A. No, the semen is stored in the ampullae which are dilatations in the lower ductus deferens prior to ejaculation.

PELVIS FEMALE PELVIS

Q. What are the muscles that make up the pelvic floor?

A. The muscles that make up the pelvic floor include the levator ani and the coccygeus. The levator ani consists of the iliococcygeus and the pubococcygeus. They both arise from the body of the pubis and insert into the perineal body. The coccygeus arises from the tip of the ischial spines and inserts into the coccyx.

Q. What is the function of the pelvic floor?

A. The pelvic floor supports the pelvic contents, in particular the bladder, uterus and anal canal. If damaged during childbirth it may lead to vaginal prolapse and incontinence.

Q. Is the uterus covered with peritoneum?

A. Most of the uterus is covered with peritoneum. Laterally the two peritoneal layers become the broad ligaments. Anteriorly, however, the peritoneum covering the uterus does not reach the upper vagina. Posteriorly, the peritoneum covers the upper vagina and forms the pouch of Douglas between the uterus and the rectum.

Q. How many parts does each Fallopian tube contain?

A. Each Fallopian tube is made up of four parts:

- Isthmus
- Ampulla
- Infundibulum
- Fimbriae.

Q. What type of epithelium lines the Fallopian tubes?

A. It is a mixture of ciliated and non-ciliated columnar epithelium that aids the movement of the ovum towards the uterus.

Q. How might an abnormality within the ovary result in pain of the inner thigh?

A. This may occur due to the fact that the ovary lies medially to the obturator nerve which, if diseased, can result in referred pain to the inner thigh.

Q. What is the round ligament?

A. The round ligament of the uterus, together with the ligament of the ovary, are embryological remnants of the gubernaculum. Originally, it began on the posterior abdominal wall and travelled through the inguinal canal towards the labium major. The ovary, however, stops its journey as it attaches to the uterus.

Q. What is its function?

A. It is debatable; however, it may possibly maintain the uterus in a position of anteversion and anteflexion.

Q. What is the lymph drainage of the ovaries?

A. The ovaries drain primarily to the para-aortic lymph nodes. They may also drain to the inguinal nodes via the round ligaments and also to the opposite ovary via the fundus of the uterus.

Q. Which branches of the internal iliac vessels leave the pelvis?

A. The obturator, pudendal and gluteal vessels.

Q. What region does the internal pudendal artery supply?

A. The internal pudendal supplies the lower rectum, anal canal and the external genitalia.

PELVIS PERINEUM AND ANUS

Q. What type of muscle makes up the anal sphincter?

A. The external anal sphincter is composed of skeletal muscle and the internal sphincter is composed of smooth muscle.

Q. What is the difference between the two sphincters?

A. The internal anal sphincter is essentially a continuation of the inner circular smooth muscular layer of the rectum. It is under involuntary control.

The external anal sphincter, however, is under voluntary control and is responsible for faecal continence. It is a continuous, funnel-shaped layer of skeletal muscle that comprises a *deep, superficial* and *subcutaneous* part. The deep end (nearest the rectum) is continuous with the puborectalis part of the levator ani muscle.

Q. What is meant by the term 'anal columns'?

A. Anal columns are layers of vertical folds of mucosal membrane present in the upper half of the anal canal. They are joined inferiorly by anal valves which contain anal glands and secrete mucus.

Q. Is there a name given to this area?

A. Yes, it is called the dentate line. The anal canal is characteristically smooth beneath this line.

Q. What are the anal cushions?

A. Anal cushions are protuberances in the anal canal that allow the anus, when closed, to be water-tight. They are known clinically as haemorrhoids when they enlarge.

Q. Where are they situated?

A. They are situated in the upper half of the anal canal, classically at 3 o'clock, 7 o'clock and 11 o'clock.

Q. What are they made from?

A. They are fleshy, subcutaneous masses consisting of connective tissue, smooth muscle and dilated capillary plexuses.

Q. If damaged, why do they result in the passage of bright red blood per rectum and not dark venous blood?

A. This is because they consist of arterio-venous anastomoses and so bright red blood is seen.

Q. What is the lymph drainage of the anal canal?

A. The upper half of the anus drains to the internal iliac nodes and the lower half drains to the inguinal nodes which can be readily palpated, if enlarged.

Q. What are the boundaries of the ischioanal fossa?

A. The ischioanal fossa is situated on either side of the anal canal.

- Lateral border – obturator internus
- Medial border – levator ani and external anal sphincter
- Base – urogenital diaphragm, sacrotuberous ligament and lower border of gluteus maximus.

The medial and lateral walls meet to form the roof of the wedge-shaped fossa.

Q. What is the purpose of this fossa?

A. This fossa allows the rectum to distend with stool and hence aids the process of defecation.

Q. Are there any disease processes specific to this area?

A. Yes, it can become infected and result in an ischioanal abscess. Occasionally infection may spread between the two.

HEAD AND NECK | THYROID GLAND

Q. What is the blood supply of the thyroid gland?

A. The thyroid gland is supplied by:

- The superior thyroid artery – a branch of the external carotid artery
- The inferior thyroid artery – a branch of the thyrocervical trunk
- The thyroid ima artery – occasionally this artery arises from the arch of the aorta or brachiocephalic trunk and supplies the isthmus.

Q. When performing a total thyroidectomy, what nerves are at risk?

A. When ligating the superior thyroid artery, the external branch of the superior laryngeal nerve is at risk. When ligating the inferior thyroid artery, the recurrent laryngeal nerve is at risk.

Q. What is the relationship of the recurrent laryngeal nerve to the inferior thyroid artery?

A. The relationship of the recurrent laryngeal nerve to the inferior thyroid artery is variable. It arises from the vagus nerve and loops around the subclavian artery on the right and the aorta on the left. It then travels lateral to the tracheo-

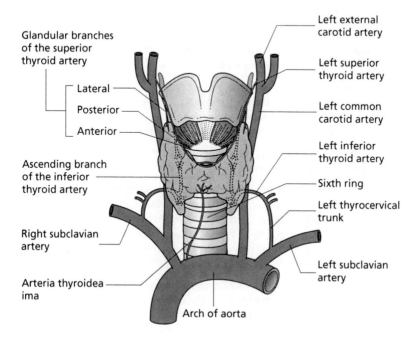

(A)

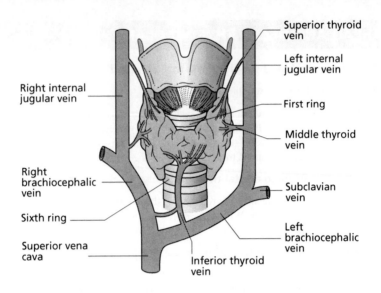

Right internal jugular vein

Right brachiocephalic vein

Sixth ring

Superior vena cava

Superior thyroid vein

Left internal jugular vein

First ring

Middle thyroid vein

Subclavian vein

Left brachiocephalic vein

Inferior thyroid vein

(B)

Fig. 3 (A) Arterial blood supply and (B) venous drainage of the thyroid gland

oesophageal groove and may pass behind, in front of or between the terminal branches of the inferior thyroid artery.

Occasionally, the nerve may arise directly from the vagus in the cervical region on the right-hand side and reach the thyroid in between the superior and inferior thyroid arteries. This is known as 'non-recurrence' and puts the nerve at risk during surgery as it may be tied off with either vessel.

Q. What clinical condition would result if this nerve was accidentally damaged during surgery?

A. The recurrent laryngeal nerve supplies motor function to all the intrinsic muscles of the larynx except the cricothyroid and sensation to the subglottic region. During thyroidectomy, the recurrent laryngeal nerve may be accidentally damaged or cut completely. If it were damaged, the cords would close in the fully adducted position. If cut completely, the cords would become paralysed and would lie in the cadaveric semi adducted position.

If unilateral, a hoarse voice would result as the opposite cord would still be able to oppose the affected cord lying in the cadaveric position. If bilateral, both cords would lie in the cadaveric position and the patient would not be able to speak at all.

Q. **What would be the clinical consequences of damaging the external branch of the superior laryngeal nerve?**

A. The external branch of the superior laryngeal nerve is motor supply to the cricothyroid muscle. It is most at risk when the upper pole of the thyroid is being mobilized. Here it lies medial to the superior thyroid artery but occasionally may wind around it.

If damaged, the voice may become husky and weak, and affected patients find it difficult to project their voice. This is obviously of some concern to opera singers or people who regularly speak in public.

Q. **Where does the thyroid gland lie in the neck?**

A. The thyroid gland consists of two lobes and an isthmus which lies over the second, third and fourth tracheal rings.

Q. **Where on the lobes does the isthmus connect?**

A. The isthmus connects the lower poles of the lobes and is positioned anteriorly.

Q. **Why is it that the whole thyroid gland moves up and down on swallowing?**

A. This is because the pretracheal fascia completely envelops the thyroid gland and is firmly attached to the second, third and fourth tracheal rings.

Q. **What is the lymph drainage of the thyroid gland?**

A. The thyroid gland usually drains to the deep cervical nodes of the neck. It may also drain directly into the thoracic duct.

Q. **What is the relationship of the parathyroid glands to the thyroid gland?**

A. There are usually four parathyroid glands known as the superior and inferior glands. The superior parathyroids can usually be found within the pretracheal capsule, posterior to the thyroid and just above the level of the inferior thyroid artery. The inferior glands are also mostly found within the pretracheal fascia. They are more variable, however, and may be found within the substance of the gland or elsewhere in the neck.

Q. **What is their blood supply?**

A. They usually obtain their blood supply from the inferior thyroid artery and drain via small veins that join the thyroid veins.

HEAD AND NECK SCALENUS ANTERIOR

Q. Where does the scalenus anterior originate?

A. The scalenus anterior arises from the anterior tubercles of the third to the sixth cervical vertebrae and attaches to the scalene tubercle on the first rib.

Q. What is its innervation?

A. It is innervated by branches of the anterior rami of C5 and 6 nerves.

Q. What is the relationship of the phrenic nerve to the scalenus anterior?

A. The phrenic nerve passes downwards on the anterior aspect of the muscle and beneath the prevertebral fascia.

Q. What other structures pass anteriorly to the scalenus anterior?

A. Other structures passing anteriorly to the scalenus include:

- Ascending cervical artery (branch of the inferior thyroid artery)
- Transverse cervical artery
- Suprascapular artery
- Vagus nerve (gives off the recurrent laryngeal nerve on the right at the level of the subclavian artery)
- Internal jugular vein
- Deep cervical lymph nodes (following the internal jugular vein)
- Subclavian vein (actually lies lower than the scalenus anterior; however, it joins with the internal jugular vein at its medial edge to form the brachiocephalic vein).

Q. What structures pass medial to the scalenus anterior?

A. Medial to the scalenus anterior is a pyramidal-shaped space bounded by the longus colli laterally, the cervical spine medially and the subclavian artery inferiorly. It contains:

- Inferior cervical sympathetic ganglion ('stellate ganglion')
- Vertebral artery and vein.

In front of this area lies the inferior thyroid artery, the sympathetic chain and the thoracic duct on the left-hand side.

Q. What is the relationship of the carotid artery to this space?

A. The carotid artery lies anterior to this space and medial to the subclavian vein.

Q. How is the subclavian artery related to the scalenus anterior?

A. The subclavian artery may be divided into three parts:

- First part – medial to the scalenus anterior, arches over pleura
- Second part – posterior to the scalenus anterior
- Third part –lateral to the scalenus anterior and ending at the lateral border of the first rib.

Q. What are their branches?

A. These are as follows:

- First part – Vertebral artery; thyrocervical trunk (inferior thyroid, transverse cervical, suprascapular); internal thoracic artery
- Second part – Costocervical trunk; dorsal scapular
- Third part – No named branch

Q. What structures can be found at the lateral border of the scalenus anterior?

A. The trunks of the brachial plexus and the third part of the subclavian artery.

HEAD AND NECK   CRANIAL NERVES

You may be shown a cadaveric brainstem and asked to point out and name the cranial nerves. It is a good idea to familiarize yourself with the appearance of each cranial nerve. You may also be asked to talk specifically about a cranial nerve. If so, it is expected that you will know the following facts:

- Nucleus
- Relevant site in the brainstem
- Site of exit through the arachnoid and dura mater
- Extracranial course including area of distribution.

If you can't get to a dissection room, familiarize yourself with the brainstem in a photographic anatomy atlas. The brainstem is as follows:

- Midbrain
- Pons
- Medulla oblongata

It contains the third to the 12th cranial nerve nuclei.

- First (olfactory) – this can be seen as a 'bulb' overlying the cribiform plate of the ethmoid bone.
- Second (optic) – this can be seen clearly as the chiasma above the pituitary gland in the middle cranial fossa. From here, it passes around the midbrain.
- Third (oculomotor) – can be seen emerging from the medial aspect of the cerebral peduncle, above the pons.
- Fourth (trochlear) – this is a very long, thin-looking nerve that emerges from the dorsal aspect of the midbrain, below the inferior colliculus. It then hitches onto the free edge of the tentorium cerebelli.
- Fifth (trigeminal) – this is made up of two roots: a large sensory one attached to the ventral pons and a motor root emerging medially to it (this is the only cranial nerve to emerge from the pons).
- Sixth (abducens) – emerges from the lower pons above the pyramid of the medulla.

- Seventh (facial) – emerges from the lower pons.
- Eighth (vestibulocochlear) – passes by the lower border of the pons.
- Ninth (glossopharyngeal) – emerges as several rootlets that merge into one from the surface of the medulla.
- Tenth (vagus) – these also emerge as rootlets that join into one from the surface of the medulla, directly below the glossopharyngeal nerve.
- 11th (accessory) – the cranial root emerges from the medulla as several rootlets beneath the vagus. The spinal root is formed from the anterior rami of the upper five segments of the cervical cord.
- 12th (hypoglossal) – also emerges from the medulla as several rootlets, positioned in a straight line between the pyramid and the olive.

Q. What controls pupillary constriction?

A. The oculomotor nerve via the Edinger–Westphal nucleus.

Q. And what about pupillary dilation?

A. Pupillary dilation is under sympathetic control from T1.

Q. How do sympathetic fibres from T1 reach the pupil?

A. Sympathetic fibres accompany the internal carotid artery to the cavernous sinus. From here they join the nasociliary nerve which is a branch of the ophthalmic division of the trigeminal nerve to reach the long ciliary nerve.

Q. What clinical condition results if this nerve is damaged?

A. Pupillary constriction, partial ptosis and reduced sweating on the affected side of the face. The clinical condition is known as Horner's syndrome.

Q. What causes Horner's syndrome?

A. Any damage to the stellate ganglion or the sympathetic chain above it such as direct trauma or carcinoma of the lung.

Q. Tell me about the course of the vagus nerve.

A. The vagus nerve is the tenth cranial nerve. It emerges as a series of rootlets from the medulla and passes through the jugular foramen. From here, it travels inside the carotid sheath alongside the common carotid artery and internal jugular vein. It has a superior and inferior ganglion just below the jugular foramen.

It gives off branches to the pharyngeal plexus, the superior laryngeal nerve and two cardiac branches on each side. It also gives off a recurrent laryngeal branch on both sides. The right hooks underneath the right subclavian artery and the left hooks under the arch of the aorta before travelling back up to the neck.

The vagi then pass behind the lung roots, supplying branches to the pulmonary and oesophageal plexuses. The nerve then divides into anterior and posterior trunks and travels with the oesophagus into the abdomen.

The vagus then supplies the foregut, midgut, biliary tree and pancreas.

HEAD AND NECK   PARANASAL SINUSES

Q. What are the paranasal sinuses?

A. Paranasal sinuses are four, paired air-containing cavities within the nasal cavity. They are connected via small channels.

Q. What lines them?

A. They are lined with ciliated respiratory epithelium which produces mucus.

Q. Where are the four paranasal sinuses?

A. The *frontal* sinuses are in the frontal bone and are separated by a bony septum. The *maxillary* sinuses are within the maxilla at the lateral margin of the nasal cavity. The *ethmoid* sinuses are a group of approximately ten air-containing cavities within the ethmoid bone, in between the upper nasal cavity and the orbit. They are called the anterior, middle and posterior groups. The *sphenoid* sinuses lie within the body of the sphenoid bone.

Q. Where do they each drain into?

A. They drain as follows:

- Maxillary sinus – middle meatus
- Anterior ethmoidal sinus – middle meatus
- Middle ethmoidal sinus – middle meatus
- Posterior ethmoidal sinus – superior meatus
- Sphenoidal sinus – sphenoethmoidal recess
- Frontal sinus – middle meatus.

Q. Which sinus is the most prone to infection?

A. The maxillary sinus, as its opening is placed high up on the nasal wall and it is therefore not efficient at draining mucus.

Q. What causes infection here?

A. Maxillary sinus infection is generally from the nasal cavity or from the upper molar teeth.

Q. How would you go about draining the maxillary sinus surgically?

A. The maxillary sinus may be drained surgically by:

- Antral puncture through the nasal cavity
- Antral drainage through the gingiolabial fold (known as the Caldwell Luc procedure)
- Through the medial wall of the sinus, below the inferior concha
- In the past, by extracting an upper molar tooth.

Q. What are the anatomical relations of the sphenoid sinus?

A. The sphenoid sinus is related to:

- Superiorly – pituitary fossa and middle cranial fossa

- Laterally – cavernous sinus and internal carotid artery
- Posteriorly – pons and posterior cranial fossa
- Inferiorly – roof of the nasal cavity.

Q. How would a maxillary sinus tumour present?

A. A maxillary sinus will usually remain symptomless until it encroaches on surrounding structures:

- Floor of the sinus – lump palpable or ulceration into palate
- Lateral wall – lump palpable in gingival or visible on the face
- Medial wall – nasal blockage or epistaxis
- Posterior wall – invasion of palatine nerves causing dental pain
- Superior spread to the orbit – diplopia.

HEAD AND NECK   TEMPOROMANDIBULAR JOINT

Q. Where is the temporomandibular joint?

A. The temporomandibular joint connects the condyle of the mandible and the squamous part of the temporal bone.

Q. What type of joint is it?

A. It is an atypical synovial joint consisting of a fibro-cartilaginous disc and fibro-cartilage on the bony surfaces.

Q. Can one temporomandibular joint move on its own?

A. No, when one moves, so does the other.

Q. How stable is the joint?

A. The joint is most stable when the jaw is closed. In this position the teeth stabilize the jaw. When open, the condyle is able to slide anteriorly over the articular eminence and may sometimes dislocate.

Q. What are the muscles that close the jaw?

A. These are the masseter, temporalis, and medial pterygoids.

Q. How would you reduce an anterior jaw dislocation?

A. When the jaw dislocates, the muscles previously mentioned go into spasm. This may be overcome by pressing firmly on the molar teeth and the joint reduced by manoeuvering back into joint or lifting up the chin.

Q. What ligaments insert into the capsule of the joint?

A. The lateral temporomandibular ligament originating from the zygomatic arch inserts into the neck of the mandible.

Q. What movements are possible at the temporomandibular joint?

A. Movements at this joint include:

- Depression of the jaw
- Elevation of the jaw
- Side to side movements
- Protrusion
- Retraction.

Q. Which group of muscles are responsible for these movements?

A. The muscles of mastication, which include:

- Temporalis (close the mouth)
- Masseter (close the mouth)
- Medial pterygoid (close the mouth)
- Lateral pterygoids (open the mouth).

Q. Which muscles are responsible for the side to side movements?

A. The medial and lateral pterygoids.

HEAD AND NECK   VERTEBRAL COLUMN

Q. How does the vertebral column develop its shape?

A. In utero the spine is flexed anteriorly and forms a 'C' shape known as the *primary curvature*. It is made up of 33 vertebrae:

- Seven cervical
- Twelve thoracic
- Five lumbar
- Nine fused in the sacrum and coccyx.

As the child learns to extend its head with sitting and standing, the spine develops *secondary curvatures* in the cervical and lumbar areas.

Q. What movements does the vertebral column allow?

A. The vertebral column allows flexion, extension, lateral flexion and rotation. The neck has a greater range of movement in that the atlanto-occipital and atlanto-axial joints allow the head to nod and rotate to some degree.

Q. What type of joint is the atlanto-occipital joint?

A. It is a synovial joint.

Q. You may be handed a vertebra, asked which region it comes from and to describe its features. For example, look at the vertebra below. Describe its features and state which area in the spine it comes from.

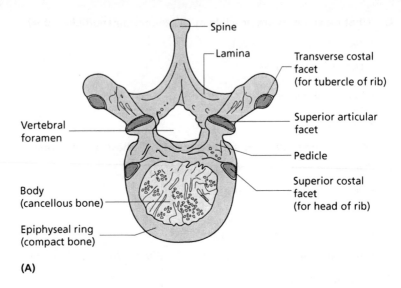

Spine

Lamina

Transverse costal facet (for tubercle of rib)

Superior articular facet

Vertebral foramen

Pedicle

Superior costal facet (for head of rib)

Body (cancellous bone)

Epiphyseal ring (compact bone)

(A)

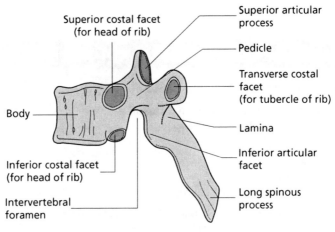

Superior articular process

Superior costal facet (for head of rib)

Pedicle

Transverse costal facet (for tubercle of rib)

Body

Lamina

Inferior articular facet

Inferior costal facet (for head of rib)

Long spinous process

Intervertebral foramen

(B)

Fig. 4 A typical thoracic vertebra (A) superior view, (B) lateral view

A. It has a heart-shaped upper and lower surface and a concave body. It may be distinguished as a thoracic vertebra by the presence of a pair of costal facets either side of the body. The facets articulate with the heads of the ribs. They also contain facets on their transverse processes for articulation with the rib tubercles. It appears that this vertebra is one of the upper thoracic vertebra. This is because their spinous processes slope downwards and become progressively more horizontal from T7 to T12.

Q. How else would you distinguish an upper from a lower thoracic vertebra?

A. The lower two thoracic vertebrae have only one facet on either side of their bodies for articulation with the rib heads. T11 and T12 don't have facets for rib tubercle articulation on their transverse processes.

Q. How does the rib head usually articulate with the body of the thoracic vertebra?

A. Each numbered rib usually articulates with the body of its corresponding vertebra and that of the one above, except for the lower two vertebrae which only articulate with their corresponding vertebrae as does the first rib with its body.

Q. How do the cervical vertebrae differ from the thoracic ones?

A. The cervical vertebrae are in the shape of a kidney bean. Their bodies are smaller. They are easily distinguishable from other vertebrae by the presence of the foramen transversarium in their transverse processes. They have small, bifid spines except for C1 and C7 which have single spines.

Q. What does the foramen transversarium contain?

A. It contains the vertebral artery, vein and some sympathetic fibres.

Q. What is special about C7?

A. C7 is otherwise known as the *vertebra prominens*. This is because it has a longer spinous process than the other cervical vertebrae, which is non-bifid and easily palpable.

Q. Which other cervical vertebrae are atypical?

A. C1 and C2 are atypical vertebrae.

C1 is called the atlas and possesses no body. It has two lateral facets on either side of the arch which articulate with the occipital condyles and carry the weight of the skull. Their lower surfaces are flat and articulate with C2 (the axis).

C2 is easily identifiable by its dens, otherwise known as the *odontoid process*. It protrudes from the superior aspect of the body of C2 and articulates with the anterior arch of the atlas. It also has a large, bifid spinous process.

Q. What ligaments attach the axis to the occiput?

A. There are several ligaments which attach the axis to the occiput:

- *Tectorial membrane* – attaches the body of the axis to the anterior foramen magnum. It is the extension of the posterior longitudinal ligament.
- *Apical ligament* – tip of the dens to the anterior foramen magnum.
- *Cruciform ligament* – this ligament is made up of a small ligament connecting the body of the axis to the occiput and the transverse ligament. This is a strong band running behind the dens connecting, from side to side, to the atlas.
- *Alar ligaments* – these lie either side of the apical ligament.

- *Anterior atlanto-occipital ligament* – extension of the anterior longitudinal ligament.
- *Posterior atlanto-occipital ligament* – extension of the posterior longitudinal ligament.

HEAD AND NECK SKULL

This section is universally feared. You will see the skull within the selection of bones on the examiner's desk and quite possibly hope that it won't be picked up. The way I dealt with this problem was to make sure that I learnt everything that I possibly could about every nook, cranny and foramen and from every angle. Also, it is a good idea once you've studied the skull to change your attitude towards it ..... for example try to think 'I really hope they ask me something about the skull' as opposed to 'if they hand me the skull it's game over!' After all, you won't be expected to know a huge amount other than the basics.

How to approach the skull

It is likely that you will be handed the skull and asked something like:

Q. Tell me what you know about this.

A. Pick the skull up in a confident manner, hold it comfortably in your hand in the anatomical position and start talking about what you know. It is worth remembering that the skull actually means that the mandible is also present. If it isn't there, it is known as the cranium. The cranium will fit comfortably onto your straightened palm, facing the examiner. Then you may begin. Some features worth mentioning include:

- The *bones* that make up the vault of the skull – frontal, parietal and occipital.
- The *sutures* – coronal (transverse suture between the frontal and parietal bones), sagittal (midline suture where the parietal bones meet) and lambdoid (transverse suture where the occipital bones meet the parietal).
- *Fontanelle* sites – bregma (the site of the anterior fontanelle, in the midline where the coronal suture meets the sagittal suture) and lambda (posterior fontanelle, where the sagittal suture meets the lambdoid).
- *External occipital protuberance* – found below the lambda, also has a palpable ridge which signifies the superior nuchal line. It is the surface marking of the tentorium cerebelli and transverse sinus and also gives attachment to the sternocleidomastoid, trapezius and other muscles to the back of the neck.
- *Pterion* – on the lateral aspect of the skull, there is an obvious 'H shape' of sutures made up from the frontal, parietal, temporal and sphenoid bones. This is the thinnest, most vulnerable part of the vault.
- *Zygomatic arch* – made up of the temporal process of the zygomatic bone and the zygomatic process of the temporal bone. Gives rise to the masseter and superficial parotid fascia.

- *Maxilla* – gives rise to the buccinator. The maxillae meet in the middle at the intermaxillary suture and form the anterior nasal spine.
- *Nasal bones* – articulate with the frontal bone and the maxilla and meet in the middle. The bony septum and conchae are visible within the nasal cavity.
- *Orbits* – house the eye, its extraocular muscles, lacrimal gland, fascia, fat, nerves and vessels. Made up of:
  - Roof – Frontal bone; lesser wing of sphenoid
  - Medial wall – Frontal process of maxilla; lacrimal bone; ethmoid bone; body of sphenoid
  - Lateral wall – Zygomatic bone; greater wing of sphenoid
  - Floor – Maxilla; Zygomatic bone; orbital process of palatine bone.
- *Superior orbital fissure* – situated between the greater and lesser wings of the sphenoid. Contains the ophthalmic division of the trigeminal nerve, oculomotor nerve, trochlear nerve, abducent nerve, ophthalmic veins and branches of the middle meningeal and lacrimal arteries.
- *Inferior orbital fissure* – arises from the medial aspect of the superior orbital fissure between the greater wing of the sphenoid and maxilla. Contains branches of the maxillary nerve (infra-orbital and zygomatic), infra-orbital veins and arteries and orbital branches of the pterygopalatine ganglion.
- *Supra-orbital foramen* – visible notch in the frontal bone within the supra-orbital margin. Transmits the supra-orbital nerve and vessels. In a vertical line drawn down from the supra-orbital foramen lies the *infra-orbital foramen* and nerve (where the maxilla and zygomatic bone meet at the infra-orbital margin) and the *mental foramen* and nerve (within the mandible, between the first and second lower premolar teeth).

Q. Alternatively, you may be handed the cranium upside down (inferior view of the base of the skull) or with the skull vault removed (superior view of the base of the skull). You may then be asked to pick a hole and talk about it.

A. All I can say is be prepared! This is actually a gift of a question as it puts the ball in your court and gives you an opportunity to show what you've learnt.

 TIP

'Holes'

Here is a list I wrote out and learnt off by heart before the exam. I was never sure if I'd ever get asked this, but I was so worried about being caught out I thought it best to be safe.

Below is a series of 'holes' and 'canals' and their contents.

- Foramen magnum – spinal cord (medulla oblongata), meninges, vertebral arteries, anterior and posterior spinal arteries, spinal root of the accessory nerve, sympathetic branches with the vertebral artery, apical ligament of dens and tectorial membrane.

✔ TIP—cont'd

- Condylar canal (behind occipital condyle) – emissary vein from sigmoid sinus to suboccipital venous plexus and meningeal branch of occipital artery.
- Hypoglossal canal – hypoglossal nerve and meningeal branch of ascending pharyngeal artery.
- Jugular foramen – jugular bulb (forms internal jugular vein), inferior petrosal sinus, glossopharyngeal, vagus and accessory nerves.
- Carotid canal – internal carotid artery with accompanying sympathetics and internal carotid venous plexus.
- Foramen lacerum – nothing actually passes through here; however, the internal carotid artery exits through its upper limits and the greater petrosal nerve reaches the pterygoid canal via its upper end.
- Internal acoustic meatus – facial nerve, vestibulocochlear nerve, nervus intermedius, labyrinthine vessels.
- Petrosquamous fissure – contains no structures.
- Petrotympanic fissure – chorda tympani, tympanic branch of maxillary artery and anterior ligament of malleus.
- Foramen ovale – mandibular nerve and meningeal branch, lesser petrosal nerve, accessory meningeal artery, emissary vein.
- Foramen spinosum – middle meningeal vessels and meningeal branch of mandibular nerve if it doesn't pass through the foramen ovale.
- Stylomastoid foramen – facial nerve and stylomastoid branch of posterior auricular artery.
- Foramen rotundum – maxillary division of the trigeminal nerve.
- Greater palatine foramen – greater palatine vessels and nerve.
- Lesser palatine foramen – lesser palatine vessels and nerve.
- Incisive foramen – greater palatine artery and nasopalatine nerve.

Q. You are handed the upturned cranium and asked 'Tell me about the inferior aspect of the base of the skull'.

A. The only way to be good at this is to get hold of a skull before the exam and familiarize yourself with its structures. It is extremely difficult to learn this from the books.

It is important not to hesitate, be confident and start with something simple that you recognize. For example, start with the foramen magnum and talk about its contents. If you can answer that correctly it may be that the examiner will be satisfied, put the skull down and move on to another subject. If he/she doesn't, then some other features to mention include:

- External occipital protuberance – superior, inferior nuchal lines and the external occipital crest in the midline which gives attachment to the ligament nuchae.
- Occipital condyles – kidney-shaped protuberances either side of the foramen magnum which articulate with the atlas.
- Hypoglossal canal – this lies above the occipital condyles and contains the hypoglossal nerve.

- Carotid canal – anterior to the jugular notch.
- Foramen ovale – in the roof of the infra-temporal fossa.
- Foramen spinosum – within the base of the sphenoid.
- Mastoid process.
- Mandibular fossa – fossa within the squamous part of the temporal bone which articulates with the mandible.
- External acoustic meatus – a bony ring made up of the squamous part of the temporal bone and the tympanic part of the temporal bone.
- Styloid process.
- Spine of the sphenoid.
- Pharyngeal tubercle.
- Pterygoid hamulus – projects from the medial pterygoid plate and provides a hook for the tendon of the tensor palati.
- Lateral pterygoid plate.

Other related questions

Q. What is the blood supply of the dura mater?

A. The dura mater is made up of a thin, outer layer and a thicker inner layer which projects into the skull to form the tentorium cerebelli and falx cerebri. The inner layer has little blood supply; however, the outer layer is supplied by nearby bone, mainly from meningeal branches:

- Anterior cranial fossa – Ophthalmic artery; anterior ethmoidal artery
- Middle cranial fossa – Middle meningeal artery; accessory meningeal artery; internal carotid artery; ascending pharyngeal artery
- Posterior cranial fossa – Vertebral artery.

Q. And what about its nerve supply?

A. The dura is mostly supplied by the ophthalmic division of the trigeminal nerve. It also receives locoregional supply from:

- Anterior and posterior ethmoidal nerves (anterior cranial fossa)
- Mandibular nerve (middle cranial fossa)
- Glossopharyngeal and vagus nerves (posterior cranial fossa).

Q. At what level in the spine does the dura mater end?

A. It commences at the foramen magnum and ends at S2.

Q. Does the pia mater also end at this level?

A. No, the pia mater extends down into the coccyx as the filum terminale.

Q. At what level is it safe to perform a lumbar puncture?

A. At L4/5.

PERIPHERAL NERVE LESIONS

Q. How may the severity of a nerve lesion be defined?

A. Nerve lesions may be classified into the following groups:

- Neuropraxia – physiological defect associated with ischaemia or focal demyelination
- Axonotmesis – axonal disruption with endo/peri or epineurium intact
- Neurotmesis – axonal and endo/peri/epineural transection.

Q. How well do these lesions usually recover?

A.
- Neuropraxia – very good prognosis, function usually recovers within 6–12 weeks.
- Axonotmesis – new axon grows from proximal stump into empty neural tube; regeneration starts after 1 month and proceeds at 1 mm/day; prognosis worsens with more proximal lesions.
- Neurotmesis – poor prognosis without repair; serial EMGs (electromyograms) may aid diagnosis and guide surgery; once neurotmesis is suspected, exploration and repair are indicated.

Whilst awaiting nerve recovery, it is vital to work with therapists to maintain joint mobility and prevent contractures.

Q. Where may the radial nerve or its branches be damaged?

A. The radial nerve (loss of wrist/finger/thumb extension with or without objective sensory loss) may be damaged in the mid third, distal third (Holstein–Lewis) or by supracondylar fractures, or by 'Saturday night palsy' (sleeping with an arm over the back of a chair).

The posterior interosseous nerve (supplies extensors of the forearm) may be damaged by compression at the Arcade of Frohse (origin of the supinator).

The superficial radial nerve (supplies dorsal hand skin, and lateral three digits up to the nail beds only; pain rather than numbness) may be damaged by blunt trauma to the radial aspect of the wrist.

Q. Where may the ulnar nerve be damaged?

A. The ulnar nerve may be damaged in the following places:

- Elbow – dislocation/condylar or supracondylar fracture
- Cubital tunnel – from the Arcade of Struther's to two heads of flexor carpi ulnaris
- Forearm or wrist – usually lacerations
- Guyon's canal – superficial and on the ulnar side of flexor retinaculum.

Q. How may the level of the lesion be assessed clinically?

A. At the wrist by intrinsic weakness (except the radial two lumbricals and the thenar muscles), and by autonomous sensory loss (pulp of little finger).

Above the elbow, as above with weakness of the flexor carpi ulnaris and flexor digitorum profundus to the ulnar two digits. There is often less clawing due to flexor digitorum profundus weakness ('ulnar paradox').

Q. Do any anastomoses between the ulnar and median nerves complicate this pattern?

A. The Martin–Gruber anastomosis in the forearm, and the Riche–Cannieu anastomosis in the palm.

Q. Where may the median nerve be damaged?

A.
- Elbow – posterior dislocation/supracondylar fracture
- Forearm – compression at the level of the pronator teres
- Wrist – laceration/distal radial fractures/carpal dislocations/carpal tunnel syndrome.

Q. What motor and sensory deficits indicate median neuropathy?

A. Abductor pollicis brevis weakness, and sensory loss over the radial aspect of the index finger pulp.

Q. Where is the common peroneal nerve most commonly injured?

A. As it curls round the neck of the fibula.

Q. What motor and sensory deficits indicate peroneal neuropathy?

A. Weakness is indicated by:

- Dorsiflexion of the ankle and extension of the hallux (deep peroneal nerve)
- Eversion of the foot (superficial peroneal nerve).

Loss of sensibility is indicated by:

- Overlying proximal fibula (common peroneal)
- Dorsum of the foot (superficial peroneal nerve)
- First web space (deep peroneal nerve).

Q. How would you investigate non-surgical causes of a mononeuropathy?

A. After history and examination, if no diagnosis is implied, first-line investigations should include:

- Full blood count (FBC)
- Urea and electrolytes (U&Es)
- Glucose
- Erythrocyte sedimentation rate (ESR)
- C-reactive protein (CRP)
- Liver function tests (LFT)
- Thyroid function tests (TFT)
- Auto-antibodies.

> **TIP**
>
> Most mononeuropathies are caused by surgically treatable causes. It is imperative to seek such a cause before committing the patient to empirical steroid or expectant therapy.

Q. What are the roots of origin of the median nerve?

A. C5/6/7/8/T1.

Note:

- Musculocutaneous – C5/6/7
- Ulnar – C8/T1
- Axillary – C5/6
- Radial – C5/6/7/8/T1
- Femoral – L2/3/4
- Obturator – L2/3/4
- Common peroneal – L4/5/S1/2.

OPERATIVE SURGERY

LYMPH NODE BIOPSY

Q. How do you classify the lymph nodes in the neck anatomically?

A. Two circles and two chains. Superficial and deep circles are located along the submental, submandibular, pre-auricular, post-auricular and occipital groups. The two chains include the superficial chain along the external jugular vein, and the deep chain along the internal jugular vein.

Q. How would you manage a young man who presents to the surgical clinic with a large painless cervical lymph node which is increasing in size?

A. The management includes taking a full history (including recent travel abroad), clinical examination, investigations and treatment.

Q. How would you examine this patient with an enlarged cervical lymph node?

A. I would examine the symptomatic lymph node and all the regional lymph nodes, including cervical, bilateral axillary and bilateral inguinal nodes. I would also examine the drainage area (i.e. head and neck region including the mouth, looking for dental causes, for example a dental abscess). Examination of other systems is necessary, including examination of the abdomen for hepato-splenomegaly etc. If the patient has any ENT-related symptoms, then they will need to have an ENT assessment.

Q. How would you investigate this patient with an enlarged cervical lymph node?

A. • Blood tests including a full blood count and differential white count, ESR or CRP if an infectious case is suspected. Viral titres might be necessary in certain cases when the patient presents early (such as glandular fever).
   • Radiological including chest X-ray to exclude pulmonary causes or mediastinal lymphadenopathy.
   • If lymph nodes in other regions are enlarged, or if a lymphoma is highly suspected, then the patient will require further investigations in the form of a CT scan of the abdomen and chest.

Q. If this patient does not have any other symptoms or signs of other lymph node enlargement, and all other investigations are normal, apart from this enlarged lymph node, then you will need to proceed to a lymph node excision biopsy. How would you carry out a cervical lymph node biopsy?

A. After carrying out all the necessary investigations preoperatively, and in a fully prepared patient who has given his/her full informed consent to undergo such a procedure, I would carry out the cervical lymph node biopsy under general anaesthesia.

The patient is positioned properly on the operating table, exposing the area of operation (using sand bags under the shoulders for example to improve the surgical exposure). The operative field is cleaned with the appropriate antiseptic agent (such as chlorhexidine 0.5% in 70% IMS or 10% bovidone iodine solution), and the patient is draped appropriately in sterile operative sheets. An appropriately sized incision is made through the skin overlying the lymph node, and the length of the incision would have to be at least twice the diameter of the lymph node to allow proper surgical exposure.

Q. Are there any precautions one has to take when making the surgical incision?

A. Yes, the incision will have to be positioned appropriately to avoid damage to important anatomical structures, such as nerves or major vessels.

Q. Can you give an example of important structures that one has to avoid when making an incision?

A. If the lymph node is located close to the inferior border of the mandible, I would have to make my incision 2 cm below the border of the mandible to avoid injury to the cervical branch of the facial nerve.

Q. Describe how you proceed after you make the skin incision.

A. I would deepen the incision to go through the skin and subcutaneous fat and fascia down to the lymph node, taking care to avoid injury to important structures. Once I reach the surface of the lymph node, I would use a blunt dissection technique, for example with a mosquito forceps, to free the lymph node from its surrounding structures. If any lymphatic vessels are encountered, I would apply an arterial forceps to these before division. I would use a meticulous technique to achieve full haemostasis, and once all the attachments of the lymph node have been freed, the node is removed for histological examination.

Q. How would you send the specimen to the pathology laboratory?

A. If lymphoma is suspected, then I would need to inform the laboratory directly, as they would need part of the specimen to be sent fresh for immunohisto-chemical staining. The rest of the specimen will need to be fixed in 10% normal saline and sent to the laboratory. If an infection (acute or chronic) is suspected (such as TB) then part of the lymph node will need to be sent to microbiology as a fresh specimen for acid-fast stain and cultures. If any pus is drained then this will need to be sent to microbiology for culture and sensitivity.

Q. How would you close the wound?

A. I would check carefully for haemostasis, and to stop any oozing or bleeding before attempting any wound closure. I would use a local anaesthetic (10 ml of 0.5% bupivacaine) to help with postoperative analgesia. The wound is closed in layers with absorbable sutures, such as vicryl 2-0. I would close the skin with an absorbable skin suture, such as vicryl 3-0 or monocryl 3-0. However, other surgeons may use other suture material such as nylon or prolene, according to personal preference.

Q. What would you do if you find the lymph node is intramuscular or is lying deep to a large muscle?

A. I would go through the muscle fibres, carefully dissecting through the fibres with blunt dissection using an artery forceps, until I reach the lymph node. I would follow the same steps of removal of the lymph node as discussed before.

Q. What would you do if you find the lymph node is firmly adherent to an important structure such as a nerve, or a major vessel like the internal jugular vein?

A. I would have to take even more care in avoiding any injury to these structures, and the best option would be to take a wedge excision biopsy of the superficial part of the lymph node but keeping the deep part undisturbed. This would still give a histological diagnosis but would prevent any serious injury to other structures.

Q. What type of diathermy would you use for haemostasis when doing a lymph node biopsy?

A. This depends on the region from where the lymph node is taken. In general, a unipolar diathermy is usually safe to use, but if one is taking out a lymph node close to important structures or in limbs, then the use of a bipolar diathermy is indicated.

Q. What would you do if your preoperative investigations revealed that the patient has ENT symptoms and that the preoperative ENT assessment has shown an ENT-related tumour? Would you proceed to do an excision biopsy of the cervical lymph node as described above?

A. No, I would have to cancel the biopsy and refer the patient to the ENT surgeons for further management. If a laryngeal tumour was found, then this patient may need to undergo a laryngectomy combined with a block dissection of the cervical lymph nodes. In such a case, any excision biopsy of an enlarged cervical lymph node could seriously compromise the long-term prognosis of the patient.

CARCINOMA OF THE BREAST

Q. A 45-year old lady presents to your out-patient clinic with a 1 month history of a lump in her right breast. What would be your initial management?

A. I would take a full history from this lady, placing emphasis on risk factors for breast cancer such as family history, age of menarche, details of pregnancies, HRT use and smoking history. Then I would fully examine her breasts to assess the size, position and mobility of the lump. I would look in particular for skin changes associated with breast cancer such as tethering, lymphatic invasion known as 'peau d'orange' and erythema. Next I would assess the axilla, palpating for any associated lymphadenopathy. To complete my examination I would check the abdomen for hepato-splenomegaly.

Q. What is the most likely diagnosis?

A. The most likely diagnosis for a lady of this age is a palpable breast cyst. It may also be an area of fibrosis or sclerosis, perceived by the lady as a discrete lump. I would, however, take caution in a lady of this age and treat the lump as a carcinoma until proven otherwise.

Q. If this lady was 25 years old, what would be the most likely diagnosis?

A. In this lady the diagnosis is far more likely to be a fibro-adenoma.

Q. How would you go about investigating this lump?

A. I would assess this lump clinically, using imaging, and obtain a fine-needle aspirate (FNA) for cytology. This is known as triple assessment and is the standard method of managing any lump in the breast. If the lady was over 30 years I would perform a mammogram and an ultrasound; however, in a lady under 30 years, the breast is too dense for mammography to be effective. In this case I would perform only an ultrasound.

If any suspicious or equivocal results were found on triple assessment, I would do a core biopsy next using a wide-bore needle in order to gain a histological diagnosis.

Q. Suppose this lump turns out to be a carcinoma, how would you manage her?

A. I would first break the bad news, preferably in quiet surroundings with a breast-care nurse and one of the patient's relatives present. I would then arrange for her to come to the clinic on another occasion in order to allow time for the diagnosis to sink in and at that stage I would discuss possible treatments. This may involve initially staging the patient using blood tests, a chest X-ray, liver ultrasound and bone scan to determine the presence of metastases. If these tests were clear, I would discuss possible surgery with her. If they were positive, I would discuss the options of chemotherapy and radiotherapy with surgery as a possibility in the future. I would discuss the need for local and systemic treatment of breast cancer in order to gain good control of the disease.

Q. What surgical treatments do you know about?

A. Surgery in breast cancer is dependent on the size, position, pathology and nodal status of the cancer. It is possible to perform breast-conserving surgery in patients whose tumours are small (preferably <4 cm), located away from the nipple and are of low histological grade. Such procedures include wide local excision or segmental mastectomy. Tumours over 4 cm treated with breast-conserving surgery are associated with a poor cosmetic result and may require a latissimuss dorsi flap in order to fill the defect.

Larger tumours and centrally placed tumours require a mastectomy. This involves removal of all the breast tissue and some of the overlying skin, including the nipple–areolar complex (although some surgeons may not agree with this).

Q. How would you manage the axilla?

A. It is important to consider an axillary procedure in both types of breast operations. If there are no nodes palpable and the tumour is less than 1 cm, it is thought to be safe to perform an axillary sample consisting of at least four nodes. Some recent evidence even suggests that this is possible in tumours less than 2 cm. Any tumour larger than this requires an axillary clearance. An axillary clearance is graded into I, II and III. Grade I involves taking all the nodes lateral to the pectoralis minor muscle, grade II involves the nodes behind the muscle and grade III involves the nodes also situated medial to the muscle, extending up to the first rib and the axillary vein. It is also possible to treat the axilla using radical radiotherapy. The rate of recurrence is similar for both treatment modalities.

Q. What are the complications of axillary treatment?

A. Both radiotherapy and surgery of the axilla may be complicated by troublesome lymphoedema. It is most common in cases of radical radiotherapy and grade III clearance. Other complications associated with surgery include wound infection and nerve damage, in particular to the intercostobrachial nerve which supplies sensation to the upper inner aspect of the arm. Both treatments may result in shoulder stiffness. Radiotherapy may also cause pneumonitis and occasionally the patient may suffer psychologically with the thought of tumour recurrence.

ABSCESS DRAINAGE

Q. What is an abscess?

A. A collection of pus.

Q. What is pus?

A. Pus is thick fluid containing inflammatory cells (such as neutrophils), bacteria/dead bacteria and dead white cells. Pus is like a battlefield of two armies: the invading soldiers of bacteria, the defending soldiers of white cells and the dead soldiers of those two armies.

Q. How would you manage a patient with an abscess?

A. After taking a full history and carrying out the appropriate clinical examination, the patient should be given adequate analgesia, which frequently is needed before a full clinical examination is completed. The patient should be prepared for surgical incision and drainage under a general anaesthetic.

Q. Name some of the common abscesses that present to the emergency surgical team.

A. Perianal and ischiorectal, pilonidal, axillary, breast, cutaneous (e.g. infected sebaceous/epidermoid cysts), pelvic, etc.

Q. What are the predisposing factors for abscesses?

A. Many factors can predispose to abscesses, but the most important include diabetes and immunosuppression. Therefore, any patient with an abscess should have a blood sugar check.

Q. How would you drain a perianal abscess?

A. In a properly prepared patient, who has undergone all the necessary emergency investigations, I would carry out the procedure under general anaesthesia. I would carry out a full examination of the region under general anaesthesia (EUA), including a sigmoidoscopy, looking carefully for any underlying fistulae-in-ano. If the EUA is satisfactory, then I would proceed to do an incision and drainage.

Q. How would you go about making your surgical incision?

A. The traditional method is to make a cruciate incision, and then to cut the corners/edges of the cruciate. However, this invariably results in a 'star-shaped' scar. A better alternative is to make a wide elliptical incision, which would heal with a better scar. I would also send swabs of pus to microbiology for culture.

Q. Why do you have to make a wide incision, removing a wide rim of skin?

A. To prevent premature healing of the skin before the abscess cavity is allowed to heal completely, as this would cause a recurrent abscess.

Q. What would happen if you do not drain the abscess?

A. The abscess may 'burst' spontaneously, and this could result in a fistula-in-ano, or a chronic abscess cavity.

Q. Why do you have to send pus to microbiology?

A. This could shed some light on the cause of the abscess. If anaerobic bacteria are grown in the culture, then a fistula-in-ano must be present, and the patient should undergo a further examination under anaesthesia and treatment of the fistula within 4–6 weeks.

Q. What would you do if you find a fistula-in-ano during the EUA and sigmoidoscopy?

A. If the fistula is low, then I would lay it open. If the fistula is high (i.e. inter-sphincteric) then I would apply a 'Seton' suture through the fistula track to drain it. (Note: this depends on the surgeon's experience. If the surgeon is not experienced enough, then a more senior surgeon who knows how to deal with a fistula-in-ano should be available.)

Q. Would you close the incised abscess wound at the time of surgical drainage?

A. Definitely not. If an attempt is made to close the incision wound, then the abscess would recur immediately, and either a fistula or a chronic abscess would develop.

Q. How would you manage the wound after surgical drainage of the abscess?

A. The abscess cavity would require debridement and irrigation (usually with antiseptic solution or hydrogen peroxide). The cavity would then need to be packed with antiseptic ribbon gauze, such as proflavin or betadine. However, I would ensure that the abscess cavity was not packed tightly, as this would cause severe pain during change of the dressing on the ward postoperatively. The next day, the abscess cavity should be dressed using simple wound dressing such as Aquacell or saline dressing gauze. Any similar sterile dressing would be good enough, as long as it keeps the skin wound open to allow full drainage of the cavity.

Q. How often would you change the dressing?

A. Usually daily, and the patient could have a bath or a shower before the dressing is changed by the district nurse. Once the dressing is comfortable enough to do with simple oral analgesia, then the patient could be discharged home for community wound care and dressing by the district or surgery nurse.

Q. Do you give the patient with an abscess any antibiotics?

A. No. Usually, most patients with abscesses do not require any antibiotics. The treatment of an abscess is surgical incision and drainage.

Q. What are the indications for using antibiotics in patients with abscess cavities?

A. If the patient has a severe degree of cellulitis around the abscess cavity, or if the patient has a very complex abscess cavity, e.g. a bad case of ischioanal abscess. Another common example of abscesses that can be treated with antibiotics is breast abscesses.

Q. How do you treat a breast abscess in a young lady?

A. If the abscess is small and if it can be drained with a needle under ultrasound scan, then all pus should be drained under ultrasound, and the patient should be admitted for intravenous antibiotics. However, the patient should be carefully monitored, and if the pus recollects then the patient should be taken to theatre for a formal surgical incision and drainage. If the pus does not re-accumulate and if the patient's condition improves dramatically, then the patient may be allowed to go home with a full course of antibiotic therapy. These patients should have a full triple assessment in the breast clinic as a follow-up to exclude any other underlying pathology (including any breast tumours), and should be treated accordingly if any breast lesions are found.

Q. Is it possible to carry out any other modified percutaneous drainage of abscesses under image guidance? Give examples.

A. Yes, localized pelvic abscesses or para-colic abscesses in the elderly and unfit. Such abscesses can be drained under ultrasound or with CT guidance, and the patient should be given combination antibiotic therapy.

Q. **Why in these patients do you try to avoid doing a full laparotomy to drain the localized abscess?**

A. Because these patients have a localized area of infection, which should respond to percutaneous drainage and antibiotic therapy. A full laparotomy would convert this area of localized abscess into generalized peritonitis, which carries added risks of morbidity and mortality. In addition, they will have all the risks and complications of a major surgical procedure. However, these patients should be carefully monitored and if they develop any signs of generalized peritonitis or uncontrolled sepsis, then the non-operative approach should be abandoned and one should proceed to a laparotomy without any delay.

Q. **Is there any place for using antibiotics by the GP?**

A. GPs rarely prescribe antibiotics in such cases; however it could be quite dangerous and detrimental to the patient's care. If the patient presents to the GP at the very early stage of cellulitis before an abscess is formed, then giving antibiotics might stop this infection from developing into an abscess, but this is rather rare. However, if the GP gives a patient with an acute abscess a course of antibiotics, then this would only makes matters worse.

Q. **How would it make matters worse?**

A. The acute simple abscess cavity will be converted into a chronic abscess cavity with trabeculations and a honeycomb appearance which is consistent with an attempt at healing with infected granulation tissue. This will make the surgical drainage of the abscess and the effectiveness of the surgical treatment much more difficult, and could result in chronic infection and extensive scarring that would require far more extensive and repeated surgical procedures to correct. It is also associated with a high risk of recurrence.

Q. **Why do antibiotics convert simple acute abscesses into chronic complex abscesses, and why do antibiotics not have much benefit in non-drained abscess cavities?**

A. Because antibiotics depend on having good blood supply and tissue perfusion. There is, however, poor blood flow in the centre of the pus within the abscess cavity and therefore the levels of antibiotics within the abscess are very low and non-functional. In addition, the inappropriate use of antibiotics would lead to the emergence of resistant bacteria, and we have many examples of these in our hospitals.

Q. **What antibiotics would you give for a patient with a perianal abscess with fistula, after surgical drainage?**

A. An antibiotic that would cover anaerobic bacteria, such as metronidazole, which is usually combined with a cephalosporin or gentamicin if the patient is septic. A similar combination of antibiotics is used for patients after drainage of pelvic abscesses.

Q. What would you do for a lady with recurrent breast abscesses and persistent discharge from a non-healing abscess wound, who also happens to be a heavy smoker?

A. It is most likely that this patient is suffering from a mammary duct fistula which is causing the sepsis, and this is usually related to heavy smoking. I would strongly advise the lady to stop smoking, and would carry out an exploration and excision of the mammary duct fistula, with a full course of antibiotics cover. I would have to warn the patient about the high risks of recurrence, especially if she continues to smoke.

Q. What would you do for a patient with severe chronic sepsis in the pilonidal area, which has been causing recurrent abscesses?

A. I would consider full surgical debridement to excise all the scarred and infected tissue, and contemplate plastic surgery (for example, in the form of a rotational flap) to cover the large defect that will result from the extensive surgical excision.

PRINCIPLES OF ANASTOMOSIS

Q. What is an anastomosis?

A. An anastomosis is the joining of two hollow organs or structures, to re-establish a lumen through which flow can continue.

Q. What is the aim of performing an anastomosis?

A. The aims are:

- To restore the continuity of a hollow organ (such as the bowel or a blood vessel) after removing a diseased section of that organ.
- To bypass an obstructed segment to divert the flow through the lumen into the distal part of that organ.

Another example of anastomoses is in transplant surgery, where the aim is to restore the inflow and outflow between the donor/grafted organ and the recipient body.

Q. Name common sites of anastomoses.

A. In the gastrointestinal tract, in the urinary tract, in vascular surgery (doing various vascular anastomoses), in transplant surgery and microvascular anastomoses in plastic surgery.

Q. Name examples of anastomoses in the gastrointestinal tract.

A. • Oesophago-gastostomy
- Gastro-jejunostomy
- Oesophago-jejunostomy
- Jejuno-jejunostomy

- Jejuno-ileostomy
- Entero-enterostomy
- Ileo-colostomy
- Colo-colic
- Colo-rectal anastomosis
- Choledocho-jejunostomy
- Cholecysto-duodenostomy
- Pancreatico-jejunostomy.

Q. What is a gastro-jejunostomy?

A. A gastro-jejunostomy is an anastomosis between the stomach and a proximal loop of the jejunum.

Q. What is an oesophago-jejunostomy?

A. An oesophago-jejunostomy is an anastomosis between the lower end of the oesophagus and a Roux-en-Y loop of the jejunum, which is carried out in patients undergoing a total gastrectomy.

Q. How is a gastro-oesophageal anastomosis performed?

A. A gastro-oesophageal anastomosis involves the joining of the stomach, after mobilization of the stomach like a tube, which is then lifted up into the chest to be anastomosed to the upper oesophagus. This is carried out in patients undergoing a distal oesophagectomy or resection of the gastro-oesophageal junction. The anastomosis can be carried out within the chest (as is the case with the Ivor Lewis operation), or in the neck (as in trans-hiatal oesophagectomy or in the McKeown's operation).

Q. What is an entero-enterostomy?

A. An entero-enterostomy is a vague term which is frequently used to refer to an anastomosis of a loop of the small bowel to another loop of the small bowel such as:

- Jejuno-jejunostomy – anastomosis between one loop of the jejunum and another
- Jejuno-ileostomy – anastomosis between a loop of the jejunum and a loop of the ileum
- Ileo-ileostomy – anastomosis between one loop of the ileum and another.

Q. What is an entero-colostomy?

A. An entero-colostomy, such as an ileo-colic anastomosis, is the anastomosis between one loop of the ileum and the colon. The commonest example is an anastomosis between the terminal ileum and the colon following a right hemi-colectomy or an extended right hemicolectomy, or the bypass of an advanced unresectable caecal cancer.

Q. What do we mean by colo-rectal anastomosis?

A. Colo-rectal anastomosis is the anastomosis between a part of the colon and the rectum, for example between the descending and the lower rectum or between the transverse colon and the rectum. This is usually carried out in patients undergoing an anterior resection of the rectum, sigmoid colectomy or left hemicolectomy.

Q. What is a choledocho-jejunostomy?

A. A choledocho-jejunostomy is an anastomosis between the common bile duct (CBD) and a proximal loop of the jejunum, or the common hepatic duct (CHD) and a proximal loop of the jejunum.

Q. What is a cholecysto-duodenostomy?

A. A cholecysto-duodenostomy is an anastomosis between the gallbladder and the adjacent duodenum.

Q. What is a cholecysto-jejunostomy?

A. A cholecysto-jejunostomy is an anastomosis between the gallbladder and a proximal loop of the jejunum.

Q. What is a panreatico-jejunostomy?

A. A pancreatico-jejunostomy is an anastomosis between the pancreatic duct and a proximal loop of the jejunum, and this is usually carried out in the form of a Roux-en-Y loop anastomosis (as in Whipple's operation)(Fig. 5).

Q. What is a Roux-en-Y anastomosis?

A. A proximal loop of the jejunum is divided, and the distal end of the divided loop is brought up to anastomose either to the oesophagus (in total gastrectomy), or to the stomach, common bile duct or pancreas. The proximal end of the divided loop is anastomosed as an 'end to side' anastomosis to the jejunum further down. The whole configuration looks like a 'Y', hence the name Roux-en-Y.

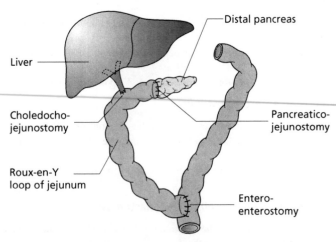

Fig. 5   Roux-en-Y anastomoses in Whipple's pancreatectomy

Q. What is Whipple's operation?

A. It is an operation designed to resect the head of the pancreas (e.g. carcinoma of the head of the pancreas). As part of the operation, a cholecystectomy and a partial duodenectomy are also performed. Anastomoses are carried out between the pancreatic duct and the jejunum, the stomach and the jejunum, and the common bile duct and the jejunum. A modified version of the Whipple's operation is pyloric preserving proximal pancreatectomy (PPPP).

Q. What are the two main rules that reduce the risks of an anastomotic leak?

A. Good blood supply to the two parts that form the anastomosis, and a careful meticulous surgical technique.

Q. What anastomoses do you perform if you are carrying out a Hartmann's operation?

A. None, as a Hartmann's operation is designed to deal with an emergency situation of either an obstructing tumour of the recto-sigmoid colon or a perforated distal colon (for example, perforated diverticulitis). Therefore, it would be considered unsafe to proceed to do an anastomosis, and accordingly the proximal end of the colon is exteriorized as an end colostomy, and the distal end (i.e. rectum) is oversewn in the pelvis. Therefore, no anastomosis is performed.

Q. In liver transplants, what anastomoses would you perform?

A. Anastomosis of the hepatic artery, the common bile duct, the portal vein and the hepatic veins/IVC.

Q. In renal transplants, what anastomoses would you perform?

A. Anastomosis of the renal artery (or arteries) usually to the iliac artery (common or external), renal vein to the iliac vein (common or external iliac vein), and the ureter to the bladder.

Q. What is microvascular anastomosis?

A. It is when you are carrying out an arterial and venous anastomosis for small vessels with the help of an operating microscope. This procedure is frequently used for flap surgery such as DIEP flap (deep inferior epigastric pedicles), or anastomosis of small digital vessels in plastic surgery.

Q. What are the main causes of anastomotic leakage?

A. Ischaemia of the two ends of the anastomosis (very important in bowel surgery), poor anastomotic technique, disease process at the level of the anastomosis (e.g. severe arteriosclerosis), infection, malnutrition, suture failure, stapler malfunction.

Q. Why do we perform fewer abdomino-perineal resections and more low anterior resections of the rectum nowadays?

A. Because of the help of the special disposable circular rectal staplers which has made low rectal surgery easier and safer in expert hands.

Q. If you are carrying out a low rectal anastomosis, what would you check if there is an anastomotic leak?

A. The anastomotic doughnuts from the surgical stapler should be carefully examined, and if any of the two rings are not complete, then an anastomotic leak is present. Also the anastomosis should be tested for air and fluid tightness and leakage, using a syringe to test the anastomosis per-anally. Postoperatively, the anastomosis could be tested for any leakage with a gentle water-soluble contrast enema, which would demonstrate the site and extent of the leakage.

Q. What would you do if you discover a leak in your low rectal anastomosis at surgery?

A. Repair the leak (if possible) with sutures, put a pelvic drain near the anastomosis, and carry out a defunctioning loop stoma to prevent faecal leakage and pelvic sepsis.

Q. What type of stoma would you carry out if there is a leak from a low rectal anastomosis?

A. The best option is to carry out a defunctioning loop ileostomy, as it has the least morbidity, and is the easier stoma to close at a later date.

Q. What would you do if the patient develops an anastomotic leak a few days after surgery, which is not defunctioned?

A. I would have to carry out an emergency laparotomy to drain the leak and to defunction the anastomosis, for example by 'taking down the anastomosis' and bringing out the two ends as stomas. A full peritoneal lavage should be carried out. The patient should be admitted to ITU postoperatively, as they might require full ventilation and multisystem support.

Q. What would happen if you have a leakage from a bowel anastomosis which is not repaired or defunctioned?

A. The patient would become septic and would develop multiorgan failure (e.g. respiratory, renal and cardiac failure).

Q. What are the signs of an anastomotic bowel leak?

A. Pyrexia and/or tachycardia, other signs of sepsis, respiratory or cardiac problems, and renal impairment. An anastomotic leak should be considered as a possibility in any patient who develops respiratory or cardiac failure problems after undergoing a colonic anastomosis.

Q. What is a Billroth I gastrectomy?

A. This is a historic operation, carried out successfully by Theodore Billroth in 1881; it involves a distal gastrectomy or antrectomy, preserving the duodenum, and an anastomosis is then made between the duodenum and the body of the stomach (see Fig. 6).

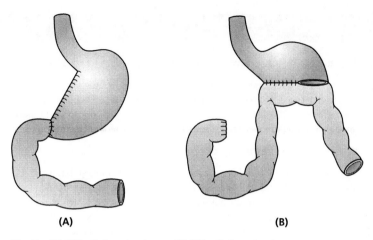

(A) **(B)**

Fig. 6 (A) Billroth I gastrectomy, (B) Billroth II gastrectomy

Q. What is a Billroth II gastrectomy?

A. This is another historic operation which was carried out by Professor Theodore Billroth in 1885; the distal two thirds of the stomach are resected, and the proximal part of the stomach is anastomosed to a loop of the jejunum, and the duodenal end is closed as a stump (see Fig. 6). Nowadays, we use a modified version of this technique in the form of a gastrectomy.

Q. What technique would you use to do a bowel anastomosis?

A. Either sutured anastomosis or stapled anastomosis (depending on experience and cost).

Q. What sutures would you use for a sutured anastomosis?

A. Any suture that I am familiar with. The commonest one is using two layers of vicryl, or a single layer of PDS or similar sutures. Nowadays, we avoid using silk sutures (which were commonly used in the past) as there is usually a severe inflammatory reaction caused by the silk.

Q. If you are using a single layer of PDS sutures for anastomosis, how would you do it?

A. I would use an interrupted sero-muscular layer of sutures.

DIATHERMY

Q. Tell me what you know about diathermy.

A. Diathermy is used commonly in surgical practice in order to cut through or coagulate tissues. This is achieved using a high-frequency alternating current of approximately 400 kHz – 10 MHz. Cutting or coagulation of body tissues is produced by the production of heat from this high-frequency current.

Q. What types of diathermy do you know of?

A. The most commonly used type of diathermy is called monopolar; however, it is also possible to use bipolar diathermy. Monopolar diathermy involves the production of a high-frequency current from a generator, which then passes through to the surgeon's forceps. The current then travels through the patient and then back to the generator via a plate electrode attached to the patient. Bipolar diathermy uses less power and is thought to be less effective; however, it is a safer option. The current from the generator passes down one limb of the forceps, through the tissue being coagulated and then travels back up the other limb of the forceps and back to the generator. In this case there is no need for the plate electrode.

Q. What is the essential difference between cutting and coagulation?

A. Cutting diathermy occurs using a continuous output of current and results in the generation of temperatures of up to 1000°C. This causes tissue disruption by vaporization of cell water. In contrast, coagulation diathermy occurs via a pulsed output of current, which desiccates tissues without causing too much tissue disruption.

Q. What are the problems with diathermy?

A. Accidental burns may occur. This is a particular hazard with laparoscopic surgery when damaged insulation may result in an accidental burn or if the diathermy is touching a second instrument holding an organ, which may produce a burn. This can have disastrous consequences particularly if the bowel is involved.

The plate electrode attached to the patient may cause accidental burns if incorrectly placed. The plate should be positioned away from metal implants, bony prominences and scar tissue. The skin underneath must also be shaved and must make good contact with the plate without skin preparation in between.

Burns may also occur if the patient is touching metal objects such as drip stands or even the metal areas of the operating table. This results in the diathermy current finding an alternative return pathway and can lead to local burns at these sites.

Q. What steps would you take to make your diathermy use safe?

A. I would always check the diathermy setting and make sure that excess alcoholic skin preparation was wiped to dryness before use. I would also check that the insulation was satisfactory. I would make sure that I placed the diathermy in a safe, insulated container when I had finished using it.

POSTOPERATIVE COMPLICATIONS

Q. Can you think of any complications that may occur as a result of a general anaesthetic?

A. There are several problems a patient may encounter as a result of having an anaesthetic. Commonly, upper airways obstruction may occur; hypoxaemia and respiratory depression also occur and may be due to opiates. This may also cause the patient to be hypotensive; similarly, waking up in excessive amounts of pain may result in hypertension. The anaesthetic agents used may also cause:

- Delayed recovery
- Liver impairment – traditionally blamed on halothane, but may be caused by various other agents
- Anaphylaxis/allergy.

Other problems may be encountered specific to the venous access:

- Thrombophlebitis
- Sepsis
- Thrombosis.

General complications include:

- Sore throat
- Nausea/vomiting
- Discomfort – nasogastric tubes, urinary catheter, central line.

Q. You are called to recovery to see a 69-year-old gentleman who has just undergone a hernia repair. He has an oxygen saturation of 89% and the nurses are concerned about his noisy breathing. How would you manage the situation?

A. My first priority would be to assess this gentleman's airway. I would check for any obstructions, such as the tongue, and perform a chin lift and jaw thrust. I would use a simple airway: a Guedel airway if the patient was still unconscious or a simple face mask/nasal cannula. I would also give oxygen, up to 100%, depending on any past history of chronic obstructive airways disease.

Q. What is the mostly likely cause?

A. It is possible that this gentleman may have a long history of smoking or chronic airways disease. This would make him at increased risk of an exacerbation of his symptoms in this scenario. It may be a result of the prolonged effects of the anaesthetic agents. This would require the use of a peripheral nerve stimulator for diagnosis and the help of the anaesthetist to reverse the effects.

Other more serious causes include: laryngeal spasm, oedema, tracheomalacia, haematoma/packs post neck surgery.

Q. Is there any way you could prevent this situation from occurring?

A. It is important to identify patients who may be at increased risk of respiratory difficulties in surgical pre-clerking. These include:

- Elderly
- History of smoking
- History of cardiac disease
- Obese
- Previous history of difficulties with anaesthetics.

In these cases, it would be a good idea to obtain further tests including a chest X-ray, respiratory function tests and perhaps an arterial blood gas. Smokers should be advised to stop, if possible. Weight loss should also be advised. If there is any evidence of respiratory tract infection, elective procedures should be postponed.

Medical therapy should be maximized preoperatively, surgery should be planned for the summer months when the patient may be less symptomatic, oxygen therapy should be administered as the patient is put to sleep and the patient should be monitored carefully postoperatively. Physiotherapy is also useful to improve atelectasis and mucous plugging postoperatively.

Q. Why are smokers at increased risk of postoperative complications?

A. Smokers have an increased risk of postoperative respiratory problems because of:

- Cardiac effects – nicotine causes hypertension, exacerbates preexisting coronary artery disease
- Carboxyhaemoglobin – decreases the oxygen-carrying capacity of haemoglobin (shifts the oxygen dissociation curve to the left)
- Impaired ciliary function and excessive production of mucus, causing mucous plugging and sputum retention
- Atelectasis and increased susceptibility to infection.

Q. Does the position of the patient on the operating table contribute to the patient's cardiorespiratory status?

A. Yes, when placed in the supine position the patient may experience changes in the ventilation–perfusion ratio whereby the dependent areas are better perfused. This can be used for beneficial purposes as in the treatment of ARDS when the patient is periodically turned to improve the ventilation–perfusion ratio.

Also, the supine position may cause a bradycardia and a decrease in cardiac output.

Q. What is the Trendelenberg position and what cardiovascular effects may occur as a result?

A. The Trendelenberg position is the 'head down' position that is commonly used by anaesthetists to insert central lines and by gynaecologists performing pelvic surgery. It causes a rise in central venous pressure and cardiac output. The respiratory effects include a reduced functional residual capacity (FRC) as a result of the pressure effects of the abdominal contents on the diaphragm. The person may also experience oedema of the head and neck.

TRAUMA

Q. What do you understand by the term triage?

A. Triage means to 'sort'. It is generally used in ATLS guidelines when referring to the sorting out of mass casualties at the scene of a major incident.

Q. What is its purpose?

A. The purpose of triage is to assess casualties according to their need for treatment:

- Immediate – i.e. relief of tension pneumothorax (RED)
- Urgent – i.e. long bone fracture (YELLOW)
- Delayed – i.e. superficial injuries (GREEN)
- Dead (WHITE).

The responsibility for triage usually lies with a designated triage officer whose only task is to triage and not to treat patients, however life threatening their condition. The clinical condition of patients may deteriorate and, as a result, the triaging process must be constantly repeated.

Q. How would you triage a patient you thought was about to die?

A. I would either triage the patient into the RED group if they had an easily reversible life-threatening condition i.e. tension pneumothorax, or I would leave them to die. The rationale behind this is that triage is for the benefit of the majority. If a patient couldn't be saved, it would compromise the care of the other patients who may survive.

Q. What do you know about the primary survey?

A. The primary survey is the initial assessment used in the management of trauma. It is intended to rapidly diagnose and treat any life-threatening conditions. It involves the following method of assessment:

- **A** – Airway and cervical spine. The patency of the airway must be immediately assessed. If there is any doubt, the oral cavity must be inspected for any blockages and a chin lift/jaw thrust used to maintain the best position for breathing. Before any manoeuvres are undertaken, care must be taken to maintain the head and neck in a neutral position and the patient should definitively be positioned on a spinal board with c-spine immobilization.
- **B** – Breathing. The whole of the chest should be adequately exposed to assess the adequacy of chest expansion and respiratory rate. The chest should be inspected for evidence of bruising, rib fractures, flail chest and open wounds. The following life-threatening conditions should be excluded: tension pneumothorax, penetrating chest injury/haemothorax, cardiac tamponade and flail chest.

- **C** – Circulation. *'Parts in the air, press on the hole'*. Direct pressure should be applied to any external haemorrhage. Intravenous access should be gained using two wide-bore cannulae (gauge 14–16), preferably in the antecubital fossa. If this isn't possible, a central line should be attempted. If this fails also, a venous cutdown should be undertaken. Once access has been obtained, blood should be sent (FBC, U+E, G+S and X-match) and fluids commenced. The type of fluids used is based on the vital signs of the patient; if the patient is shocked, colloids should be commenced, otherwise Hartmann's solution can be given.
- **D** – Dysfunction of the central nervous system. This involves a quick assessment of the patient's neurological status: pupil reflex, ability to respond to command etc.
- **E** – Exposure. Full exposure should be obtained using a large pair of scissors. Care must be taken to avoid hypothermia.

Q. What clinical features would suggest to you that your patient is shocked?

A. These include:

- Hypotension, reduced pulse pressure
- Tachycardia
- Tachypnoea
- Sweaty, cool peripheries
- Poor capillary refill
- Poor urine output (less than 0.5 ml/kg/hour)
- Reduced level of consciousness.

It is also possible to predict the degree of shock by the injuries, i.e. fractured femur can result in 2 l of blood loss.

Q. A 30-year-old man is brought into your Emergency Department having been involved in a road traffic accident. He is aggressive and has an open fracture of his left lower limb. He also has lots of bruises on the left side of his chest wall. You find that his blood pressure is 100/60 mmHg and his pulse 125 bpm. How much blood do you think he has lost and how would you classify this degree of shock?

A. It is likely that this gentleman has lost approximately 1.5 – 2 l of blood. His vital signs and aggressive behaviour classify the degree of shock as class III. If he doesn't respond to a rapid infusion of colloids, he may be continuing to bleed into his chest as indicated by the bruises on his chest.

Classification of hypovolaemic shock

	Class I	Class II	Class III	Class IV
Pulse (bpm)	80–100	100–120	120, weak	>120
Systolic BP	Normal	Normal	Reduced	Low
Diastolic	Normal	Raised	Reduced	Low/not recordable
Urine output (ml/hour)	>30	20–30	10–20	<10
Capillary refill	Normal	Reduced	Reduced	None
Respiratory rate	Normal (~15/min)	15–20	>20	>20
Colour	Normal	Pale	Pale	Grey, clammy
Consciousness	Alert	Anxious	Drowsy, aggressive	Confused, unconscious
Estimated blood loss	Up to 0.75 l (~15%)	0.75 – 1.5 l (15–30%)	1.5 – 2 l (30–40%)	>2 l (>40%)

Q. Can you describe to me how you would perform a venous cutdown?

A. I would perform a venous cutdown if I was unable to establish venous access peripherally or centrally. I would call my registrar if I had never performed the procedure before. Then I would clean and drape the area of skin over the long saphenous vein, anterior to the medial malleolus. I would then make a transverse incision, approximately 2 cm in length, anterior to the medial malleolus. Using blunt dissection, I would explore the area and locate the long saphenous vein. Then I would ligate the distal end of the vein using a silk tie (2/0) and place a tie around the proximal end as a controlling sling. Then I would make a transverse incision over the vein, large enough to admit a 12 gauge cannula, and tie in place using the silk tie. I would then connect the cannula to a giving set and commence a litre of intravenous fluids.

Q. Can you think of any other sites where a venous cutdown may be performed?

A. The basilic vein in the antecubital fossa and the femoral vein in the groin.

Q. Is there any other technique that can be used in children if intravenous access cannot be obtained?

A. Yes, interosseous. This involves the insertion of an interosseous trocar into the anteromedial aspect of the tibia, approximately two fingers distal to the tibial tuberosity. The cannula is inserted through the cortex of the bone and into the bone marrow where fluids may be administered rapidly.

CHEST TRAUMA

Q. You are called urgently to see a 37-year-old man in the Emergency Department who has been involved in a fight in the street. He has been stabbed in the second intercostal space on the left-hand side of the chest. He doesn't seem to be responding to resuscitation. What is the most likely cause?

A. It is likely that this gentleman has a laceration of the heart, great vessels or main bronchus. As a result, it is highly likely that he has cardiac tamponade/ haemothorax.

Q. Would you consider performing an emergency thoracotomy?

A. I would consider performing an immediate thoracotomy if the patient's cardiac rhythm was electromechanical dissociation (EMD) and if I had the skills to undertake such a procedure. If the rhythm was asystole, the chances of survival would be very slim.

Q. If the gentleman had not arrested, but came to you with a sucking chest wound, how would you manage this?

A. I would immediately assess his airway, breathing and circulation. Then I would cover the wound with a sterile dressing that was occluded on three sides. I would then insert an intercostal drain at a site away from the wound and arrange for the wound to be surgically explored when the patient had been stabilized.

Q. What might occur if a large sucking chest wound is left uncovered?

A. If a sucking chest wound is left uncovered, the intrathoracic pressure equilibrates with atmospheric air and as a result air will pass preferentially through the wound. The increasing amount of work required to adequately ventilate the lungs may result in respiratory failure.

Q. Tell me how you would go about inserting a chest drain.

A. Firstly, I would take a full history and examine the patient. Then I would reassure myself of the indication for the chest drain and confirm the side by looking at the chest X-ray. Then I would obtain informed consent, explaining all the risks associated with the procedure and the alternative treatment options, if any.

I would sit the patient in a comfortable position on the bed, preferably at 45° with their arm hanging normally by their side, exposing the area beneath the axilla. I would clean and drape the area and infiltrate with 1% local anaesthetic, making sure to anaesthetize the pleura. I would aim to use either the fourth or fifth intercostal space, just anterior to the mid-axillary line. Once the local anaesthetic has taken effect, I would make a transverse incision, approximately 4–5 cm long over the fourth or fifth intercostal space. Using blunt dissection, I would open the wound to the level of the rib and once at the rib, would further dissect through the intercostal muscle making sure to dissect above the rib so as to avoid the neurovascular bundle. Once in the pleura, there is usually a rasp of air or gush of fluid depending on the pathology; at this point I would insert a finger into the hole and gently sweep around the entry site ensuring no danger will come to the lung. Then I would remove the trocar from an appropriately sized chest drain and insert it, clamped, into the chest using large surgical artery forceps. Once in position, I would attach the end of the drain to an underwater drainage kit and release the clamp. If I was happy that the drain was swinging/ bubbling satisfactorily, I would suture the drain to the chest wall using silk in a purse string fashion. I would cover the drain insertion site with a clear dressing, such as tegederm, for future inspection of the wound and request a chest X-ray.

Q. Can you tell me any complications that may occur during this procedure?

A. Complications may occur with:

- The procedure – inserting into the wrong side of the chest, injury to the inter-costal bundle, injury to the chest wall, injury to the lung/heart/oesophagus.
- The chest drain – failing to drain due to incorrect position, incorrect size of drain, blocked lumen. Tension pneumothorax as a result of accidental clamping. Erosion into nearby structures, fracture of the end of the drain and hence a foreign body requiring removal.
- The drainage system – accidental disconnection, placing above the level of the patient's chest and the water travelling into the chest.
- Infection.

Q. What diagnosis would you suspect if you were shown a chest X-ray with a widened mediastinum?

A. Firstly, I would check that the chest X-ray was a P–A (posterior–anterior) and not an A–P as this often gives the impression of a widened mediastinum due to the anterior position of the heart in the chest and the posterior position of the X-ray plate.

I would suspect a diagnosis of an injured or ruptured aorta, particularly if there was a history of a deceleration-type injury.

Q. How would you manage this patient?

A. I would like to fully resuscitate this patient, aiming to keep his/her blood pressure less than 100 mmHg. I would then request further imaging providing the patient was stable enough; a CT scan or aortogram. The definitive treatment would be surgical repair by direct repair or interposition of a graft; however, the injury is usually fatal.

HEAD INJURY

Q. What is a coma?

A. A coma may be defined as the inability to obey commands, open eyes or speak. This corresponds to a Glasgow Coma Score (GCS) of less than 8.

Q. Can you explain the GCS for me.

A. The Glasgow Coma Score is a method of assessing consciousness. It is usually recorded as part of the secondary survey and is also useful in monitoring the progress of patients who have sustained head injuries.

It comprises the following parameters.

Eye opening	Spontaneously	4
	To speech	3
	To pain	2
	None	1
Verbal response	Orientated	5
	Confused	4
	Inappropriate	3
	Incomprehensible	2
	None	1
Motor response	Obeys commands	6
	Localizes to pain	5
	Flexes to pain	4
	Abnormal flexion	3
	Extension to pain	2
	None	1

A total score is obtained out of 15, and may be used to monitor deterioration or improvement after a head injury.

Q. Are there any other clinical observations that may be recorded in the management of a head injury patient?

A. It is a good idea to record the pulse, arterial blood pressure, temperature, respiratory rate, pupillary diameter, pupillary reflex and also movement of all the limbs.

Q. Why is it so important to record the arterial blood pressure?

A. It is important to record the blood pressure because:

$$\text{Cerebral blood flow} = \text{Mean arterial pressure (MAP)} - \text{Mean intracranial pressure (ICP)}$$

If the mean arterial pressure drops to less than 60-70 mmHg in the presence of a raised intracranial pressure, neuronal ischaemia occurs very rapidly.

Q. How can the body prevent this occurring?

A. The cerebral circulation is usually autoregulated. The muscular walls of the cerebral arterioles are independent of nerve supply and maintain the cerebral blood flow at a constant flow despite changes in arterial blood pressure. In patients who are unconscious due to a head injury, this ability to autoregulate is lost.

Q. What causes a raised intracranial pressure and what are the consequences?

A. A raised intracranial pressure may be caused by:

- Intracranial haemorrhage
- Cerebral oedema
- Increase in intracranial blood volume (as a result of loss in vascular tone).

As intracranial pressure increases, cerebrospinal fluid (CSF) is forced out into the spine to compensate. If the pressure continues to increase, the brain 'shifts' within the cranial cavity and herniation may occur. The falx cerebri is able to resist a certain amount of mass movement; however, with increasing pressure 'coning' occurs. This involves herniation through the brainstem resulting in a reduced conscious level, an initial pupillary constriction followed by a fixed dilation as a result of third nerve compression. The brainstem compression results in respiratory and cardiovascular dysfunction that is invariably fatal.

Q. Why is the initial management of a head injury so important?

A. This is because failure to diagnose and treat complications such as intracranial haematomas can lead to an increase in head injury mortality.

Q. How would you manage a 22-year-old gentleman who has been brought to your Emergency Department, unconscious, with a history of a head injury?

A. Immediately, I would attend to his airway, breathing and circulation.

- Airway – endotracheal intubation may be necessary, taking care to stabilize the neck, and a rapid sequence induction performed.
- Breathing – adequate oxygenation must be ensured by administering oxygen, and positive pressure ventilation may be instituted immediately in order to control $P\mathrm{CO_2}$ and reduce the possibility of intracranial hypertension.
- Circulation – hypotension must be avoided and hence fluids should be commenced. Blood pressure should be carefully restored. Some centres advocate the use of intravenous mannitol which is a strong osmotic diuretic in order to control intracranial hypertension.
- Dysfunction of the CNS – GCS should be recorded, pupil size and reflexes, and limb movements.
- Exposure – a full body examination should be undertaken. X-rays of the skull, cervical spine and chest should be obtained and a CT scan of the head, if indicated.

After initial stabilization of the patient, every effort should be made in order to obtain information regarding the mechanism of injury, and prophylactic intravenous antibiotics should be prescribed in case of a basal skull fracture, CSF leak, a compound or depressed fracture.

Q. When would you consider performing a burr hole?

A. I would first discuss the case with a neurosurgeon. Then I would consider performing a burr hole in an emergency situation if a patient with a head injury, who was previously alert, rapidly deteriorated with a fixed dilated pupil on the same side as a skull fracture and I felt adequately confident to perform the procedure.

Q. What would you do if you didn't find a clot beneath the dura?

A. I would call for expert neurosurgical help and consider siting another burr hole in the frontal and parietal regions.

BURNS

Q. What different types of burns do you know about?

A. Burns may be thermal, due to either extreme heat or extreme cold. They may also be chemical or electrical.

Q. How would you classify burns?

A. Burns have two important features used in their classification. These are the extent, or size of the burn area, which is usually expressed as a percentage of the body area they cover. The palm of the hand including the fingers is approximately equal to 1% of a patient's total surface area. The second characteristic which is used to assess burns is the depth a burn has penetrated.

Q. What is the 'rule of nines'?

A. The rule of nines is a quick method of assessing the size of a burn.

- 9% head
- 9% one arm
- 18% one leg
- 36% trunk
- 1% palm.

Given that the palm is approximately 1% of the body's surface area, it may be useful to measure burns. If severely burnt, it may be easier to calculate the unburned area using the palm and subtract from 100.

Q. What is the significance of the size of the burn?

A. Mortality is proportional to the size of the burn and also worsens with age.

Q. How would you clinically assess the depth of a burn?

A. The presence of erythema and blistering indicates a partial thickness burn. Partial thickness burns are then further divided into superficial and deep dermal. Grey or white discoloration is seen with full thickness burns. They may have a leathery texture. Loss of pain sensation also indicates a full thickness burn.

Q. What is the pathophysiology involved with burns?

A. The increase in heat that occurs with the initial burn causes an increase in capillary permeability. This allows proteins to escape into the extravascular compartment resulting in tissue oedema and fluid loss. This may be sufficient to cause circulatory collapse.

Platelets and neutrophils are attracted to the area and erythrocytes may also be haemolysed (microangiopathic haemolytic anaemia – MAHA). There is an overall increase in the body's oxygen consumption, associated with an increase in metabolism and a negative nitrogen balance. Elevated levels of serum cortisol result in an increase in gluconeogenesis and protein catabolism. Insulin resistance also develops and the elevated serum levels of catecholamines contribute to the overall catabolic state.

Q. What commonly leads to death in burns victims?

A. Infection and fluid loss.

Q. What would go through your mind when assessing the airway of a burns patient?

A. An immediate priority is correct management of the airway. Burns patients can suffer burns to the oropharynx and upper airway. Smoke inhalation can lead to laryngeal oedema, therefore leading to hypoxia and carbon monoxide inhalation. It also predisposes to ARDS.

Features from the history of the burn are important. A fire in a confined space, burns to the face or a hoarse voice indicate the possibility of a compromised airway. Immediate intubation and ventilation may be appropriate if the burn is severe or there is indication of upper airway involvement.

Q. In a case of smoke inhalation, what clinical features would lead you to suspect involvement of the airway?

A. I would look for the following:

- Reduced conscious level
- Facial burns/singeing of nostril hairs or eyelashes
- Black carbon deposits in/around mouth or nose
- Stridor
- Hoarseness.

Q. Once the airway was secure what would be your immediate management of a severely burned patient?

A. Assessment of the circulating volume is the next priority. This usually requires insertion of a central venous catheter. Skin loss and inflammation are the reasons for large volumes of water being lost to the air.

Pulse, blood pressure and haematocrit should all be regularly monitored.

Adequate intravenous fluid replacement is very important. Any adult with over 10% burns, or a child with over 5% burns will require fluid replacement. Fluid replacement regimes vary between units and individual consultants. Common formulas include the Mount Vernon formula and the Parkland regime (see Teaching note).

✻ TEACHING NOTE

Mount Vernon formula

Plasma is given 0.5 ml/kg/% burn in the following time periods after the burn:

- 4 hours
- 4 hours
- 4 hours
- 6 hours
- 6 hours
- 12 hours.

Totalling 36 hours after the burn.

Parkland formula

Ringer's lactate is used.

- First 8 hours – 4 ml/kg/% burn (give half)
- Give the other half over the next 16 hours.
- Second 24 hours – 2 l of 5% dextrose + colloid 0.5 ml/kg/% burn.

Adequate fluid replacement will help to minimize acute tubular necrosis, which is exacerbated by the circulating myoglobulin, leading to rhabdomyolisis. To optimize renal management an in-dwelling urinary catheter needs to be inserted.

Analgesia is essential, usually with intravenous opiates.

Any adult or child burnt badly enough to require fluid replacement should also be referred to a specialist burns unit.

Stress ulcer prophylaxis, antibiotics in the presence of sepsis and nutritional support should be started at an early stage.

Q. Do you know of any other complications which might occur to a burns victim?

A. Due to the large fluid volume disturbances, burns patients are susceptible to electrolyte disturbance.

The skin loss makes temperature regulation difficult and hypothermia needs to be considered and treated, with regular core temperature measurement.

The large-scale physical insult predisposes patients to coagulopathies such as disseminated intravascular coagulation and systemic inflammation response syndrome.

Sepsis can occur at any time and should always be considered

Q. What role does surgery play in the management of a burns patient?

A. Circumferential eschars causing respiratory or limb compromise may need to be released in the short term.

The longer-term management also varies between units and consultants. Skin will require grafting in areas of either deep dermal or full thickness burning. Grafting can occur either immediately or wait for up to 2 weeks when shave and autologous grafting can be attempted. Eventually cosmetic reconstruction may be appropriate for disfiguring scars.

PERIPHERAL VASCULAR DISEASES

Q. You are the duty surgical registrar, and you get called by the medical registrar to see a 75-year-old man who is recovering on ITU from a myocardial infarction which he sustained 5 days previously. He is now complaining of severe acute pain in his right leg, which is now feeling quite cold and pale. How would you manage this patient?

A. After taking a history and carrying out a detailed clinical vascular examination, I would need to establish whether this is an acute embolic disease and, if so, where the source of his embolus is.

Q. You found the patient to be in atrial fibrillation, and that he has all the '6P' signs of acute limb ischaemia. What are the '6Ps' and how would you proceed with the management?

A. The '6Ps' are:

- Pain
- Pallor
- Pulseless
- Paraesthesia
- Paralysis
- Perishingly cold.

I would liaise with my medical colleague in starting the treatment for the patient's atrial fibrillation (such as digoxin therapy) after confirmation by an ECG. I would start immediate treatment for arterial embolism in the form of intravenous analgesia, such as morphine, and intravenous heparinization. I would contact the on-call radiologist for an emergency angiogram and start TPA therapy to restore the arterial flow. The patient will then have to be heparinized and also commenced on warfarin. Further cardiac investigations will be needed, such as an echocardiogram, etc.

Q. Where would you expect the level of the embolus to be?

A. Clinically, one could predict the level of the embolus depending on the symptoms and clinical signs. Acute ischaemic changes in the leg would indicate a femoral embolus, and ischaemic changes up to the thigh level would indicate an embolus in the iliac artery.

Q. What would you do if you do not have the facilities for an emergency angiogram and TPA therapy available at your hospital, and the patient's cardiac status would not allow him to be transferred to another hospital where such a facility could be delivered?

A. I would inform theatres to prepare for an emergency arterial embolectomy under local anaesthesia and low-dose intravenous sedation. I would also inform the duty anaesthetist and ask him/her to be in theatre while the procedure is being carried out. I would explain the procedure to the patient, outlining the risks and complications and obtain an informed consent. The patient will have to be prepared for emergency surgery.

Q. What intravenous sedation and local anaesthesia would you give and how much?

A. A small dose of midazolam, such as 2 mg, for sedation. For local anaesthetic, I would use a mixture of 0.5% lignocaine and 0.25% bupivacaine, 10–20 ml of each to infiltrate the groin/femoral region, and I would mark the area of skin infiltrated by the local anaesthetic. I would keep some of the local anaesthetic mixture available to be used for top-up during the surgical procedure, if needed.

Q. How would you proceed then?

A. I would clean and drape the patient in the appropriate manner, exposing both groins, and the whole of the affected lower limb. I would also use a sterile clear plastic bag to cover the affected foot, to allow easy palpation of the foot pulses or application of a hand-held Doppler probe.

Q. How would you proceed with the surgery?

A. I would make the incision in the groin on the affected side, along the course of the common and superficial femoral artery. I would deepen the incision carefully, to get to the artery, which should be easily palpable, and carefully dissect around the artery and its main branches, exposing the femoral artery at its bifurcation. I would use further infiltration of local anaesthesia as necessary to make sure that the patient remains as comfortable as possible during the procedure.

Q. What would you do if the patient has an iliac artery embolus, and you cannot feel the femoral pulse?

A. I would still make my incision along the anatomical landmarks of the femoral artery, over the mid-inguinal point and below the inguinal ligament. I would proceed carefully to feel for the artery, which can be felt as a hard cord as one gets through the layers of dissection.

Q. **You've exposed the femoral artery at its bifurcation, what would you do next?**

A. I would gently apply vascular slings around the common femoral artery, the superficial femoral artery and the profunda femoris artery, and I would also apply suture slings around the smaller branches to prevent back bleeding when performing the arteriotomy.

Q. **You've put all the vascular slings around all the appropriate branches and around the main trunk of the femoral artery, what would you do next?**

A. I would apply non-traumatic vascular clamps (cushioned, if available) around the common femoral, the superficial femoral and the profunda femoris arteries. The clamps are applied carefully to give enough area of arterial exposure in order to perform the embolectomy with ease. I would then proceed to perform the arteriotomy on the common femoral artery at the level of the bifurcation.

Q. **In what direction would you place the arteriotomy, and what are the choices?**

A. I would place my arteriotomy incision longitudinally, but it may also be placed transversely.

Q. **What are the benefits and problems associated with the position of the arteriotomy incision?**

A. In a longitudinal arteriotomy, narrowing of the lumen (stenosis) may occur when the arteriotomy is closed; however, a saphenous vein patch may remedy this problem. With a transverse arteriotomy, an intimal dissection may occur requiring an endarterectomy which may prove difficult in the presence of atheromatous plaques.

Q. **You've performed the arteriotomy, and despite your arterial clamps, you are still getting some back bleeding. What would you do?**

A. I would look for any other small arterial branches that I have missed, and I would put a sling tie around its origin to stop the back bleeding.

Q. **What would you do next?**

A. I would hold the sling around the common femoral artery carefully, and I would temporarily release the clamp around the common femoral artery (which was applied a fair distance higher than my arteriotomy) to assess the inflow of arterial blood. If there is no flow, then there is an embolus in the iliac artery, and I would need to pass an arterial Fogarty's catheter up into the common femoral artery into the iliac to clear the inflow.

Q. **What size of Fogarty's catheter would you use for this?**

A. I would pass a size 4 Fogarty's catheter, and I would gently fill the balloon with saline to extract the embolus very gently. Once the lumen is clear, then I would flush the common femoral artery with heparinized saline, and reapply the arterial clamp.

Q. What would you do next?

A. I would then explore the superficial femoral artery, by removing the clamp from the artery and then pass an arterial Fogarty's catheter down the superficial femoral artery to the leg/foot. I would use a size 3 catheter to do so, and apply very gentle pressure with the syringe to fill up the catheter balloon gently in order to extract the embolus. I would repeat the process again until all parts of the embolus have been extracted. I would then flush the artery with heparinized saline, and reapply the clamp. I would carry out the same procedure to the profunda femoris artery, and then flush it with heparinized saline. I would then close my arteriotomy.

Q. What sutures would you use to close the arteriotomy?

A. A 4/0 or 3/0 Prolene suture continuous, taking care not to damage the intima or dissect the arterial wall. I would keep all arterial clamps on until the arteriotomy is closed.

Q. What would you do next?

A. I would perform the 'internal flushing manoeuvre', by removing the clamps and the suture slings from the smaller branches first, and then from the profunda femoris artery before removing the clamp off the common femoral artery. The last clamp to be removed would be from the superficial femoral artery. I would apply gentle pressure with surgical gauze on the arteriotomy site to stop any blood oozing. I would then examine the leg and foot for change of colour and the appearance of palpable arterial pulses, which would take a couple of minutes (or less). Once the circulation to the affected limb has been restored, and the foot becomes hyperaemic and warm, and when all the oozing from the arteriotomy site stops, I would close the wound in layers, using absorbable vicryl sutures. I would close the skin with a subcuticular suture, such as monocryl, and I would also leave a suction drain in the wound (for example a Redivac drain).

Q. Do you have to use a drain in the wound? Why?

A. It is a personal preference, but I would prefer to use a suction drain as the patient will be on heparin infusion and then warfarin therapy, and so the risk of wound haematoma and its complications is high.

Q. What would you do if you find that you have restored the blood flow into the affected limb, but that the other leg has become pale, cold and ischaemic after you have passed the Fogarty's catheter up into the iliac artery?

A. This indicates that there was a saddle embolus at the aortic bifurcation or within the iliac artery, which has been pushed down into the other leg. This is the reason why I would have exposed and prepared the other groin (and leg). I would do exactly the same procedure on the other groin, exposing the other femoral artery and proceed to carry out a femoral embolectomy on the other leg in exactly the same manner as the first leg.

Q. What is the long-term management of this patient?

A. I would commence him on warfarin, and once his INR (international normalized ratio) is within the therapeutic range, I would discontinue the heparin treatment.

Q. How long would you keep the patient on warfarin?

A. For a minimum of 6 months, but usually for life or until the atrial fibrillation/ underlying cardiac disease has been treated.

Q. What would you do if the patient has a brachial artery embolus instead of a femoral embolus?

A. I would do the same as for the femoral embolus.

Q. If you had to perform a brachial artery embolectomy, and there were no facilities for TPA, where would you make your surgical exploration incision?

A. Either over the medial aspect of the arm, to explore the brachial artery in its mid-arm section, where the risks of damaging nerve tissue can be significant, or in the antecubital fossa. The Fogarty's catheter is passed up to the axillary artery and down into the radial and ulnar branches in the same manner as with the femoral artery.

Q. A 65-year-old man is referred to you, as the duty surgeon, with abdominal and back pain of 2 hours' duration. He also complains of painful cold legs. What is your main differential diagnosis?

A. A leaking aortic aneurysm.

Q. You examine the patient, and you cannot feel any palpable abdominal aortic aneurysm, but the patient has no palpable pulses in either groin, and has cold legs, with all the signs of acute ischaemia. While you are examining the patient, the pain disappears and all the patient's pulses return to normal. The patient feels much better. What do you think has happened?

A. This patient has a dissecting aortic aneurysm, which usually involves the thoracic aorta.

Q. Why do you think that the arterial pulses disappeared in the groin and then reappeared?

A. The aortic dissection has progressed further down, and as it does so, it may temporarily or permanently occlude the arterial orifices of some of the aortic branches, including the iliac vessels.

Q. How would you manage this case?

A. I would need to contact the on-call cardiothoracic team urgently, and to arrange for an emergency CT scan of the abdomen and chest. I would also have to control this patient's blood pressure, as hypertension is a major contributing factor. The CT scan would tell us what grade the dissection is, and this would outline the method of treatment.

Q. Suppose that the same patient did not recover his pulses, and that his blood pressure was low (80/50). On examination he has tenderness and fullness in the epigastrium. He is obese and you find it difficult to feel his abdominal aorta. What would you do?

A. I think he might still have a leaking abdominal aortic aneurysm, and accordingly I would manage him as an emergency with a provisional diagnosis of a leaking aneurysm.

Q. How would you manage a leaking aortic aneurysm?

A. I would assess and resuscitate the patient simultaneously (i.e. assessment and treatment run concurrently) until the patient's condition has been stabilized. I would insert two intravenous cannulae, at least one of which should be a wide-bore cannula or a central line. I would give the patient intravenous analgesia, and commence intravenous fluids gently to maintain the blood pressure around 90–100 systolic. I would also insert a urinary catheter. I would carry out urgent blood tests such as FBC, U&E, glucose, amylase, LFT and clotting screen, and contact the blood bank to ask for an immediate cross-match of ten units of blood with at least four units of FFP. I would arrange for an emergency CT scan of the abdomen to confirm the diagnosis (providing the patient is stable enough), and I would contact the anaesthetist and theatre staff immediately. I would contact the senior surgeon (or the vascular surgeon on-call in some hospitals) to inform them about the patient, and book an ITU bed.

I would also speak to the patient and his relatives to let them know what is happening. Once the CT scan confirms the diagnosis, then the patient may be transferred to theatre for an emergency laparotomy, and grafting of the ruptured aorta. The anaesthetist will have to be present while the patient is having the CT scan. If the patient is very unstable, an emergency laparotomy may be carried out (in the presence of the appropriate senior surgeon) without a CT scan.

Different scenario

Q. An 80-year-old diabetic lady is referred to you as an emergency with pain and gangrene of the toes on one leg. During your clinical examination, you find that she has bilateral chronic leg ischaemia, but has a dry gangrene of the toes of one foot, and absent pulses in both feet. What would you do?

A. I would carry out a full clinical assessment, and admit the patient for further investigation and management. I would give the patient adequate analgesia (such as morphine). If the patient's pre-morbid condition is good, then a full vascular assessment of her peripheral vascular disease using Doppler is required. However, if the patient is moribund and normally bedridden, then full vascular investigations can be considered unnecessary.

Q. **This lady's diabetes is out of control, she lives in a nursing home and is bedridden. What would you do next?**

A. I would control her diabetes, by using insulin sliding scale for example, and I would prepare the patient for an amputation of the gangrenous foot. I would explain the situation to the patient and her family, and I would get an informed consent for this treatment.

Q. **What type of amputation would you do? Would you just amputate the gangrenous toes and if so why?**

A. No, I would not amputate just the toes, as the circulation is poor. She also has diabetes which would reduce the chance of healing after amputation of the toes. I would do a below-knee amputation, or consider an above-knee amputation, which would make it easier to nurse the patient afterwards, as she is already bedridden.

Q. **What are the problems of doing a below-knee amputation in such a patient with pre-morbid mobility problems?**

A. It is most likely that the patient would develop flexion contractures of the knee which would make nursing the patient very difficult and may result in wound breakdown.

Q. **How would you carry out an above-knee amputation?**

A. In a fully prepared and consented patient, I would perform the procedure under general or spinal anaesthesia. The patient should be given full antibiotic cover (including penicillin) in view of the presence of ischaemia, gangrene and diabetes.

The patient is positioned supine on the operating table. The whole lower limb is cleaned and draped appropriately and the gangrenous foot is covered with disposable sterile drapes. The flaps are measured and marked with a sterile tape measure and a marker pen. I would measure the anterior and posterior flaps, with the level of the bone division at 13–14 cm from the knee-joint line. I would make the anterior flap 1–2 cm shorter than the posterior flap, which would position the wound a fraction anteriorly and therefore prevent pressure on the wound when the patient is lying in bed postoperatively. This would facilitate the wound healing, and reduce the risk of wound breakdown. I would make my skin incisions along the markings of the anterior and posterior flaps, cutting through the skin, subcutaneous fascia, fat and muscles down to bone (femur). I would need to identify the main vessels (femoral artery and vein) and to clamp them with arterial forceps before dividing them. I would also need to identify the sciatic and femoral nerves, and divide them with a scalpel, making sure to apply diathermy to any accompanying vessels. I would need to avoid applying ligatures to the nerves, as this could cause severe postoperative phantom pains and neuromas. Once the main vessels and nerves were divided, I would carry on with the dissection to the bone, cutting through the periostium at the appropriate level (usually 13–14 cm above the knee-joint line). I would apply the metal protector to protect the soft tissues around the femur, and then use the saw to cut the bone, bevelling the anterior edge of the bone. Once the bone is cut completely, the amputated leg is now completely disconnected from the patient's thigh and is discarded appropriately into a special bag for tissue disposal. The edge of the bone is filed to smooth the rough border, and bone wax is applied to stop any oozing from the cut end of the bone. The main vessels are transfixed or ligated with heavy absorbable sutures, and full haemostasis is achieved with ties and diathermy.

A trial approximation of the flaps is made to make sure that the flaps are not tight and, if in any doubt, the bony end is trimmed further as needed. The anterior and posterior flaps are sutured together using absorbable sutures (such as vicryl), suturing the edges of the muscle and fascia together. I would use two suction drains to the wound/flaps, and would then apply the skin sutures. I personally use subcuticular vicryl or monocryl sutures, but other surgeons may prefer interrupted Prolene sutures. A loose gentle dressing is applied to the wound.

I would continue with antibiotics for a minimum of 5 days, and inspect the wound at 24–48 hours. Proper nursing care is required for these patients.

Once the wound has healed completely, and all the swelling has gone, the patient can be assessed for prosthesis if mobility is desirable.

Similar steps are used for a below-knee amputation, but the flaps are measured and marked either as a 'Skew-flap' or as a 'long posterior Burgess Flap'.

TRACHEOSTOMY

Q. What are the indications for a tracheostomy?

A. The most common indication is the need for long-term mechanical ventilation in patients with chest or head injuries. Other indications include respiratory muscle paralysis, such as myasthenia gravis, poliomyelitis, polyneuritis or cervical cord lesions.

Airway obstruction above the level of the vocal cords is another indication for tracheostomy, such as a huge goitre or an advanced malignancy of the larynx. In a very large goitre that is causing tracheomalacia, a tracheostomy can be carried out at the time of thyroidectomy, and in the case of laryngeal cancer a laryngectomy is also carried out.

Tracheostomy is rarely carried out as an emergency, and although it can be a life-saving operation, it should be performed as an urgent semi-elective procedure in a properly prepared operating theatre.

Q. How would you carry out a tracheostomy?

A. In a properly prepared patient, I would check the indications for such an invasive procedure and that the appropriate informed consent has been obtained, if possible. I would then carry out the tracheostomy under general anaesthetic as a planned procedure with usual operating conditions and in the presence of fully devoted and experienced staff who are trained in dealing with these cases (including the anaesthetist).

Last-minute emergency tracheostomies performed on the ward generally have disastrous consequences.

The patient is positioned supine on the operating table, with full extension of the neck and a sand bag or folded blanket positioned under the shoulders. All the necessary tracheostomy equipment (with the tubing and all the connections) is checked before starting the procedure, including the availability of the correct size of tube and other spare parts. I would clean and drape in the appropriate fashion, and would then proceed to make my surgical incision over the trachea.

Q. How would you make your incision and how would you then proceed?

A. I would make a transverse skin incision just below the cricoid cartilage (patient's one finger breadth below it), and then deepen the incision down to the deep cervical fascia. Once the skin and the platysma have been divided, I would stop all bleeding and then proceed with the dissection strictly in the midline (as few vessels will be encountered and this will reduce the bleeding and other complications). I would get my assistant to retract the edges of the wound upwards and downwards to expose the deep fascia. I would then cut through the deep fascia vertically, separating the strap muscles layer by layer (between the sternohyoid and sternothyroid muscles) and retract these muscles sideways using two small retractors, until the tracheal rings are exposed.

Q. How would you deal with the thyroid isthmus and how would you proceed afterwards?

A. Once the trachea is exposed, I would free the thyroid isthmus using blunt dissection. I would then clamp, cut and ligate the isthmus and I may use transfixing sutures in order to achieve full haemostasis. I would then insert a hook below the cricoid cartilage to pull the trachea proximally upwards into the wound.

I would have to take great care with children, as the child's trachea can be pulled a long way out of the chest, so choosing the level of the cut should be against the trachea and not the suprasternal notch. It is therefore necessary to palpate the cricoid cartilage and count down the tracheal rings before making the cut in the trachea.

Q. How would you make your cut into the trachea and how would you insert the tube?

A. Many types of tracheal stomas have been described, for example in infants a short vertical incision is preferable. Most people perform either a flap or a circular window incision. Before I make my incision into the trachea, I would warn the anaesthetist that I am going to do so, and I would make a 1.5 cm three-sided rectangular cut between the second and third rings and through the third ring of the trachea to make a flap based inferiorly. I would take care not to puncture the balloon of the endotracheal tube, but if a puncture is made then I would need to inform the anaesthetist. I would pass a stitch through the upper part of the flap, to prepare for the insertion of the tracheostomy tube. I would now ask the anaesthetist to withdraw the endotracheal tube, and I would insert the tracheostomy tube and connect it to the anaesthetic machine (making sure that my tube connector fits the anaesthetic tubing).

The hook and the stitch usually open the trachea sufficiently to pass the tube, but I could use a dilator if necessary (although this is not usually necessary). I would now inflate the cuff of my tracheostomy tube and I would then achieve full haemostasis of any residual bleeding. I would then close the wound in layers around the tube, and then tie the tapes with the knot near the front, and apply light wound dressing.

Q. What is the most important part of doing a tracheostomy?

A. The postoperative care is the most important part of performing a tracheostomy. This includes the nursing care in looking after the tracheostomy tube and keeping the airway clear. Therefore, the availability of devoted nursing staff is the most important aspect in order to reduce the morbidity and mortality. The tracheostomy will need careful and regular care, including regular suction of bronchial secretions. Any shortcomings in such care would result in the patient's death.

Q. What are the complications of tracheostomy?

A. Immediate operative complications include:

- Bleeding (for example from the thyroid isthmus or from injury to major vessels)
- Mechanical tracheal obstruction (rare)
- Using the wrong size of tracheostomy tubing
- Malfitting connection to the anaesthetic machine (incompetent staff).

Postoperative complications include:

- Tracheal stenosis (caused by badly planned incision in the tracheal wall or trauma from the inflatable cuff)
- Displacement of the tube
- Tracheal obstruction with bronchial secretions due to poor nursing care.

The patient is deprived of the ability to cough and talk, the inspired air is no longer humidified by the upper air passages, and the patient will be fully dependent upon the insertion of suction catheters to clear bronchial secretions.

Q. How do you deal with the problem of inability to talk?

A. Once the scar tissue has healed, one could use a special voice box which can be fitted to the tracheostomy tube, or the patient can be taught to put his/her finger on the tracheostomy opening to be able to speak. In the early postoperative period, the patient will have to be provided with a pad of paper and a pen to be able to communicate with staff and relatives, and this should have been explained to the patient preoperatively.

Q. **If the patient no longer needs the tracheostomy, what would you do to it?**

A. No further action is required, as once the tube has been removed, the tracheostomy hole will close with scar tissue spontaneously with time.

Q. **Are there any other ways to perform a tracheostomy?**

A. Yes, one could perform a tracheotomy, with a 'mini-tracheotomy' tube. This is the process of inserting a small tracheotomy tube with a guiding trocar, which can be carried out under local anaesthesia on ITU. However, the full tracheotomy set is required, including experience of the operator. This procedure is a short-term method of relieving airway obstruction at the level above the vocal cords, where a small plastic tube is inserted through the fascia above the cricoid cartilage. Tracheotomy tubes are usually available in ITU and A&E departments.

THYROID SURGERY

Q. **A patient attends your clinic with a large swelling in the anterior triangle of the neck of 2 years' duration. How would you manage this patient?**

A. The most likely diagnosis is a goitre. I would take a full history and carry out a full neck and relevant clinical examination including:

- Examination of both triangles of the neck on each side and the regional lymph nodes
- Examination of the eyes (for signs of thyrotoxicosis such as Graves' disease, exophthalmos, lid retraction or lid lag)
- Cardiovascular examination (for example looking for atrial fibrillation, resting tachycardia, bruit over the thyroid gland or the neck vessels)
- General examination (for example thyroid tremor).

The general examination would elucidate whether or not the patient has any clinical signs of hyper-, hypo- or euthyroid status. I would then carry out further investigations to determine the nature of the goitre.

Q. **What investigations would you carry out if you find that the patient has a large nodule affecting part of the thyroid gland?**

A. These would include:

- Blood tests – including thyroid function (T4 and TSH), thyroid auto-antibodies, serum calcium, basic biochemistry, and full blood count
- Radiological tests – ultrasound scan of the neck (and guided fine-needle aspiration (FNA) cytology if any large solid nodule is seen), chest X-ray with thoracic inlet (in cases of suspected retrosternal extension), thyroid isotope scan (if solid nodules are found), and a CT or MRI scan of the neck and chest (if the patient has any retrosternal extension of the goitre) to assess the intrathoracic component of the goitre

- An ENT assessment of the vocal cords would also be necessary if surgery is contemplated or if malignancy is suspected.

Different scenarios with different results of investigations

Q. **You've arranged all of the above investigations and the ultrasound scan shows a multinodular goitre with a large solid nodule, which is a 'cold nodule' on isotope scan. The FNA cytology revealed follicular cells. What would you do then?**

A. I would explain these results to the patient, indicating that he/she would require thyroid surgery and that there is a small risk of the presence of a tumour in the gland for which treatment will be needed.

Q. **What does it mean when the cytologist says that there are follicular cells and therefore a malignancy cannot be excluded?**

A. This means that the patient has a solid nodule, which could be reactive changes in a multinodular goitre, or a benign follicular adenoma or a follicular carcinoma. However, it is not possible to differentiate these on cytology, and the histology can only be confirmed after surgery (i.e. thyroidectomy).

Q. **You've explained the results to the patient and told the patient that surgery is needed. What sort of surgical treatment would you advise for this patient?**

A. I would advise a total or near total thyroidectomy.

Q. **What would you tell the pathologist before you carry out the operation?**

A. I would ask the pathologist for urgent (e.g. 48 hours) histology results, and the specimen should be sent to the pathology laboratory urgently.

Q. **Would you ask for a frozen section?**

A. If this facility is available, then yes. However, frozen-section histological examination of the thyroid (especially a carcinoma) is usually inaccurate and difficult. Therefore, I would prefer a full urgent histology.

Q. **How would you perform a total thyroidectomy?**

A. In a fully prepared patient, who has been properly investigated with an ENT assessment and informed consent, I would carry out the procedure under general anaesthesia. The patient may need potassium iodide (Lugol's solution) and/or anti-thyroid medications preoperatively (if thyrotoxic). I would check that these issues had been addressed in surgical pre-clerking.

I would position the patient supine on the operating table with full neck extension, using a sand bag or folded blanket under the shoulders. I would clean and drape in the appropriate manner (using head towels for example). I would avoid using iodine-based skin cleansing agents.

Q. Where would you make your incision and how would you proceed afterwards?

A. I would make my collar incision along the skin crease, approximately a finger breadth above the suprasternal notch. I would then extend my incision through the platysma, down to the fascia covering the strap muscles. I would raise the upper flap to a level above the cricoid cartilage, and the lower flap to the level of the upper margin of the sternum. I would carefully stop any subcutaneous bleeding, as full haemostasis is very important.

I would then apply the Joll's retractor to expose the strap muscles. I would make a vertical incision through the midline raphe, between the strap muscles of both sides down to the thyroid gland.

I would stand on the right-hand side of the operating table to deal with the left lobe of the thyroid gland, and on the left side to deal with the right lobe. I would then position my assistant's Langenbeck retractors to retract the strap muscles in order to expose the thyroid gland. I would need to decide at this point whether or not I need to divide the strap muscles.

Q. Why would you need to divide the strap muscles?

A. If the goitre is very large, then I would need to divide the strap muscles to make the surgery and the surgical exposure much easier. It would also reduce the morbidity.

Q. How would you divide the strap muscles, at what level, and why?

A. I would divide the strap muscles between two clamps and would transfix the divided ends to allow repair at the end of the procedure. I would then divide the muscles high, because of the entry of nerve supply through the ansa cervicalis, which enters the muscles from below. I would repair the muscles with interrupted PDS at the end of the procedure.

Q. How would you proceed afterwards?

A. I would then proceed with gentle dissection, laterally dividing the branches of the middle thyroid vein and using the assistant's retractor to provide adequate surgical exposure.

With gentle and blunt dissection, I would free the upper border of the thyroid gland and then use the thyroid dissector to loop around the superior thyroid vessels. I would then apply double ligatures around the superior thyroid pedicles using the thyroid dissector and mounted aneurysm needles, for example using vicryl ties. Once the vessels have been doubly ligated, I would divide the superior pedicle to free the upper border of the gland. This would allow further mobilization of the lateral part of the gland and I would then begin lifting the gland forward, with gentle and blunt dissection.

I would look carefully for the recurrent laryngeal nerve and the parathyroid glands. The nerve usually lies behind the parathyroid gland close to the inferior thyroid artery. Once the nerve and the parathyroid glands have been identified and carefully preserved, I would ligate the inferior thyroid artery in continuity (or ligate its branches close to the gland). I would then start lifting off the thyroid gland from the trachea, using gentle dissection and vicryl ties for haemostasis.

The gland is then lifted off the trachea and freed, using ligatures or bipolar diathermy for haemostasis, making sure to avoid any diathermy near the nerve. The thyroid isthmus is then freed from the trachea, and the dissection is resumed on the other lobe.

I would have to change to the other side of the table before dissecting on the opposite lobe. I would carry out the same technique as before. If I find any lymph nodes, then I would take them out as a biopsy. Full haemostasis should then be achieved. A suction drain is used to drain each side (i.e. two Redivac drains). I would then infiltrate the skin flaps with local anaesthesia, such as bupivacaine, as part of postoperative pain relief. I would then close the wound in layers using 2/0 and 3/0 vicryl. The skin closure is either carried out using Mitchell's skin clips or subcuticular sutures (surgeon's preference).

Q. What would be your postoperative care of this patient?

A. I would monitor the patient's serum calcium postoperatively, and correct any hypocalcaemia as required. Even when the parathyroids have been left intact, they may occasionally become ischaemic. The patient may then develop hypoparathyroidism, which would require medical treatment. I would ask for an urgent 48 hour histology, and if this shows a benign pathology, then the patient may be commenced on thyroxine replacement prior to discharge from hospital.

Q. What would you do if the histology reveals a follicular carcinoma?

A. I would not need to perform a completion thyroidectomy, as the patient had a total thyroidectomy. I would discuss the need for radioiodine therapy followed by thyroxine replacement with the patient. If the carcinoma extends through the thyroid capsule, then radiotherapy to the neck may be necessary, especially if there are any positive lymph nodes.

A different scenario

Q. Supposing the preoperative investigations had revealed a single nodule affecting one lobe of the gland with the rest of the gland looking normal. What would you do then?

A. I would explain the situation clearly to the patient and would advise the patient to undergo a hemi-thyroidectomy. I would need to remove the thyroid isthmus with the affected lobe, and I would still ask for urgent histology. If the histology shows any evidence of malignancy, then I would have to proceed to a completion thyroidectomy as soon as is feasible.

Q. What would you do if the preoperative investigations demonstrated a multinodular goitre without any cold nodules?

A. I would discuss with the patient the choice of having a subtotal or a near total thyroidectomy, and I would proceed the same way as described before.

Q. What are the complications of thyroidectomy?

A. The complications include:

- General – bleeding, infection, risks of general anaesthesia, keloid scar
- Specific – recurrent laryngeal nerve injury, superior laryngeal nerve injury, hypoparathyroidism causing hypocalcaemia, hypothyroidism and recurrence of the goitre (in partial thyroidectomy).

Q. How would you deal with a retrosternal goitre?

A. The extent of the goitre should be fully assessed preoperatively, with chest X-ray and CT scan (or MRI scan) of the chest and thoracic inlet.

I would inform the patient that a sternotomy might be necessary in order to remove the thoracic/mediastinal part of the goitre. I would inform them that thoracic surgical cover may therefore be necessary at the time of thyroidectomy. I would prepare the patient preoperatively as I would for a thyroidectomy; however, ITU back-up will be required postoperatively.

I would request a cross-match of four units of blood for the time of surgery. I would clean and drape the neck and the chest, as I would for a sternotomy. I would proceed with the thyroidectomy through a collar/neck approach as usual, since it is usual to remove the mediastinal component through the neck. I would start with the thyroidectomy through the neck as described above. However, if it is not possible to perform the thyroidectomy through the neck incision, I would proceed to a sternotomy with the help of the thoracic surgeons.

A median sternotomy is carried out as usual (after the superior thyroid pedicles have been doubly ligated and divided, as this would reduce the blood loss). I would open the chest and use a bone wax to stop any bony oozing from the edge of the sternotomy, and I would achieve haemostasis from the edges of the wound. I would then open the upper anterior mediastinum and assess the mediastinal component of the goitre. I would try to free this part of the goitre with gentle and careful dissection and avoid injury to any of the major vessels.

Once the mediastinal component is freed, I would then perform a total thyroidectomy in the usual manner. I would then achieve full haemostasis, and insert two suction drains into the neck wound and two chest/mediastinal drains into the chest wound.

I would close the wounds in layers using vicryl in the neck, and stainless steel wire (or no.1 nylon) to the sternotomy wound. The subcutaneous and skin layers are then closed accordingly. The patient should be transferred to ITU postoperatively and should be kept ventilated overnight or when respiratory function is satisfactory.

The postoperative care is similar to that of total thyroidectomy. The drains (chest and neck) are usually removed in 24–48 hours, when the drainage is minimal. Thyroxine replacement is given, depending on the histology.

HERNIAE

Q. A 20-year-old man presents at the surgical clinic with a swelling in the left groin. It is causing him some local discomfort. How would you manage this patient?

A. I would take a full history and carry out a full clinical examination, including examination of the abdomen and genital area.

Q. You found that he has an easily reducible swelling with a cough impulse in the groin. How would you differentiate between an inguinal and a femoral hernia?

A. If the swelling is above and medial to the pubic tubercle, then it is an inguinal hernia. If it is below and lateral to the pubic tubercle, it is a femoral hernia.

Q. Which is more common in a young man, an inguinal or a femoral hernia?

A. An inguinal hernia is far more common.

Q. What types of inguinal herniae are there?

A. Indirect, direct and combined (Pantaloon hernia).

Q. How would you differentiate between a direct and an indirect inguinal hernia?

A. I would put my finger over the mid-point of the inguinal canal (over the deep ring). If I could control the swelling then it is an indirect hernia, but if the hernia bulges medial to my finger (i.e. through the muscle wall of the inguinal canal) then it is a direct hernia.

Q. How would you repair an indirect inguinal hernia in this man?

A. I would ensure that the patient was properly prepared for surgery including obtaining the appropriate informed consent (including explanation about the possible side effects and risks).

I would then undertake a mesh repair of the hernia, under general anaesthesia. The procedure may be carried out as a day case, and it may also be carried out under local anaesthesia. My personal preference, however, is to repair the hernia under general anaesthesia (GA).

The patient is positioned supine on the operating table. The patient should be given one dose of antibiotics, as prophylaxis (although this is a personal preference). The patient is cleaned and prepped in the appropriate fashion. A skin incision is made in the groin skin crease overlying the hernia. The wound is deepened through the subcutaneous fascia and fat, down to the external oblique muscle. The superficial ring is exposed and the inguinal canal is opened to expose the spermatic cord and its contents. The cord is then examined carefully to identify the hernial sac and also to confirm the diagnosis of a direct, or indirect sac, or both.

Once the hernia sac has been identified, it can then be carefully dissected off the spermatic cord whilst avoiding injury to the contents of the cord (including the vessels and the vas). The cremasteric vessels may need to be ligated and divided to gain access and to achieve full haemostasis. After the hernial sac has been freed, the sac must then be carefully opened to identify any bowel or omentum contents within it (sliding hernia).

If the sac is empty, it is then transfixed and excised (herniotomy). If there is a large direct sac, then the sac can be invaginated and plicated using a Prolene or nylon suture. If a direct sac is found, I would have to see if the patient also has an indirect sac (as pantaloon herniae are present in 5–10% of cases, and can be responsible for early cases of recurrent hernia).

Once the sac is transfixed and excised, I would then repair and reinforce the weakened posterior wall of the inguinal canal using a mesh (such as a Prolene mesh) in a modified Lichtenstein technique. I would tailor it appropriately to cover the weakened posterior wall, and to allow an opening for the spermatic cord to pass through. I would apply interrupted or continuous sutures to fix the mesh in position and then ensure that haemostasis is achieved. I would then close the wound in layers using absorbable sutures (such as vicryl). I would use local anaesthetic (such as bupivacaine) for postoperative pain relief and subcuticular sutures to close the skin.

The patient may then be discharged home when comfortable, although policy at most units is to wait until the patient has passed urine (as acute urinary retention after hernia repair is a rare possibility).

I would advise the patient to avoid heavy lifting or strenuous exercise for the early postoperative period so as to avoid risks of early recurrence.

Q. Can you always use a mesh for repair of inguinal hernia?

A. No, in cases of a strangulated or gangrenous hernia, I would use a suturing technique. Unfortunately, this technique carries a higher incidence of recurrence.

Q. What other techniques do you know of that can be used to repair an inguinal hernia?

A. Other well known techniques include Bassini's repair (with or without Tanner slide), Darn and Shouldice repairs. One can use a combination of these techniques, such as a Bassini repair with a Darn reinforcement.

Q. Describe how you would perform a Bassini's repair.

A. The hernia sac is transfixed and excised in the same way as described above. I would then identify the firm tissue which will be used for the repair, and I would use a 0 or 1 monofilament nylon, or Prolene, to suture the aponeurosis and muscles to the inguinal ligament. I would start medially and take a good bite of the aponeurosis and the periostium over the pubic tubercle. I would carry the union laterally, behind the cord as far as the internal ring, where the emerging spermatic cord is enclosed snugly.

I prefer to combine this technique with another layer of Darn reinforcement by using a similar suture to go back from the internal ring towards the pubic tubercle (which reduces the risks of hernia recurrence). Other techniques are used according to personal preference.

Q. What are the risks of hernia repair?

A. The risks include:

- Recurrence
- Infection (which could be a contributing factor for recurrence)
- Haematoma
- Damage to structures of the spermatic cord (such as the testicular vessels and the vas)
- Testicular atrophy
- Hydrocoele
- Injury to deeper structures (such as injury to the iliac or femoral vessels, catching loops of bowel, etc.)
- Urinary retention
- Chronic pain syndrome (due to injury to the ilioinguinal or iliohypogastric nerves).

In addition, there are also the risks of general or local anaesthesia.

Q. What type of repair would you consider in a child with a congenital inguinal hernia? Would you use a mesh?

A. No, I would not use a mesh for a hernia repair. I would carry out a herniotomy only, as a herniorrhaphy is not required in children. The inguinal canal has not fully developed in children, and is much shorter than in adults. As the child gets older, the superficial and the deep rings will grow apart, thus reducing the risk of future recurrence. If the child does not have a full hernia, but has a patent processus vaginalis (PPV), then ligation of the PPV is all that is required.

Q. How would you deal with a 13-year-old boy with a large inguinal hernia?

A. I would carry out a herniotomy similar to that in adults, but as the inguinal canal is partially developed, then the boy would also require a herniorrhaphy.

Q. Would you do a mesh repair or a sutured (e.g. Bassini's) repair for this boy?

A. I would not use any mesh or any continuous sutured repair, as the child is still growing and such a repair might impede further growth. Accordingly, I would use interrupted PDS sutures to carry out a modified Bassini's repair. As the child continues to grow, the inguinal canal continues to develop and the interrupted PDS sutures will absorb or will grow apart as the inguinal canal gets longer.

Q. If a 1-year-old child presents with a left congenital inguinal hernia, would you explore both groins and why?

A. As the left testis reaches the scrotum earlier than the right one, theoretically the child might have bilateral inguinal herniae. I would examine the child carefully looking for any signs of bilateral herniae and I would carry out a bilateral herniotomy if he had evidence of bilateral herniae. However, I personally would not explore both groins, although some surgeons might adopt this option.

I would warn the parents that the child has a higher incidence of having a right-sided hernia in the future, and that we would need to repair it if he develops one.

INTESTINAL OBSTRUCTION

Q. What are the cardinal symptoms of intestinal obstruction?

A. The cardinal symptoms of intestinal obstruction include:

- Abdominal pain
- Vomiting
- Abdominal distension
- Absolute constipation.

Q. Can you describe the pain?

A. The pain is classically colicky and severe.

Q. Is it always associated with vomiting?

A. No, vomiting is generally a feature of small bowel obstruction. The vomitus also differs according to the level of obstruction:

- At the pylorus – very watery
- High up in the small bowel – bile-stained vomit
- Lower down in the small bowel – brown, thicker vomit, often described as 'faeculent'.

Q. Are there any other differences in the clinical features of small and large bowel obstruction?

A. Other differences include:

- Less abdominal distension is seen in small bowel obstruction
- Pain – in small bowel obstruction, it tends to be worse in the epigastrium/umbilicus, in large bowel obstruction it is worse in the lower abdomen/left or right iliac fossae
- Onset of symptoms – small bowel obstruction tends to present with pain, vomiting and little distension. Large bowel obstruction presents with pain, absolute constipation and distension. In such cases, vomiting tends to occur late.

Q. What about the radiological differences?

A. Radiological differences include:

- Valvulae conniventes – continuous across the wall of the small bowel
- Haustra – characteristic of large bowel and do not travel all the way across the bowel wall.

Q. How would you classify the causes of intestinal obstruction?

A. I would classify as follows:

	Small bowel	Large bowel
In the lumen	Foreign body	Faecal impaction
	Bezoar	Bezoar
	Gallstone	
In the bowel wall	Lymphoma	Carcinoma
	Inflammatory stricture	Diverticulitis
		Inflammatory mass
		Ischaemic colitis
		Anastomotic stricture
		Hirschsprung's disease
		Endometriosis
External	Adhesions	Volvulus
	Herniae	Intussusception
	Intussusception	Megacolon
	Congenital bands	Pseudo-obstruction
		Adhesions
		Congenital bands

Q. In large bowel obstruction, how would you know if the iliocaecal valve was competent?

A. If the iliocaecal valve was incompetent, it would prevent reflux into the small bowel and hence the obstruction would be confined to the large bowel. With time, pressure builds up in the caecum and it rapidly distends. It is associated with severe right iliac fossa pain and visible peristalsis may be seen. Eventually the blood supply to the caecum is compromised and may perforate.

Q. How would you investigate a patient who you suspected had intestinal obstruction?

A. After taking a full history and performing a full abdominal system examination, I would perform the following investigations:

- Full blood count
- White cell count
- Amylase
- Urea and electrolytes
- Liver function tests

- Pregnancy test, if appropriate
- Abdominal and erect chest X-rays.

If I had a high suspicion of intra-abdominal pathology, I would arrange an abdominal CT scan.

Q. **You are a surgical registrar on call and you have been called to see a 60-year-old gentleman on ITU. He underwent a CABG 3 weeks ago and has developed renal failure requiring dialysis since. You are called to see him as he has had increasing abdominal distension for 2 days. What is the most likely diagnosis?**

A. It is likely that this gentleman has developed pseudo-obstruction secondary to his renal failure. He has also undergone major cardiac surgery which can commonly result in the development of an ileus postoperatively.

Q. **How would you manage him?**

A. First, I would take a full history and examine the patient. I would also arrange limited contrast imaging, depending on his cardiovascular stability, in order to exclude a possible obstructing lesion. I would then advise conservative management and correction of any predisposing factors such as sepsis.

Q. **You have a 75-year-old lady presenting with all the symptoms and signs of bowel obstruction. How would you manage this lady?**

A. I would take a full history and carry out a full relevant clinical examination, looking for an underlying cause for the obstruction.

Q. **Name the four most common causes of bowel obstruction.**

A. Herniae, adhesions, volvulus and tumours.

Q. **Imagine that this lady has not had any previous operations and she does not have any palpable external herniae. What would you do?**

A. After resuscitating the patient and carrying out a full assessment, I would prepare the patient for an exploratory laparotomy, as the underlying cause is obscure.

Q. **How would you do that?**

A. Under general anaesthesia, in a prepared patient who has received intravenous fluids, analgesia, and has a nasogastric tube and a urinary catheter prior to surgery.

I would position the patient supine on the operating table. If the preoperative clinical assessment suggests a distal bowel obstruction, then I would carry out a rigid sigmoidoscopy before the laparotomy. If I discovered any rectal pathology, I would position the patient on the table in the Lloyd–Davies position. With a small bowel obstruction, a supine position is adopted.

I would make a long midline incision, cutting through the skin, fat and linea alba, taking great care not to damage any loops of bowel upon entering the peritoneal cavity. Once the peritoneal cavity has been entered, I would then follow the dilated loops of bowel distally until the area of obstruction is reached, where there will be some loops of collapsed bowel distal to it. I would deal with the cause of obstruction (such as hernia, adhesion or tumour etc.) and free the obstructed loop. I would then assess the viability of the obstructed segment of the bowel and any non-viable segments would be excised. If the obstruction involves the small bowel, if there is no peritonitis or if there is evidence of contamination, then a primary bowel anastomosis can be carried out (provided the ends of the anastomosed loops have good blood supply). If there is any doubt, or if the obstructed part involves the distal large bowel, then a stoma should be considered, and a Hartmann's resection can be carried out.

Q. Imagine that this lady has not had any previous surgery to cause any adhesions and there were no palpable herniae. You find, however, that she is in atrial fibrillation and has a distended silent tender abdomen with minimal other clinical findings. What is the most likely cause of her symptoms?

A. It is most likely that she has a mesenteric artery embolism causing mesenteric infarction, and she would need an emergency laparotomy.

Q. You've carried out an emergency laparotomy, and you've found a superior mesenteric artery embolism. What would you do?

A. I would assess the viability of the affected part of the bowel. If the bowel is ischaemic but not gangrenous, then I would carry out a superior mesenteric artery embolectomy (or call the vascular surgeons to do it if I do not have the experience of doing this procedure). I would then heparinize the patient, and commence warfarin when she starts an oral diet.

Q. What would you do if you find that only half of the small bowel is gangrenous?

A. I would resect the affected part, and I may bring the two ends of the bowel as stomas, if there is any concern about the blood supply of the remaining loops of the bowel.

Q. What would you do if you find the whole midgut section gangrenous (i.e. the whole of the small bowel and proximal colon)?

A. This would be incompatible with survival, and I would close the abdomen and start the patient on a diamorphine pump. I would speak to her family immediately and treat her as a terminally ill patient, keeping her comfortable until she dies.

Q. Suppose that the patient presents with bowel obstruction but no palpable herniae can be felt. The patient has pain, however, and paraesthesia over the skin of the upper inner aspect of one of her thighs. What is the most likely cause of her bowel obstruction?

A. The most likely cause is an obstructed or a strangulated obturator hernia. The cause of pain and paraesthesia over the upper inner thigh is due to pressure on the obturator nerve which has its cutaneous distribution over that part of the thigh.

I would carry out a laparotomy and I would free the obstructed loop of the bowel. I would also repair the hernia from the inside, during the laparotomy.

Q. If you have a patient with an obstructed femoral hernia as the cause of the bowel obstruction, how would you deal with this operatively?

A. I would carry out exploration and repair, either through a low approach or through a high approach.

Q. Which one would you choose and why?

A. I would do a high approach, such as a McEvedy's or Henry's approach, as the high approach gives better control and access to inspect the affected loop of the bowel and it is also easier to resect the bowel, if required.

In the low approach, it is sometimes difficult to identify the sac in the fatty lump, and it is more difficult to perform the bowel resection.

Q. Would you use any drains when you carry out an emergency laparotomy for bowel obstruction?

A. No, not usually. However, if the patient has a pelvic or paracolic abscess, then I would consider using a drain. Usually, if a drain is required during an emergency laparotomy, then one has to reconsider if a primary anastomosis is advisable or not.

ANAL AND PERIANAL DISEASE

Q. What can you tell me about fissure in ano

A. Fissure in ano is a longitudinal tear in the lower third of the anal canal. It is common (up to 15% of referrals to rectal clinics) and seen mainly in young adults. Over 80% are situated posteriorly. Constipation is thought to be the primary cause; however, there is no actual evidence for this and constipation may be the result of the fissure rather than the cause.

The aetiology is unknown.

Anal fissures are the most common anal abnormalities seen in Crohn's disease and ulcerative colitis. Symptoms include:

- Pain, immediately after defecation
- Bleeding (blood on the paper after wiping)
- Pruritis
- Watery discharge
- Constipation.

Skin tags or papilla may develop if the fissure is chronic.

Treatment is generally conservative, using topical glyceryl trinitrate and local anaesthetic to control anal spasm and pain. This leads to healing in approximately 50% of cases.

Lateral sphincterotomy is the surgical option. This leads to healing in 95% of cases after 2–3 weeks.

Q. How would you perform a lateral sphincterotomy?

A. The operation is best performed under general anaesthetic. I would divide the distal internal sphincter up to the level of the dentate line. I would make my incision lateral and away from the fissure.

Q. What are the causes of pruritus ani?

A. The causes of pruritus ani include:

- Eczema
- Psoriasis
- Moisture
- Faecal soiling
- Localized infection
- General medical conditions i.e. diabetes mellitus, obstructive jaundice and lymphoma.

Q. How do sexually transmitted diseases affect the anal region?

A. Sexually transmitted diseases can affect the anus in both sexes, although homosexual males are most commonly affected. Many sexually transmitted conditions can be present in the rectum and may be asymptomatic.

Gonorrhoea usually presents with symptoms of constipation, tenesmus and a mucopurulent discharge; treatment is with penicillin.

Anal chlamydia trachomatis may produce ulcers and friable mucosa, sometimes leading to fissures and rectal strictures. Tetracycline is the usual treatment.

Primary syphilitic chancres may be seen in the anus, which may progress to a generalized proctitis or mucosal polyps. Penicillin is still the treatment of choice for syphilis.

Pain, severe ulceration, constipation and discharge are seen with anorectal herpes simplex. Early oral or topical acyclovir helps to shorten the duration and severity of attacks, although recurrence is likely.

Anal warts, caused by human papilloma virus types 6 and 11, produce typical warty lesions and may grow to a large size. Excision or cryotherapy can be used as treatment, although recurrence is still possible.

Acquired immune deficiency syndrome has several anal manifestations, including fissures, severe ulceration, rectal lymphoma or Kaposi's sarcoma.

Q. What causes haemorrhoids?

A. Haemorrhoids are primarily seen in Western societies. They are due to a refined Western diet which is low in fibre and this is the primary cause. This leads to straining at stool and engorgement of the anal cushions. As the hard stool is forced out, shearing forces disrupt the anal cushions leading to piles.

Q. What are the anal cushions?

A. The normal anus contains three cushions of vascular tissue underlying the mucosa of the upper third. These are vascular spaces in between the fibrous stroma.

Q. What symptoms do haemorrhoids present with?

A. Mostly haemorrhoids are completely asymptomatic and so require no treatment. Other symptoms include:

- Painless fresh blood after wiping, sometimes resulting in anaemia
- Mucous discharge
- Prolapse of the haemorrhoid
- Acute strangulation/thrombosis associated with pain.

Q. How would you treat haemorrhoids?

A. Asymptomatic haemorrhoids do not require treatment. Small non-prolapsing symptomatic haemorrhoids can be treated with bulking agents or injection sclerotherapy. Prolapsing piles which arise above the dentate line should be banded. Prolapsing piles which cross the dentate line which are too large to band or have a large external component should be treated by haemorrhoidectomy.

Q. How would you perform a haemorrhoidectomy?

A. I would ensure that the indications for the operation were correct and obtain full, informed consent. I would also ensure that the patient had been adequately prepared for surgery with a phosphate enema.

I would perform the operation under general anaesthetic, with the patient in the lithotomy position. I would sit facing the perineum and insert a proctoscope into the rectum to visualize the area. Using haemostatic forceps, I would draw the haemorrhoid towards me and make a 'V'-shaped incision in the anal skin at the base of the haemorrhoid. I would then raise the haemorrhoid towards the lumen and away from the internal sphincter. The haemorrhoid is then transfixed, ligated and divided approximately 5 mm distal to the ligation. This is repeated for the other haemorrhoids present, ensuring that adequate mucocutaneous bridges are left between them. This prevents an anal stricture forming. The wounds should be left open and packed with gauze to keep the mucocutaneous bridges flat against the internal sphincter.

Q. Would you perform this procedure as a day case?

A. It is possible to perform this procedure as a day case; however, I would be worried about the postoperative analgesia as it is generally associated with a lot of pain.

Q. What are the complications associated with this procedure?

A. The complications include:

- Bleeding
- Infection/abscess formation
- Fissure

- Constipation, usually as a result of pain/fear of opening the bowels
- Incontinence/sphincter damage
- Recurrence
- Anal stenosis.

Also included are the risks associated with a general anaesthetic.

APPENDICECTOMY

Q. An 18-year-old lady is referred to you, as an emergency, with right iliac fossa pain. What are the five common causes of such pain in a young lady of this age group?

A. These include:

- Appendicitis
- Salpingitis, pyosalpynx and tubovarian abscess (PID)
- Urinary causes such as cystitis/pyelonephritis (UTI) or ureteric colic
- Mittelschmerz's syndrome (ruptured luteal cyst causing severe period pain)
- Ectopic pregnancy (although it is far less common than the above causes, it is very important to exclude it in this age group, as it will be fatal if missed).

Q. How would a patient with acute appendicitis usually present?

A. Central abdominal pain which then localizes to the right iliac fossa. This is associated with loss of appetite, and occasionally nausea (and vomiting). The patient may get other bowel symptoms, such as constipation or diarrhoea, and occasionally symptoms that mimic cystitis (if the patient has a pelvic appendix, the inflammation may irritate the bladder).

The patient will have some degree of tachycardia, and low-grade pyrexia in the early stages. There is tenderness with guarding and rebound tenderness in the right iliac fossa. Occasionally pain is felt in the right iliac fossa when pressure is applied to the left iliac fossa (Rovsing's sign). The patient may also be dehydrated with foetor oris.

The white cell count is usually elevated, but the patient may have neutropenia in perforated appendicitis with peritonitis.

Q. What is the most reliable method of diagnosing appendicitis?

A. Clinical examination; the presence of tenderness, guarding and rebound tenderness in the right iliac fossa.

Q. What is the least reliable method to diagnose appendicitis?

A. A white cell count elevation is the least reliable.

Q. How would you perform an appendicectomy in this lady of 18 years old?

A. I would take a full history and examine the patient. Then I would prepare the patient fully for theatre, after obtaining informed consent. I would then perform the procedure under general anaesthesia. The patient should be positioned supine on the operating table. I would clean and prepare the whole abdomen (in case further procedures are deemed necessary). The patient should be given antibiotics in the Emergency Department or in the anaesthetic room prior to surgery (such as metronidazole).

Q. Where would you make your incision?

A. Traditionally the incision is made over McBurney's point, as a 'grid-iron incision'. However, in a young lady, I would do a Lanz incision which gives better cosmetic results since it runs along the skin lines of Langer.

Q. Where would you position your Lanz incision and how would you proceed after you make the skin incision?

A. I would commence my incision 1–2 cm medial to the anterior superior iliac spine, and continue it transversely. I would then deepen my incision through the subcutaneous fat and fascia, down to the external oblique muscle. I would then use wound retractors to expose the external oblique muscle.

I would split the fibres of the external oblique along its fibres using blunt dissection to get to the internal oblique. I would then split the fibres of the internal oblique and transversus abdominis muscles again using blunt dissection in order to get to the peritoneum. No muscle fibres are divided, however, as this is a muscle-splitting procedure. I would then apply two artery forceps to hold the peritoneal layer up. I would then use a scalpel to gently divide the peritoneal layer, taking care not to catch or damage any loops of the bowel.

Once the peritoneum has been opened, I would adjust my assistant's retractors in order to achieve a good operative exposure. I would take a swab for microbiology of any peritoneal fluid (for culture) and I would inspect the caecum and small bowel for any other pathology (such as a Meckel's diverticulum or caecal tumours). I would then inspect the ovaries and tubes in order to rule out pelvic inflammation, an ectopic pregnancy or a pelvic abscess.

I would then gently mobilize the caecum to look for the appendix. Once found, I would examine it to confirm the diagnosis and begin mobilization of the appendix. I would then clamp and divide the mesoappendix to de-skeletonize the appendix. I would then apply a Dunhill forceps at the base of the appendix. I would then apply a surgical tie to its base and then divide the appendix, at its base.

I would use diathermy to the exposed mucosa of the appendix stump in order to prevent the possibility of a mucocele forming, and then I would apply a purse string suture to the caecum, around the appendix stump, in order to bury it inside the caecum. I would ensure that the instruments used to divide the appendix are not used again so as to avoid contamination.

I would then carry out peritoneal lavage using normal saline, and if any pelvic collection is found, then I would drain it and carry out full pelvic lavage. I would close the wound, in layers, using absorbable sutures (such as vicryl), and perform a betadine wound lavage to reduce the risk of wound infection. I would ensure that full haemostasis is achieved, and close the skin using a subcuticular suture (such as vicryl or monocryl). I would not use any drains unless there is a large abscess collection, which would then require proper drainage. I would give the patient two more doses of antibiotics postoperatively.

Q. What would you do if you find the appendix is not badly inflamed on the outside?

A. I would then cut through the appendix wall along its longitudinal access on its antimesenteric border to inspect its lumen. If the mucosa is inflamed, then the diagnosis is confirmed. If the mucosa is normal, then I would have to search for another cause for the patient's symptoms.

Q. What would you do if you found that the appendix was normal; however, there was an ectopic pregnancy?

A. I would ask for the gynaecologist to come to theatre, and inform the anaesthetists about the findings. I would then request a cross-match. I would avoid disturbing the ectopic pregnancy sac, as this may trigger a tremendous haemorrhage. Once the gynaecologist is in theatre, I would hand over the patient to their care; however, I would stay to assist with the surgery, which usually involves an excision of the affected Fallopian tube.

Q. What are the complications of an appendicectomy?

A. Complications include:

- Infection
- Wound abscess
- Bleeding
- Pelvic abscess
- Peritonitis
- Keloid scar
- Peritoneal adhesions
- Incisional hernia (rare)
- Damage to other structures (such as ovaries, Fallopian tubes, caecum and small bowel).

In addition, there are the risks associated with general anaesthesia.

WOUND CLOSURE

Q. What types of wound closures do you know of?

A. Primary, delayed primary and secondary closures.

Q. How would you decide whether to close a wound or not?

A. This depends on:

- The type of wound
- The condition of the patient
- The surrounding environment (i.e. most battle wounds are left open).

When there is any doubt about closure, I would leave the wound open.

Q. What is delayed primary wound closure?

A. This is when the closure of the wound is carried out 2 – 7 days after injury. This allows for any infection to declare itself and for oedema to subside. When the wound is clean, dry, pink or with a thin layer of fibrin/early granulation, it is suitable for delayed primary wound closure. If there is purulent exudate, residual necrotic tissue, oedema, redness of the margins or lymphangitis, the closure must then be delayed.

Q. What is secondary wound closure?

A. This is when the wound is not closed and is regularly dressed. This allows the wound to stay open in order that healing may occur by secondary intention (with the help of granulation tissue).

This is the usual course of wound closure in cases of severe wound infection, or in the presence of an abscess cavity. A greasy dressing should be avoided. The wound should be filled, and not packed, with dry gauze topped by a light dressing of gamgee, and the whole dressing is held in place by adhesive tape.

Irrigation with saline permits the dry dressing to come away, without starting bleeding.

Q. What are the factors that affect wound healing?

A. These include local and general factors:

- Local factors include poor blood supply, adhesions to bony surfaces, conditions predisposing to continued tissue breakdown and inflammation (such as infection and foreign bodies), movement that subjects the wound to persistent trauma, neoplasm, exposure to ionizing radiation, and lack of exposure to light (such as ultraviolet light). Poor surgical technique can influence wound healing (for example, sutures applied too tightly that cause ischaemia to the wound edges).
- General factors include age (healing is faster in the young), nutrition (protein deficiency, lack of vitamin C and zinc), hormones (such as glucocorticoids), temperature (healing is slower in cold weather).

COMPARTMENT SYNDROME

Q. What is compartment syndrome?

A. Compartment syndrome is an increase in pressure within a fascial compartment that usually occurs as a result of muscle swelling and oedema post-injury. It may occur anywhere in the body, but is particularly common in the forearm and lower leg.

It may be defined as an increase in compartment pressure above capillary pressure resulting in ischaemia.

Q. What is the pathophysiology?

A. A soft tissue injury causes a rise in tissue pressure. Areas most at risk include the lower leg and forearm due to their inflexible fascial coverings (muscles are enclosed in fascial sheaths and bounded by bone). Tissue ischaemia results and with a sustained increase in pressure, necrosis of the underlying nerves and muscles eventually occurs.

Q. Who is most at risk of developing compartment syndrome?

A. Those most at risk include patients with:

- Open/closed fractures, any soft tissue injury
- Crush injuries – trapped under a large object/within a car after a road traffic accident
- Pressure injuries as a result of prolonged unconsciousness.

Q. What symptoms and signs would lead you to a diagnosis of compartment syndrome?

A. Firstly, a history of a crush or compression injury and symptoms affecting the lower leg or forearm. Symptoms would include increasing pain, altered sensation in the sensory distribution of nerves that may be involved, palpable muscular stiffness and tenderness and pain on passive stretch of the muscles. It is classically stated that loss of pulses is a late sign; therefore pulses are often still palpable. There is also a weakness or paralysis of the affected muscle groups.

Q. If you were to try to measure the inter-compartmental pressure, what would convince you of the diagnosis?

A. The normal resting pressure within a compartment is approximately 3–4 mmHg. Compartment syndrome is thought to occur when pressures reach 30 mmHg.

Q. What complications may occur particularly in severe crush injuries?

A. Crush syndrome may occur as a result of a crush injury. Crush syndrome is where rhabdomyolysis develops as a result of muscle necrosis. There is a release of myoglobin and potassium into the circulation when the limb is released and reperfusion occurs. If severe, hypovolaemia, acute renal failure and cardiac arrest may occur as a result of the toxic effects of myoglobin.

Q. How would you treat an unconscious patient on ITU whom you suspected to have compartment syndrome?

A. A patient who is unconscious on ITU would be very difficult to assess. I would have a high threshold of suspicion given a history of a soft tissue or crush injury. I would examine the affected area and have a low threshold for performing an emergency fasciotomy. I would undertake this procedure by placing a vertical incision over the affected area, incising through the fascial covering until I reached muscle. I would then ensure adequate haemostasis, thoroughly wash and clean the area with betadine and dress the wound with gelonet and gauze.

Q. Would you excise any necrotic muscle you came across?

A. Necrotic muscle may result in sepsis if left; however, if I was unsure as to the viability of the muscle, I would leave it alone and reassess the next day as the muscle may recover once the compartment has been released.

Q. How would you close the wound in the long term?

A. Primary closure is unlikely due to the size the wound inevitably becomes. It is likely that the patient will need skin grafting.

Q. Can you think of any long-term sequelae of an untreated compartment syndrome?

A. Untreated compartment syndrome may result in permanent paralysis, ischaemic contractures (similar to Volkmann's contractures – compartment syndrome was first described by Volkmann) and gangrene.

CERVICAL SPINE INJURIES

Q. What is whiplash?

A. Whiplash is the term given to a neck injury. It is a soft tissue injury that occurs as a result of a sudden hyper-extension of the neck, for example being thrown forward in a road traffic accident. It is associated with pain and stiffness and treated with analgesics only.

Q. How would you exclude a possible underlying fracture?

A. I would take a full history and examine the patient. The mechanism of injury, clinical symptoms and signs and neurological status of the patient may lead me to suspect a possible spinal fracture. Ultimately, X-rays would help me to definitively diagnose a fracture.

Q. If a patient with multiple injuries was brought to you in the Emergency Department and you suspected a possible cervical spine injury, what precautions would you take to minimize the damage?

A. My main priority would be to check the airway, breathing and circulation whilst maintaining control of the cervical spine. I would achieve this by maintaining the neck in a neutral position and transferring the patient onto a spinal board. Then I would place a hard collar around the patient's neck and maintain it in the neutral position using sand bags either side of the neck, taped to the spinal board.

Q. What would you do if the patient started vomiting?

A. I would either apply suction to the mouth or arrange for the entire spinal board to be tilted to allow the patient to vomit into a kidney dish.

Q. What X-rays would you request?

A. I would request cervical spine (anteroposterior and lateral), chest X-ray and pelvis X-rays in a multiply injured trauma patient.

Q. What features what you look for to exclude a c-spine fracture?

A. Firstly, I would ensure that the films were adequate; that all seven cervical vertebrae were visible (C7–T1). Then I would check for:

- Correct alignment of the vertebrae, along the spinous processes, anterior and posterior marginal lines and the anteroposterior diameter of the vertebral canal
- Individual vertebrae for defects/obvious fracture lines (>25% forward displacement of one vertebra on another indicates unifacet dislocation, >50% indicates bifacet dislocation, the height of each vertebra should be equal anteriorly and posteriorly)
- Abnormalities of the disc spaces or facet joints
- Predental space – <3 mm in adults, <5 mm in children
- Soft tissue swelling in the prevertebral region – <7 mm above the larynx, <22 mm below it.

Q. What would you do if you felt that the views didn't adequately show the C7–T1 vertebrae?

A. I would request further views depending on which vertebrae weren't clearly visualized. If it were the lower cervical vertebrae, then I would request a 'swimmer's view' which involves placing one arm above the head, or I would repeat the original views with as much traction as could be tolerated on both arms. Other views include oblique and odontoid peg (through the open mouth), if suspicion is high.

Q. What other radiological features may help you diagnose cervical instability?

A. Other features of cervical instability include:

- Widening of the facet joints
- Angulation of the vertebrae (>10%)

- Loss of normal cervical lordosis
- Compression of the body of the vertebrae (>25%).

If the clinical features don't match the radiological ones, it is worth consulting a radiologist for their opinion and further views.

Q. What is the usual mechanism of injury for c-spine injuries?

A. C-spine injuries are usually sustained in hyper-extension and hyper-flexion injuries. These may occur in road traffic accidents where the patient is thrown forwards or backwards suddenly.

Q. How would you manage a patient whom you suspected to have a c-spine injury?

A. If I suspected a cervical spine injury, I would urgently obtain an expert orthopaedic opinion. After stabilizing the c-spine initially with a hard collar and sand bags, I would take a full history, perform an examination and arrange for the relevant X-rays. I would then stabilize the patient according to the type of injury sustained:

- Atlanto-occipital dislocations i.e. Jefferson 'burst' fracture of C1 – stabilize in a hard collar if displacement is <7 mm, reduce with halo traction if >7 mm.
- Odontoid peg fractures – Philadelphia collar, occasional internal fixation if significant displacement.
- Traumatic spondylolisthesis/Hangman's fracture – Philadelphia collar or halo traction depending on the degree of displacement.

Q. What would be the consequences of a missed unstable cervical injury?

A. This may result in spinal cord injury if not managed properly.

CHOLECYSTECTOMY

Q. A 50-year-old lady is admitted as an emergency with nausea, pain and guarding in the right hypochondrium. She also has a pyrexia. You have made a diagnosis of cholecystitis. How would you manage this patient?

A. After full clinical assessment, I would commence the patient on intravenous antibiotics (a cephalosporin), and treat her dehydration with intravenous fluids. I would ask the nurses for regular observations. I would then arrange for an urgent ultrasound scan of the abdomen.

I would monitor the patient's condition, including taking blood tests such as a full blood count, amylase, liver function tests and basic biochemistry.

Q. An abdominal ultrasound scan shows an inflamed gallbladder which is full of stones, but the diameter of the common bile duct (CBD) is 7 mm. The blood tests were all normal, apart from a white cell count of 14. How would you proceed then?

A. The diameter of the CBD is within the normal range, and the results confirm that the patient has cholecystitis. I would then continue with the treatment for cholecystitis, and would prepare the patient for an urgent elective cholecystectomy.

Q. When would you perform the surgery?

A. Historically, many surgeons would wait for 4–6 weeks before performing a cholecystectomy. The rationale behind this is that the inflammation should subside in this time, thereby making the surgery technically easier. However, many surgeons would proceed with the surgery sooner than this.

Q. What are the indications for an emergency procedure?

A. The indications for an emergency procedure include:

- An acute infective episode that does not settle down with antibiotic therapy
- Jaundice
- An empyema of the gallbladder, which does not respond to non-operative management.

Q. How would you treat empyema of the gallbladder?

A. Intravenous antibiotics and ultrasound-guided percutaneous transhepatic drainage of the gallbladder.

Once the patient recovers from the acute episode, then an urgent elective cholecystectomy should be arranged. If the ultrasound drainage is not successful, then an emergency laparotomy and a cholecystostomy or a cholecystectomy should be carried out. This is an open procedure, although it can be carried out laparoscopically in experienced hands.

Q. Imagine the patient had a simple acute cholecystitis which responded to antibiotics, and you admitted the patient for an urgent elective cholecystectomy. How would you proceed?

A. In the properly prepared patient, who has been fully assessed and investigated prior to surgery, I would carry out the procedure under general anaesthesia. The patient is positioned supine on the operating table, and the operating table is positioned to enable the access of intraoperative X-ray imaging/fluoroscopy. I would clean and prepare in the appropriate fashion (for laparoscopic as well as an open approach).

I would infiltrate a small dose of local anaesthetic/adrenaline mixture (e.g. 1% lignocaine with 1:100 000 adrenaline) to the site of insertion of the umbilical port. I would make an adequate length of incision in the umbilical/para-umbilical region (1.5 cm length incision) and I would then dissect down to and through the linea alba.

I would insert my laparoscopic trochar, under direct vision, through the umbilical incision. This is a safer technique than using an insufflation needle inserted blindly. A special, safe laparoscopic trochar can be used to minimize the risk of injury to the bowel or other structures.

Once the port is through the abdominal wall, CO_2 gas may be insufflated and a laparoscope is introduced through the port. A routine laparoscopy is carried out to confirm the diagnosis and to identify any other pathology, including any possible injury to the bowel during insertion of the port.

Once the laparoscopy is satisfactory, other ports may then be inserted under direct laparoscopic vision. I would use a four-port technique, using two 10 mm and two 5 mm ports (although some surgeons use a three-port technique). Once all the laparoscopic ports are inserted, I would then start dissection of the gallbladder. This may be performed in several ways:

- Retrogradely from the fundus downwards.
- Retraction of the body of the gallbladder above the liver and dissection around the gallbladder neck, thereby exposing Chalot's triangle. The junction of the cystic duct and the common bile duct may then be visualized.

I would need to identify the cystic artery and apply double ligaclips (or lockable PDS special clips) prior to dividing the cystic artery, close to the gallbladder wall. Once the cystic duct is identified, I would make a small incision into the lumen of the cystic duct and I would insert a cannula into the cystic duct. I would secure it in place using a ligaclip, gently applied, and I would then irrigate with the cannula using normal saline. I would then carry out an intraoperative cholangiogram in order to confirm the anatomy and also to identify any stones in the CBD. If the cholangiogram is satisfactory, I would then proceed to apply double ligaclips or a loop ligature to the cystic duct. I would then divide the duct.

I would then dissect the gallbladder off the bed of the liver, using careful dissection with a diathermy hook. If any accessory ducts or bleeding vessels are identified, I would apply ligaclips. Once the gallbladder is dissected off the liver completely, I would then inspect the gallbladder bed within the liver, the ligaclips that I have already applied to the cystic artery and duct, to ensure full haemostasis and no bile leak.

I would then insert the laparoscopic retrieving bag through one of the large ports (for example, the umbilical port, after changing the camera position to the epigastric port), and I would put the freed gallbladder into the bag. Then I would take the gallbladder out through the port site. If the gallbladder (in the retrieval bag) gets stuck, I would make the umbilical wound larger to allow safe delivery of the gallbladder through the wound.

I would then inspect all laparoscopic wounds for any bleeding, and I would close the two large wounds with interrupted PDS sutures. This reduces the risk of a port site incisional hernia. The two 5 mm ports do not require any muscle closure. Skin closure of all wounds is carried out (using vicryl rapide, for example) after further infiltration of local anaesthetic.

If any difficulties are encountered, such as bleeding or a bile leak that cannot be controlled laparoscopically, then I would have a low threshold of conversion to an open procedure.

Q. What are the risks and complications of laparoscopic cholecystectomy?

A. These include:

- Injury to the common bile duct, (this can result in stricture or jaundice)
- Bile leak
- Bleeding
- Injury to the hepatic artery
- Injury to other structures (such as the bowel and stomach)
- Abscess
- Diathermy injury to the CBD (can cause delayed stricture formation)
- Missed CBD stones.

If the patient has preoperative jaundice, a dilated CBD on preoperative ultrasound or a history of pancreatitis, then a preoperative endoscopic retrograde cholangiopancreatogram (ERCP) is indicated, especially if the operating surgeon has little experience with intraoperative choledochoscopy.

An ERCP would add to the risks and complications.

PERITONITIS

Q. What is peritonitis, and how would you classify it?

A. Peritonitis is inflammation or infection affecting the peritoneum and its cavity. It is classified into localized and generalized.

Q. How would a patient with peritonitis present?

A. The patient presents with:

- Hypotension
- Tachycardia (pulse >120 bpm)
- A low blood pressure
- A constricted periphery
- A characteristic 'drum-like' and tender abdomen.

Q. A 70-year-old man is referred to you, as the duty surgical registrar, with peritonitis and septic shock. His abdominal pain started in the left iliac fossa, 24 hours ago. How would you manage this patient?

A. After obtaining an initial history and carrying out the initial essential clinical examination, I would treat the patient for septic shock by inserting two wide-bore intravenous cannulae and commencing resuscitation. I would then obtain the following blood tests:

- Full blood count
- Biochemistry
- Liver function tests
- Clotting screen
- Blood glucose
- Blood group
- Cross-match
- Blood cultures.

I would commence intravenous antibiotics, such as gentamicin and metronidazole, after taking into consideration any history of drug allergies. As this patient is in septic shock, resuscitation of the patient and continued clinical assessment should run concurrently until the patient's condition has been stabilized. I would resuscitate the patient with intravenous fluids in the form of colloids as plasma expanders, such as gelofusin or haemaccel, and treat the dehydration with crystalloid fluid (to replace the lateral compartmentalization of fluids into the peritoneal cavity and bowel lumen).

I would prescribe adequate analgesia, such as intravenous morphine, and arrange for all the necessary emergency investigations. These would include:

- Erect chest X-ray,
- Abdominal X-ray
- ECG.

I would also insert a nasogastric tube in order to drain the stomach prior to any anaesthesia, or to reduce further leakage, for example from a perforated peptic ulcer.

I would insert a urinary catheter to carefully monitor fluid balance. In view of the patient's age and increased risk of morbidity and mortality, he would probably need admission to ITU for preoperative stabilization and resuscitation prior to any surgical intervention. He may require central venous monitoring and early multisystem support which would be best dealt with on a high-dependency unit or on ITU.

To rush in and deal with the underlying cause without careful, speedy, attention to this patient's general state may have disastrous consequences. A few hours should be spent on improving this gentleman's clinical condition, prior to surgical intervention.

Q. You've managed to resuscitate the patient adequately, and he is now ready for surgical intervention. How would you proceed?

A. I would prepare the patient for an emergency laparotomy, particularly if the source of the peritonitis is still uncertain.

I would explain this to the patient and the relatives, including the possible need for a stoma and I would obtain informed consent. Once the patient is anaesthetized, I would re-examine the abdomen, by palpation, on the operating table. Then I would prepare and drape the abdomen for the emergency laparotomy.

Q. How would you make your incision?

A. I would do a long midline incision, to allow full exposure for a full exploratory laparotomy.

Q. You come across a perforated diverticulitis of the sigmoid colon associated with faecal peritonitis. How would you proceed in this case?

A. I would use suction to wash out all of the leaked faecal fluid. I would send some of the fluid for microbiology. Then I would carry out an extensive peritoneal and pelvic lavage using warm saline or water. I would apply a gentle bowel clamp to the area of perforation whilst I am carrying out the lavage. I would begin mobilizing the diseased segment of the colon, and I would perform a Hartmann's resection of the affected sigmoid colon.

I would bring out the proximal end of the colon as an end-colostomy and I would close the distal end. Alternatively, I could bring it out to the surface as a double-barrel colostomy, providing it is long enough to reach the abdominal wall. I would then repeat the peritoneal lavage and I would close the abdomen in layers. I may consider leaving the abdominal wound open as a laporostomy, if the contamination is heavy. This will then require a delayed primary closure at a later stage, when the patient's condition is more stable.

Drains are not normally necessary, unless there is a pelvic cavity with an abscess. In this case, the abscess cavity requires drainage.

I would then transfer the patient to ITU and I would keep the patient on combination antibiotics. I would seek advice from the microbiologist for the appropriate antibiotic therapy.

The patient would require careful and intensive monitoring on ITU postoperatively, as he would most likely require multiorgan support.

Q. What are the complications of peritonitis?

A. These include:

- Septicaemia
- Septic shock
- Multiorgan failure – cardiac, respiratory and renal
- ARDS
- Abscesses – for example, subphrenic or pelvic
- Wound infections
- Incisional hernia
- Coagulopathy
- Death.

TESTICULAR TORSION

Q. A 4-year-old boy is referred to you as an emergency with right groin and hip pain. What are the important differential diagnoses that you will need to exclude?

A. I would need to fully assess the child (including taking an adequate history and doing a clinical examination). My differential diagnosis would be:

- Acute appendicitis
- Testicular torsion
- Inflammation
- Congenital hip abnormality.

Q. You've examined the child; he has the full range of movement in his hip, but he gets severe groin pain when he stands up. The abdomen is soft and non-tender, but he has severe tenderness on examination of the scrotum. This makes it impossible to palpate the testes properly. What is your main concern?

A. I would suspect a testicular torsion until proven otherwise.

Q. What would you do next?

A. I would prepare the patient for an emergency surgical exploration and an orchidopexy.

Q. Imagine that the time is 9 p.m., and the child had something to eat an hour earlier. The anaesthetist asks if you could delay the operation until the next morning. Would you agree?

A. Definitely not, as this child will need an emergency surgical exploration as soon as possible, and we should not wait until the child is fully fasted for surgery. Any delay could result in necrosis or gangrene of the affected testis, and therefore is not acceptable.

Q. How long would it take for the testis to survive after the torsion has taken place?

A. Ideally, surgery will have to be carried out less than 4 hours after the onset of symptoms. Gangrene or permanent ischaemic damage to the testis occurs within 4–6 hours.

Q. You took the child to theatre that evening, and on exploring the testis you confirmed that there is torsion of the testis. What would you do?

A. I would untwist the testis, correct the torsion and inspect the viability of that testis. I would then wrap the affected testis with gauze soaked in warm saline (and I would ask the anaesthetist to increase the ventilated oxygen). If the testis is viable, then I would carry out an orchidopexy. If the testis is gangrenous,

I would perform an orchidectomy. This would have been fully explained to the parents, and the full consent for an orchidopexy or orchidectomy should have been obtained prior to surgery.

Q. What is the underlying pathology that would make you carry out an orchidopexy?

A. The patient would have the 'bell-clapper' deformity, which makes the testis quite mobile and susceptible to torsion on its spermatic cord (from where it derives its blood supply).

Q. Suppose you find the testis to be viable. How would you perform an orchidopexy in a 4-year-old child?

A. I would create a dartos pouch between the scrotal skin and the dartos muscle; then I would carry out a dartos pouch orchidopexy. I would use absorbable sutures to do so and to close the scrotal skin (for example plain catgut).

Q. Why wouldn't you perform another type of orchidopexy, such as a Jaboulay technique?

A. The safest, quickest method and the one more guaranteed to prevent future recurrence of the torsion is a dartos pouch orchidopexy. It also has fewer side effects.

Q. If the testis were gangrenous, for example if there was a delayed referral by the GP, and you've already missed the boat, what would you do, and why?

A. I would carry out an orchidectomy on the affected side and I would also explore the other side to carry out an orchidopexy on the other testis. This is because the congenital abnormality (the bell-clapper deformity) would normally be bilateral. I would explain the situation to the parents in full.

Q. In a different scenario, you explore the painful testis, and you find the testis to be normal, but you find that the child has a torsion of the testicular appendix. What do you call this and what would you do?

A. This is called torsion of the hydatid of Morgagni. I would excise the torted hydatid of Morgagni and I would carry out an orchidopexy, as before.

Q. Would you explore the other non-symptomatic side?

A. Yes I would, as this is usually a bilateral anomaly and a similar occurrence could affect the other testis in the future. This is not clear-cut, and some surgeons would not explore the other side. However, as the child is having surgery for one side, it would make sense to deal with the other testis prophylactically.

Q. If you have a 22-year-old man with one-sided scrotal pain, what would you do?

A. I would assess the patient in the same way as for the child, and I would explore the testis and perform an orchidopexy. However, I would probably carry out a combination of a modified Jaboulay and dartos pouch orchidopexy and I would also explore the other side.

Q. If this 22-year-old man has other urinary symptoms such as pyuria and epididymal tenderness, and you suspect that he has epididymo-orchitis, what would you do to confirm your diagnosis?

A. I would test the patient's urine and I would perform a Doppler examination of the affected testis, by applying the probe on the body of the testis. Then I would do the cord compression test by applying finger pressure to the spermatic cord and then releasing the pressure to observe the interruption to the blood flow – this confirms whether or not there is a blood flow to the testis. However, this technique is dependent on the experience of the operator and may not be quite accurate.

If in doubt, I would explore the testis to confirm the diagnosis. If there is no evidence of torsion, I would only carry out a Jaboulay orchidopexy on the explored testis.

Q. What is the age limit for testicular torsion?

A. Torsion is far more common under the age of 20.

Q. Can you still get testicular torsion in men of 40 or 50 years of age?

A. Yes, you can.

CIRCUMCISION

Q. What are the common indications for a circumcision?

A. These include:

- Phimosis
- Paraphimosis
- Recurrent severe ballanitis
- Religious reasons
- Tumours.

Q. You have a 10-year-old boy with recurrent ballanitis, preputal adhesions and severe phimosis with ballooning of the foreskin during micturition. How would you carry out a circumcision?

A. The child should be fully prepared for surgery. I would carry out the operation as a day case, with the availability of an experienced paediatric anaesthetist. The child is given a general anaesthetic and positioned supine on the operating table.

I would clean and drape the operating field, using gentle antiseptic solution such as Savlon. I would use a small artery forceps to dilate the pinpoint narrowed foreskin, and I would then use a probe and a Savlon-soaked gauze to divide all the preputal adhesions and free the adherent foreskin from the glans penis. I would then clean the glans penis with antiseptic solution (Savlon) and I would hold the dorsal and ventral edges of the foreskin with small artery forceps.

I would then divide the foreskin on the dorsal border, making sure not to cut too much skin (i.e. not to de-glove the penis).

I would excise the affected foreskin around the whole of the glans penis. I would then achieve full haemostasis, using small artery forceps and catgut ties. Some surgeons use bipolar diathermy. Unipolar diathermy should never be used. Once the haemostasis has been achieved, I would apply 4/0 interrupted catgut (or vicryl rapide) to suture the skin over the distal part of the penile skin to the frennular skin at the base of the glans penis 'in a figure of 8 fashion'. I would then apply interrupted catgut sutures between the distal penile skin and the skin at the base of the glans penis. I would apply topical lignocaine (lidocaine) 2% gel to the distal part of the penis, and local marcain injection to the dorsal base of the penis (for postoperative analgesia).

A loose Vaseline dressing is then applied. I would cover the surgery with antibiotics, to reduce the incidence of wound infection, since the child had ballanitis. I would give the patient adequate analgesia and would advise the parents to give their son a bath daily.

Q. What are the risks and complications of circumcision?

A. Infection, bleeding/haematoma, excision of too much skin, injury to the glans penis, breakdown of the wound.

Q. You've carried out a circumcision on a 20-year-old adult, and the patient asks you if he is allowed to have intercourse. What would you advise?

A. I would advise him to avoid any sexual activity until the wound is fully healed, which is a minimum of 2–3 weeks.

Q. You are called to deal with an elderly and unfit patient, who now has a severe and painful paraphimosis. This is the result of failure to pull the foreskin back to its normal position after a urinary catheterization the day before (by the house surgeon). You have tried to reduce the paraphimosis, but it was not possible and quite painful. What would you do?

A. I would proceed to perform a dorsal penile slit, under local anaesthesia, using aqueous lignocaine cream (Emla cream) and local injection of local anaesthesia at the perineal membrane (at the dorsal base of the penis, below the symphysis pubis where the nerve supply emerges through the fascia). This would allow immediate release and I would then reduce the foreskin. I would then overrun the cut edge of the dorsal slit to achieve full haemostasis, as bleeding from the swollen edge of the cut foreskin can be problematic.

I would carry out the procedure under full aseptic technique, which can be carried out in the Emergency Department.

Q. Would the patient need full circumcision at a later date?

A. No, as this can be used as an alternative to circumcision in the elderly and unfit.

CLINICAL PATHOLOGY

CELL GROWTH

Q. What is cell differentiation?

A. Differentiation is where a cell develops a specialized function that distinguishes it from its parent cell. This occurs as a result of increased expression of selective genes whose products result in the formation of such a cell.

Q. What is the effect of hormones and growth factors on normal growth?

A. Hormones are produced in specific glands, released into the circulation and exert their effects on a distant organ. Growth factors tend to be produced in various tissues throughout the body and may act on the cell that produced them (autocrine effect) or on a cell close by (paracrine effect). Commonly, growth hormone and insulin-like growth factor-I (IGF-I) control postnatal growth.

Q. What is the cell cycle?

A. The cell cycle is the progressive steps a cell moves through in order that DNA (deoxyribonucleic acid) may be synthesized and cells may divide. It is made up of several phases:

- G_0 – resting phase
- G_1 – first gap phase (main determinant of the cell cycle)
- G_2 – second gap phase (variable length)
- M – mitosis (nuclear division and cytoplasmic division)
- S – synthesis (DNA).

The time taken for cells to divide varies; for example, intestinal epithelium divides much more rapidly than liver cells. The main determinant of the time taken to divide is the time spent in the G_1 phase of the cell cycle. The S, G_2, and M phases are usually of constant length. G_0 indicates a resting phase. Cells which stay here permanently die at the end of their lifetime and do not divide (permanent cells e.g. neurones).

Q. Can you name any agents that influence the progression of the cell cycle?

A. Factors that influence cell cycle progression include:

- p53, p27, p21
- Cyclins and cyclin-dependent kinases (CDK)
- Retinoblastoma and related genes.

Q. What is hypertrophy?

A. Hypertrophy is an increase in the size of an organ by an increase in cell size without division.

Q. What is hyperplasia?

A. Hyperplasia is an increase in the size of an organ by an increase in cell number.

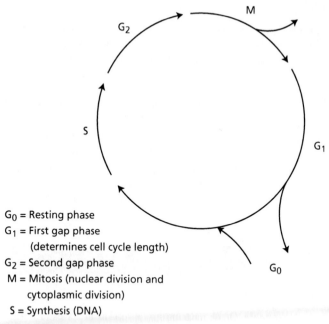

G_0 = Resting phase
G_1 = First gap phase
     (determines cell cycle length)
G_2 = Second gap phase
  M = Mitosis (nuclear division and
     cytoplasmic division)
  S = Synthesis (DNA)

Fig. 7   The cell cycle. G_0 resting phase, G_1 first gap phase
(determines cell cycle length), G_2 second gap phase, M mitosis
(nuclear division and cytoplasmic division), S synthesis (DNA)

Q. Can you name any examples of each of these?

A. They may be a physiological or a pathological response to a stimulus.

Hypertrophy

- Physiological – muscle hypertrophy in athletes, uterine hypertrophy in pregnancy
- Pathological – cardiomyopathy, muscular dystrophy.

Hyperplasia

- Physiological – thyroid hyperplasia in puberty and pregnancy
- Pathological – Graves' disease, endometrium with oestrogen use.

Q. When might hypertrophy and hyperplasia occur together?

A. They may occur together in Graves' disease, prostate enlargement and adrenal hyperplasia.

Q. What cell growth factors are important in wound healing?

A. The principal factors are platelet-derived growth factor (PDGF) and transforming growth factor beta (TGF-β).

PDGF:

- Stimulates proliferation of the epithelial cells in the epidermis with the help of epidermal growth factor and insulin-like growth factors I and II
- Stimulates proliferation of myofibroblasts in the dermis.

TGF-β:

- Stimulates production of collagen and fibronectin from myofibroblasts
- Collagen is laid down and fibronectin encourages epithelial migration.

The healing process requires the presence of oxygen and is influenced by epidermal growth factor from saliva (when the wound is licked), hormones such as thyroxine, nutrients and growth factors. Angiogenic factors encourage the formation of new capillaries, which increases the concentration of inflammatory cells reaching the necrotic area and speeds up the healing process.

APOPTOSIS

Q. What is apoptosis?

A. Apoptosis (from the Greek meaning 'to fall off' as in leaves of a tree) is programmed cell death or 'cell suicide' and is a normal, physiological part of growth and development. It is also a mechanism for removal of cells that contain abnormal DNA.

Q. What is necrosis?

A. Necrosis is cell death as a result of cell injury or exposure to cytotoxic agents. It is therefore pathological and has no part in normal tissue homeostasis. It is generally associated with an inflammatory reaction which is not seen in apoptosis.

Q. What are the biological features that are specific to apoptosis?

A. Apoptosis, or 'programmed cell death', is characterized by the following:

- Loss of plasma membrane asymmetry and attachment
- Condensation of the cytoplasm and nucleus
- Internucleosomal cleavage of DNA (digested into smaller fragments)
- Cell eventually fragments into 'apoptotic bodies'.

The resultant apoptotic bodies are then removed by phagocytes and this process is not associated with inflammation.

Q. How is apoptosis measured?

A. Generally, apoptosis is assessed by detecting biological events or morphological features associated with the process of programmed cell death. For example, the commonest method of detecting apoptosis is measurement of caspases, proteases induced in apoptosis.

It is extremely difficult to measure the process of apoptosis itself as it is generally not detected as it occurs. It is therefore only possible to pick up markers that indicate when it has occurred.

Q. What is the physiological importance of apoptosis?

A. Apoptosis is an essential part of tissue homeostasis. The constant production of cells by mitosis and removal by apoptosis allows for a continuous cell turnover able to cope with environmental change. For example, apoptosis occurs in the endometrium as a natural part of the hormonal cycle when levels of hormones drop. It is also responsible for the degeneration of the thymus after childhood.

It is of most importance in embryological development where three types of apoptosis are seen to occur:

- Morphogenic apoptosis – where tissue/organ structural change occurs i.e. cell death of the skin separating fingers, cell death in the dorsal neural tube during tube closure.
- Histiogenic apoptosis – where tissues/organs undergo differentiation i.e. the hormonal influence on the Müllerian/Wolffian ducts causing female/male genital tracts to develop.
- Phylogenetic apoptosis – where embryological vestigial structures are removed i.e. the pronephros.

Q. Can you give any examples of inappropriate induction of apoptosis?

A. Some examples of inappropriate induction of apoptosis include:

- Transplant rejection
- Graft-versus-host diseases
- Autoimmune disorders i.e. AIDS
- Malignancy
- Alzheimer's disease
- Hodgkin's disease.

Q. What genes are involved in the regulation of apoptosis?

A. Genes that activate apoptosis include p53 and c-myc. Genes that inhibit apoptosis include bcl-2.

DISORDERS OF CELL GROWTH

Q. What is the definition of metaplasia?

A. Metaplasia involves the transformation of one fully differentiated cell type into another.

Q. Why does it occur?

A. It is a reversible change that occurs in response to an environmental stimulus and is an adaptive process. It may be classified into connective tissue and epithelial metaplasia. It is thought that an underlying genetic process results in the transformation and that the final differentiated cell type is better able to withstand the new environmental stimulus.

Q. Can you give some examples of each type?

A. Examples of each include:

Epithelial metaplasia

The commonest example of epithelial metaplasia involves a change to squamous epithelium. For example:

- Bronchi – ciliated respiratory epithelium in smokers
- Bladder/kidneys – transitional epithelium in the presence of stones and infection such as schistosomiasis
- Prostate – in response to hormonal treatment/trans-urethral resection
- Endocervix – in response to hormonal surges i.e. puberty
- Salivary glands/bile ducts/pancreas – due to the presence of stones.

Other examples include:

- Barrett's oesophagus – replacement of squamous epithelium by gastric epithelium in patients with reflux oesophagitis
- Breast – apocrine metaplasia
- Stomach – replacement of gastric epithelium with intestinal epithelium in response to the pathogen *Helicobacter pylori*
- Gallbladder – in response to the presence of stones.

Connective tissue metaplasia

The commonest variant is osseous metaplasia, for example:

- Bronchial cartilage – tracheopathia osteoplastica
- Vascular system – calcium deposits within atheromatous arterial walls
- Eye – in response to chronic uveal tract disease.

It is less common to develop chondroid metaplasia, which involves the formation of metaplastic cartilage and myeloid metaplasia, which involves the formation of bone marrow.

Q. Why does metaplasia concern us?

A. Metaplasia is of some concern due to the possibility of progression into dysplasia and eventual malignancy. For this progression to occur, however, there would need to be a persistent environmental stimulus. It is unlikely that a metaplastic lesion would progress to a malignant one of its own accord.

Q. What is dysplasia?

A. Dysplasia is a pre-malignant condition characterized by:

- An increase in cell growth
- An increase in the number of mitoses

- Presence of abnormal mitoses
- Abnormal cellular differentiation
- Loss of cellular cohesion
- Cellular atypia including pleomorphism, hyperchromatism and a high nuclear/cytoplasmic ratio.

It may be caused by prolonged environmental stress to a tissue, longstanding inflammation and also by carcinogens. Examples of these include alcohol, smoking, viral infection, e.g. human papilloma virus, and chronic inflammatory conditions.

Dysplastic lesions are of concern as they may progress to malignant lesions. This may occur in areas of metaplasia such as bronchial epithelium in smokers.

Severe dysplasia essentially resembles a neoplastic lesion apart from the fact that it hasn't invaded the basement membrane. It may also be referred to as carcinoma in situ.

Q. Can you give any examples of dysplasia?

A. Some examples include:

- Cervix – cervical intra-epithelial neoplasia (CIN) grades I, II and III.
- Oesophagus – Barrett's oesophagus due to longstanding oesophagitis
- Bronchus – as a result of long term smoking
- Large bowel – as a result of longstanding active ulcerative colitis.

Q. What is the definition of neoplasia?

A. Neoplasia is the development of an abnormal mass of tissue which grows excessively and in an uncontrolled manner. Its growth also persists after the removal of the initial stimulus to grow. Neoplasms may be benign or malignant.

WOUND HEALING

Q. What do you understand by the term granulation tissue?

A. The formation of granulation tissue is a process involved in tissue repair. It involves proliferation of capillary endothelial cells to 'fill in the gap' caused by the initial injury or tissue loss. They result in the production of new vascular channels or capillary 'loops' which are classically seen in the base of a healing ulcer. There is also production of myofibroblasts which secrete collagen in order to aid wound contraction.

Q. Does the same process occur in all tissues?

A. Granulation tissue is thought to aid the repair of all tissue injuries; however, different tissues have different regenerative capacities. Not all cells are able to replicate themselves, for example, specialized tissues such as glomerular tissue are unable to reform their architecture and neural tissues do not regenerate at all. They are known as permanent cells. Other examples of such cells include striated muscle and myocardial cells.

Q. Explain the process of healing by primary intention in skin wounds.

A. Healing by primary intention occurs when skin is cleanly incised with a scalpel. There is little trauma to the surrounding tissues and minimal tissue loss. If the edges are then opposed accurately by suturing, healing occurs rapidly. In the first 24 hours fibrin is produced in order to form the initial link between the two opposed skin edges. Over the next few days, fibroblasts migrate across the area followed by proliferation of capillary blood vessels. Across the surface of the wound a scab forms, initially followed by migration of epidermal cells resulting in scar formation. It is usually possible to remove the sutures by day 10.

Q. How does this differ from healing by secondary intention?

A. Healing by secondary intention occurs in wounds where there is tissue loss and the wound edges are far apart. There is formation of granulation tissue into the wound and dead tissue is removed by neutrophils and macrophages. Myofibroblasts within the granulation tissue produce collagen which results in the formation of a scar and wound contraction. In wounds with a high degree of skin loss, a considerable amount of epithelial regeneration needs to occur in order to cover the defect. The end result may be a cosmetic deformity.

Q. Do you know of any factors controlling wound healing?

A. Haemorrhage occurs at the time of tissue injury resulting in aggregation of platelets and thrombus formation. Platelets degranulate and release platelet-derived growth factor (PDGF) and transforming growth factor beta (TGF-β). These are both growth factors and attract inflammatory cells such as neutrophils and macrophages to remove any bacteria, debris or necrotic tissue from the wound. PDGF also acts within the epidermis to promote epithelial regeneration with the help of epidermal growth factor (EGF) and insulin-like growth factors I and II (IGF). PDGF also stimulates the myofibroblasts in the dermis to proliferate; similarly, collagen production is stimulated by TGF-β.

The rate of wound healing is also dependent on a new blood supply and vascular proliferation is stimulated by angiogenic growth factors.

Q. What factors may delay wound healing?

A. Factors delaying wound healing may be general or local. Local factors include excessive tissue loss, site of wound (for example, neck of femur fractures), the presence of a foreign body and excessive movement at the wound site. General factors include age, poor nutrition (e.g. amino acid or vitamin deficiencies), infection, poor circulation to the area, drugs (e.g. corticosteroids, cytotoxic agents) and diabetes.

AMYLOID

Q. What is amyloid?

A. Amyloid is the deposition within tissues of a group of pathological proteins which form characteristic β pleated sheets. It has a fibrillar ultrastructure and is made up of proteins such as serum amyloid proteins A and P, peptide hormones and immunoglobulin light chains. It may be local or systemic and interferes with the affected tissue or organ, usually by accumulation on the basement membrane.

Q. What are the differences between local and systemic amyloidosis?

A. Systemic amyloidosis involves the deposition of amyloid in various organs. It commonly affects the spleen, liver and heart but may affect any organ. It results in enlargement of the affected organ and can cause organ failure as the tissue hardens. Systemic amyloidosis may be further classified into secondary, hereditary, haemodialysis-related, myeloma-related and senile amyloidosis.

Secondary amyloidosis results from a chronic inflammatory disease process, e.g. bronchiectasis, rheumatoid arthritis and TB. The commonest protein involved is serum amyloid protein A which is an acute phase reactant commonly elevated in chronic inflammatory conditions. It is classified as *AA amyloid*.

Hereditary amyloidosis is extremely rare. It includes familial Mediterranean fever and Portuguese nephropathy. It may also be associated with some forms of neuropathy.

Haemodialysis may result in amyloidosis due to deposition of β_2 microglobulin which is characteristic of this condition. It may also result in arthropathy and carpal tunnel syndrome. It is also known as *AH amyloid*.

Myeloma-related amyloidosis is otherwise known as *AL amyloid*. It is derived from the excessive amount of light-chain monoclonal immunoglobulins produced by myelomas. The amyloidosis that results typically affects multiple organs.

Senile amyloidosis is common. It is thought to be derived from serum pre-albumin and is found in small amounts in the heart and arterial system. It is rarely symptomatic and is known as *AS amyloid*.

Local amyloid can occur in any organ. It may be the result of tumours which produce peptide hormones, for example medullary carcinoma of the thyroid which affects the calcitonin-producing C cells. This type of amyloidosis is known as *AE amyloid*. Local amyloid is more commonly seen in the cerebrum of people affected by Alzheimer's disease. It manifests as senile plaques and deposits within cerebral arteries.

Q. What would lead you to suspect a diagnosis of amyloidosis?

A. Amyloidosis is associated with certain clinical conditions:

- Carpal tunnel syndrome
- Organomegaly especially hepatosplenomegaly

- Renal failure
- Cardiac failure
- Macroglossia
- Purpura.

If a patient presented with any of these conditions and had an underlying condition such as myeloma, I would suspect amyloid as the cause. If a patient presented with cardiac or renal failure alone, I would think it unlikely that the cause would be amyloidosis. There are far more common causes that I would want to exclude first, for example hypertension.

Q. How is a diagnosis of amyloid made?

A. Amyloid is usually diagnosed by rectal biopsy which is stained with Congo or Sirus red dyes that turn a characteristic orange and exhibit green birefringence under polarized light. It may also be diagnosed by biopsying the affected organ and demonstrating β pleated sheets under the electron microscope. It is also possible to determine exactly where the amyloid originated from using special techniques.

THROMBOEMBOLIC DISEASE

Q. What is a blood clot?

A. A clot is a solid mass of blood constituents that forms when blood is allowed to coagulate outside the body or post-mortem. Activation of the clotting cascade results in an initial elastic mass comprising alternating white and red layers surrounding a fibrin mesh.

Q. What is a thrombus and what causes it?

A. A thrombus is a mass of blood constituents that occurs within blood vessels in the living body. It occurs within the vascular system when blood flow is slow, when there is damage to the vessel wall and when there is increased coagulability of the blood. These predisposing factors are known as Virchow's triad.

Q. What is the difference between thrombi that form in arteries and veins?

A. The essential difference between the two is that arterial thrombi tend to form on atheromatous plaques and deep vein thromboses tend to arise from valves. The stimulus to thrombus formation in both cases is turbulence within the vessel wall. In the case of atheromatous plaques, the plaque enlarges causing turbulence within the vessel, and also ulcerates with loss of the endothelial lining. The exposed collagen then attracts platelets and thrombus forms as fibrin is deposited and red cells are incorporated.

In deep vein thrombosis the valves may become damaged by trauma or the vein may be occluded by stasis following surgery, immobilization or hypotension. The result is the development of a thrombus in a low-pressure system which may then embolize to the lungs.

Q. What is an embolism?

A. An embolism is usually derived from a thrombus. It consists of a mass of blood constituents that has broken off a main thrombus, travelled within the vascular system and blocked a lumen elsewhere. An example of this is a pulmonary embolism which is derived from a deep vein thrombosis originating in the calf veins.

Q. Do you know of any other examples of emboli?

A. Emboli may be made from solid, liquid or gas. Examples of these include amniotic fluid, fat embolus as a result of long bone fracture, tumour metastases, infective emboli (e.g. vegetations from infected heart valves), atheromatous plaque rupture, nitrogen gas emboli in caisson disease ('the bends') and foreign bodies secondary to intravenous injection.

Q. What are the risk factors for deep vein thrombosis (DVT)?

A. General risk factors include:

- Age (increased risk with advancing age)
- Immobility
- Hypercoagulable states (e.g. malignancy)
- Smoking
- Pregnancy
- Oral contraceptive pill/HRT
- Obesity
- Family history
- Thrombophilia (e.g. protein C, S and anti-thrombin III deficiency).

Specific risk factors include:

- Pelvic surgery
- Pelvic or lower limb fractures
- Any form of major surgery.

Q. Describe the clinical presentation of a thrombosis.

A. The clinical presentation varies depending on the site of the thrombosis and whether or not the vessel lumen has been fully occluded. A complete occlusion of an artery by a thrombus would result in a pale, cold pulseless leg distal to the occlusion. This would eventually lead to gangrene if the circulation was not restored.

In the case of a DVT, the patient presents with a swollen, painful lower limb. There may also be a red–blue discoloration of the skin and extreme pain may be elicited on squeezing the calf (Homan's sign).

MICROBIOLOGY

Q. What laboratory methods are used in order to diagnose bacterial infection?

A. Most bacterial infections are diagnosed by culture of the organism involved. Other laboratory tests involved include:

- Microscopy
- Serology
- Bacterial identification
- Tests of antimicrobial drugs.

Q. What does microscopy involve?

A. Microscopy involves the preparation of stained and unstained (wet) films. A stained film is heat fixed or a dye is used to fix the specimen. The slide is then assessed using microscopy for staining characteristics, the shape and arrangement of cells and the presence of polymorphs (pus cells).

A wet film is where specimen fluid is placed on a slide and covered with a slip. Microscopy is then used to look for bacteria and cells.

Q. What do you know about gram staining?

A. Gram staining is a widely used bacteriological method used to distinguish gram negative and gram positive organisms. The process involves the addition of crystal violet and iodine solution. The solution is then decolorized with acetone or alcohol and counterstained with carbol fuchsin. The results are:

- Gram positive – bacteria resist decolorization – stains BLUE–BLACK
- Gram negative – bacteria decolorized – stains PINK.

Q. Can you give me any examples of gram negative and positive organisms?

A. Gram positive cocci

- *Staphylococcus aureus, epidermis*
- *Streptococcus pneumoniae* (α), *viridans* (α), *pyogenes* (β), *faecalis*

Gram negative cocci

- *Neisseria meningitidis, gonorrhoea*
- *Branhamella catarrhalis*

Gram positive rods

- *Corynebacterium diptheria, diphtheriods*
- *Clostridia tetani, perfringens, botulinum, difficile*
- *Listeria monocytogenes*

Gram negative rods

- *E. coli*
- *Campylobacter*
- *Klebsiella*
- *Yersinia*
- Enterobacteria
- *Haemophilus*
- *Proteus*
- *Legionella*
- *Pseudomonas*
- *Bord. pertussis*
- *Salmonella*
- *Brucellus*
- *Shigella*
- *Vibrio cholera*
- Anaerobes, Bacteriodes, *H. pylori*
- *Mycobacterium tuberculosis, leprae*
- Spirochaetes, *Treponema, Borrelia, Leptospira*

Q. Are there any other types of staining used in bacteriological diagnosis?

A. Yes, it's possible to stain for acid-and alcohol-fast bacilli. These are useful in the diagnosis of TB. The Ziehl–Neilson stain involves heating carbol fuchsin, decolorizing with acid and alcohol and then counterstaining with methylene blue. If TB is present, there will be red bacilli evident against a blue background.

The auramine stain involves the addition of auramine-phenol, decolorizing with acid and alcohol and then adding potassium permanganate. If positive, the bacilli stain fluorescent yellow against a dark field when viewed under UV light.

NECROSIS

Q. What is the definition of necrosis?

A. Necrosis is pathological cell death.

Q. What types of necrosis do you know of?

A. There are several types of necrosis:

- Coagulative necrosis – this type of necrosis occurs in most organs in the body. Soon after tissue death, coagulation occurs. Initially the affected area retains its shape; however, with advancing necrosis it may weaken as the dead area becomes phagocytosed. After the dead area has been removed, repair can then occur according to the tissue's ability to regenerate.
- Colliquative necrosis – this type of necrosis occurs in the brain and results in liquefaction of the dead neural tissue. The end result is a fluid- filled cyst.

- Gangrene – this is irreversible tissue death characterized by putrefaction. It may be dry or wet and tends to follow arterial occlusion particularly of the lower limb. This can result in eventual auto-amputation of the affected area.
- Fat necrosis – this condition occurs after trauma to fat tissue or when adipose tissue is broken down by lipases. It occurs commonly in the breast and can also occur in pancreatitis. When it occurs in the breast, it may present clinically with a lump. It eventually heals by fibrosis.
- Caseous necrosis – this is classically associated with tuberculosis. It results in dead tissue which has completely lost its original structure. Histology may demonstrate an eosinophilia. There may also be an associated inflammatory reaction.
- Fibrinoid necrosis – this occurs in the walls of arteries that are subjected to high pressures as in malignant hypertension. The muscular wall undergoes necrosis and is associated with deposition of fibrin.

Q. What is the difference between necrosis and infarction?

A. Infarction is death of tissues specifically caused by ischaemia or loss of blood supply. Necrosis refers to generalized tissue death due to toxins, trauma or vascular occlusion.

Q. Tell me about gangrene.

A. Gangrene is the result of gradual vascular occlusion and is irreversible. It may be wet or dry. Dry gangrene is the result of ischaemia. The affected area, commonly the lower limb, becomes black as a result of iron accumulation from degraded haemoglobin. There is a characteristic line of demarcation. It then may undergo mummification and auto-amputate with healing above the affected area. This type of gangrene is commonly seen in gradual atherosclerotic diseases such as diabetes mellitus.

Wet gangrene is essentially dry gangrene complicated by infection. It is characteristically dusky with a spreading erythema and a rotten smell. It is difficult to treat with antibiotics due to the poor surrounding circulation and may result in a progressive gangrene leading to generalized septicaemia. It presents with pain and is associated with circulatory collapse.

Treatment of arterial occlusion involves medical therapy for diseases such as diabetes and surgical intervention in order to restore vascular inflow; or established gangrene may be treated by amputation.

Q. What is the difference between this condition and gas gangrene?

A. Gas gangrene is specifically caused by the anaerobic spore-forming organism *Clostridium perfringens*, which produces a toxin causing characteristic crepitus of the affected area from formation of gas bubbles in the tissues.

Q. What other clostridial infections are there?

A. Other *Clostridia* include:

- *Clostridium tetani* (causes tetanus)

- *Clostridium difficile* (causes pseudomembranous colitis)
- *Clostridium botulinum* (causes botulism).

Other clostridial infections can cause gas gangrene, such as *Clostridium septicum* and *novyi*. They are also anaerobic gram positive bacilli.

Q. What is the treatment of gas gangrene?

A. The treatment involves prompt diagnosis, radical debridement of the affected area and intravenous penicillin.

IMMUNODEFICIENCY

Q. What is the immune system?

A. The immune system is the body's defence mechanism against infection. It is specific and has memory.

Q. What is immunodeficiency?

A. Immunodeficiency is a defective immune system resulting in the state of being immunocompromised. It is characterized by infections caused by organisms which are usually non pathogenic such as cytomegalovirus and *Pneumocystis carinii* and may result in overwhelming sepsis. The defect may involve any component of the immune system, for example stem cells, phagocytes, neutrophils or T cells.

Q. What types of immunodeficiency are there?

A. Immunodeficiency may be primary or secondary. Primary or congenital immunodeficiency is extremely rare. It can affect any component of the immune system. Secondary or acquired immunodeficiency usually occurs later in life as a result of another disease process, for example infection by human immunodeficiency virus (HIV).

Q. What types of primary immunodeficiency do you know of?

A. Primary immunodeficiency is genetic and more common in children. It can cause neutropenia as a result of stem cell deficiency. It may also result in neutrophil and complement defects.

Specific defects in B cell production occur in Brutons disease. This disease is characterized by a total lack of B cells and no antibodies. Di George syndrome results in a lack of T cells due to an absence of the thymus. It is also possible to develop abnormalities of both T and B lymphocytes. This rare condition is known as severe combined immune deficiency (SCID).

The most common inherited immunodeficiency is a selective IgA deficiency which is usually asymptomatic.

Q. How do these differ from acquired immunodeficiency?

A. Acquired immunodeficiency is significantly more common than primary immunodeficiency. The commonest cause of this condition is malnutrition. Other causes include:

- Malignancy – for example, haematological malignancies such as leukaemia and lymphoma where normal marrow cells are replaced by malignant ones.
- Infections – acute viral infections such as glandular fever caused by Epstein Barr virus can result in depressed immunity. Other infections such as malaria and HIV also result in immunodeficiency.
- Drugs – for example, cytotoxic agents damage stem cells and lymphocytes and are used to inhibit tumour growth. Radiotherapy can cause a similar effect. Other immunosuppressive drugs include corticosteroids, azothiaprine and cyclosporin.
- Chronic renal failure – patients receiving regular dialysis are at risk of developing a combined T and B cell immunodeficiency. This is thought to be due to the accumulation of toxic metabolites.
- Loss of components of the immune system – for example, antibodies lost in nephritic syndrome and lymphocytes lost through the bowel in intestinal lymphangiectasia.
- Splenectomy – patients who undergo splenectomy are susceptible to bacterial infection, particularly from pneumococcal and meningococcal septicaemia.

Q. If you found out that one of your patients was immunocompromised, how would this affect your management?

A. The significance of detecting immunodeficiency in a patient is that they are at increased risk of developing overwhelming sepsis from opportunist pathogens. Opportunist pathogens are organisms that wouldn't normally result in illness. For example, in HIV-positive patients, opportunistic pathogens resulting in disease include *Candida*, *Herpes simplex* and *Cryptosporidium*. Other pathogens include *Pneumococcus* and *Meningococcus*, particularly in splenectomy patients.

Management of these types of patients includes aseptic technique and broad-spectrum antibiotic cover for all procedures, barrier nursing and specific antibiotic therapy for microorganisms as required.

Other treatments include passive gammaglobulin therapy for specific antibody deficiencies, bone marrow transplantation and eventually gene replacement therapy in the case of inherited primary immunodeficiency.

Q. How does HIV result in immunodeficiency?

A. HIV is an acquired retroviral infection and is characterized by a significant deficiency in cell-mediated immunity. Receptors for the HIV virus are known to be CD4 and are expressed by T helper cells. The virus attaches to CD4 and is thought to induce apoptosis. CD4 T helper cells are vital for the immune system because they activate B cells to produce antibodies and themselves produce cytokines to help kill microbes.

The end result is a falling CD4 T cell count which can be measured periodically to monitor disease progression.

ACUTE INFLAMMATION

Q. What is inflammation?

A. Inflammation is the body's normal response to an insult/injury. It has characteristic phases. It is designed to combat the infection/insult that has caused it and should only last from a few days to a few weeks. If the affected area does not heal, the inflammation becomes chronic.

Q. What are the causes of acute inflammation?

A. The causes of acute inflammation may be classified into:

- Infections – mostly bacterial and viral
- Ischaemia
- Tissue trauma e.g. thermal, cold, irradiation
- Toxins e.g. acids, corrosives
- Allergy e.g. hypersensitivity reactions to antigens such as pollen

Q. What does the acute inflammatory response consist of?

A. Inflammation is provoked by damage from heat, trauma, infection or toxins and an acute inflammatory response occurs. This is largely mediated by the degranulation of mast cells which contain histamine granules. The release of histamine results in vascular dilatation and hence there is an increase of blood flow to the area. Mast cells also degranulate in response to IgE antibody and other components of the complement system.

The increase in blood supply to the affected area results in an increase in leucocytes and neutrophils. There is also an extravasation of plasma proteins resulting in the formation of oedema within the damaged tissue. There is a resultant increase in intravascular blood viscosity and hence the blood flow slows down. This allows neutrophils, which would normally travel in the central stream of the blood vessel and not make contact with the vessel wall, to extravasate into the affected tissues.

Q. What is the role of the neutrophil in acute inflammation?

A. The neutrophil polymorph is one of the characteristic histological features of acute inflammation. They are attracted to the scene of tissue injury by the presence of other neutrophils and other components of the complement system. They are able to pass through the vessel wall via an increase in vascular permeability and plasma viscosity. Their main function is to bind to microorganisms and later ingest them by a process called phagocytosis.

Q. What are the clinical signs of acute inflammation?

A. The clinical signs are classically redness, warmth, pain, swelling and loss of function:

- Rubor – redness, due to dilated blood vessels
- Calor – warmth, due to an increase in vascular flow to the area
- Dolor – pain, due to the pressure from surrounding oedema and from inflammatory mediators such as prostaglandins
- Tumor – swelling, from the sudden accumulation of fluid.

Q. What inflammatory mediators are involved that you know of?

A. Inflammatory mediators include:

- Leukotrienes – derived from arachidonic acid and result in vasodilatation
- Prostaglandins – also derived from arachidonic acid, cause an increase in vascular permeability and can result in platelet aggregation
- Serotonin – released from mast cells and causes vasoconstriction
- Lymphokines – released from lymphocytes and are used to attract other inflammatory mediators.

There are also four cascade systems in plasma that are activated during the acute inflammatory response. These include:

- Coagulation system – activation of this system results in the production of fibrin from fibrinogen which is a major part of the inflammatory exudates.
- Fibrinolytic system.
- Kinin system – primarily bradykinin results in an increase in vascular permeability and causes the pain associated with inflammation.
- Complement system – components of this system are essential for chemotaxis of neutrophils, opsonization of bacteria and an increase in vascular permeability.

Q. Which two components of the complement system are mostly responsible for mediating the inflammatory response?

A. It is mostly C3a and C5a.

Q. What is the end point of the acute inflammatory response?

A. Neutrophils are primarily responsible for mediating the acute inflammatory response. They have a life span of approximately 1–4 days. Once the toxins have been diluted and phagocytosed, macrophages appear to help clear up the debris that remains. If the tissues then return to normal, complete resolution is said to have occurred. If pus accumulates in the tissues, an abscess may develop which becomes walled off, making it difficult to treat with antibiotics. This process is known as suppuration.

Alternatively, the affected area may organize which results in the formation of granulation tissue and eventually fibrosis.

Persistence of the toxin that caused the initial acute inflammatory response results in the development of chronic inflammation.

Q. Do you know of any circumstances where acute inflammation can cause more harm than good?

A. Yes, an acute inflammatory response results in a sudden onset of tissue swelling which may compromise an airway, cause a mass effect intracranially or result in ischaemia and necrosis e.g. a burst appendix.

CHRONIC INFLAMMATION

Q. How does chronic inflammation differ from acute inflammation?

A. Chronic inflammation is characterized by different cells to those seen in acute inflammation. Classically, macrophages, lymphocytes and plasma cells are involved as opposed to neutrophils. Chronic inflammation is also characterized by the formation of granulation tissue and fibrosis.

Q. What causes the development of chronic inflammation?

A. Chronic inflammation may develop *de novo* or from acute inflammation that has failed to resolve. Common examples include:

- Foreign bodies
- Inflammatory conditions e.g. ulcerative colitis
- Resistant intracellular organisms e.g. mycobacteria
- Autoimmune disease e.g. rheumatoid arthritis
- Primary granulomatous diseases e.g. Crohn's disease, syphilis
- Organ transplant rejection.

If chronic inflammation does develop from acute inflammation, it tends to occur secondary to abscess formation. Healing then occurs with the formation of granulation tissue and fibrosis.

Q. What is the role of macrophages in chronic inflammation?

A. Macrophages are essentially scavenging phagocytes. They are initially attracted to the area by lymphokines and other macrophages. They develop from monocytes which are present in the blood and become macrophages as they migrate into the inflamed tissues. They then become 'activated' by increasing in size and mobility, ready to ingest the offending microorganism/particle. They have a longer life span than neutrophils.

If a particle/microorganism is too large for one macrophage, several may accumulate, resulting in granuloma formation. When two or more macrophages join together to digest a large particle, their membranes may actually fuse and a multinucleate giant cell is formed. Giant cells are said to have an increased digestive capacity; once they have been ingested, microorganisms are then killed by lysosomal enzymes.

Q. Are there any organisms that are able to avoid being killed by macrophages?

A. Yes, classically *Mycobacterium tuberculosis* and *M. leprae* are able to resist the intracellular killing and remain within the macrophages for many years. This persistence of infected macrophages results in a delayed-type hypersensitivity reaction which is T cell mediated and can result in widespread tissue damage when the macrophages die and release their lysosomal enzymes.

Q. What is the role of lymphocytes in chronic inflammation?

A. Lymphocytes are usually involved where infectious organisms are present. Initially, the natural immune system (neutrophils and macrophages) produces a non-specific response. Lymphocytes enable the immune system to mount a more specific defence; however, it has a much slower onset. B lymphocytes are stimulated by antigens to become plasma cells which secrete antibodies. They may also act as antigen-presenting cells (APCs) to T lymphocytes by binding to the antigen to be destroyed.

T lymphocytes are part of the cell-mediated immune response which is specific to the antigen and has memory. The next time it meets the same antigen, it is therefore able to mount a very rapid and specific defence. T lymphocytes may be subdivided into helper T cells which stimulate B lymphocytes into producing antibody and cytotoxic T cells which produce cytokines and kill antigens such as viruses.

Q. How might this immunological defence be harmful to the patient?

A. Cytokines produced by T lymphocytes attract inflammatory cells such as macrophages and neutrophils. When a large defence is mounted against a resistant microbe, the granuloma formation can be so extensive that organ function becomes impaired. In some cases, the immune system does not mount a response at all, as in schistosomiasis; this is equally harmful to the patient as liver failure develops.

Q. What clinical features are associated with chronic inflammation?

A. Chronic inflammation may be associated with ulceration, formation of granulomas, caseation (characteristic of TB), abscess cavity formation (classically thickening of the wall/affected tissue) and fibrosis.

CARCINOGENIC VIRUSES

Q. Can you name any viruses that induce malignancy?

A. Examples of viruses that induce malignancy include:

- Human papilloma virus (HPV) – causes cervical intra-epithelial neoplasia (CIN) and later cervical cancer
- Hepatitis B virus – liver cancer

- Epstein Barr virus (EBV) – Burkitt's lymphoma, nasopharyngeal cancer
- Human immunodeficiency virus (HIV) – Kaposi's sarcoma
- HTLV1 – T cell leukaemia.

Q. How do these viruses induce malignancy?

A. There are several mechanisms by which viruses induce malignancy:

- Viruses can directly cause malignancy by becoming integrated into a cell's genome and also by activation of cellular oncogenes
- They may indirectly cause malignancy through diseases such as chronic hepatitis which predispose to malignancy (liver cancer).

CARCINOGENESIS

Q. What is a carcinoma?

A. A carcinoma is a malignant epithelial tumour. It may be derived from the endoderm, mesoderm or ectoderm.

Q. What do you understand by the term carcinogenesis?

A. Carcinogenesis is the process by which tumours develop. This may involve benign and malignant stages; however, the term carcinogenesis is generally applied to the development of malignant tumours.

The process of carcinogenesis begins with a single cell. That cell undergoes a mutation as it divides and by a subsequent multistep process becomes malignant. This enables it to grow autonomously without normal cellular growth control.

Q. What causes the initial mutation?

A. This may be environmental or genetic. Carcinogenesis may occur as a result of:

- Exposure to chemical carcinogens e.g. smoking and lung cancer
- Environmental carcinogens e.g. radiation
- Inherited disease e.g. retinoblastoma, familial adenomatous polyposis
- Certain viruses (q.v.).

There are also several environmental factors that may place an individual at increased risk of carcinogenesis occurring:

- Diet e.g. fat and colorectal cancer
- Race e.g. breast cancer is less common in Africa
- Transplacental e.g. diethylstilbestrol and vaginal cancer in female babies
- Pre-malignant disease e.g. ulcerative colitis and colorectal cancer
- Inherited risk associated with conditions such as Li-Fraumeni syndrome and multiple endocrine neoplasia (MEN) syndromes.

Gender and family history also play a large part in determining the risk of carcinogenesis; for example women with first-degree relatives affected by breast cancer are at a higher risk of developing the disease than other women.

Environmental factors or exposure to carcinogens are by far the commonest causes of cancer worldwide.

Q. What is a carcinogen and how does it cause a genetic mutation?

A. A carcinogen is an agent that is thought to induce malignancy. Carcinogens have been identified by epidemiological evidence, as a result of exposure and through testing on laboratory animals.

They interact with DNA resulting in functional abnormalities in the genes that it encodes. The result is a genetic mutation that causes a dividing cell to act abnormally and grow beyond all normal control mechanisms. It is thought that further mutations occur by a multistep process to allow a malignant tumour to acquire the properties it needs in order to invade the basement membrane and metastasize.

Q. How do chemical carcinogens act?

A. Chemical carcinogens are usually hydrocarbons which form charged molecules known as epoxides. Epoxides then bind to DNA and RNA to cause a genetic mutation.

Q. Can you give me any examples of chemical carcinogens?

A. Examples include:

- B-naphthylamine (aromatic amines) – used in the rubber/dye industry and causes bladder cancer
- Nitrosamines – used in fertilizer and cause gastrointestinal tract cancers
- Soot (polycyclic aromatic hydrocarbon) – causes scrotal cancer
- Aflatoxin (mycotoxin from *Aspergillus flavus*) – causes liver cell carcinoma
- Azo dyes – cause liver and bladder cancer
- Alkylating agents – cause leukaemia
- Arsenic – causes skin cancer
- Asbestos – causes pleural plaques and mesothelioma
- Nickel – causes lung cancer.

Q. What is the difference between 'initiation' and 'promotion?'

A. Initiation and promotion are both involved in the early stages of carcinogenesis. Initiation is the process by which cellular DNA is altered, and hence as the cell divides it has the potential to become carcinogenic. Promotion is the next step in the process. It induces proliferation of the altered cell and hence the development of the carcinoma. It is due to further genetic mutations occurring spontaneously or following exposure to promoters. Initiators and promoters allow the carcinoma to develop to a level where it can grow autonomously.

Q. What is an oncogene and what is its role in the development of a carcinoma?

A. Cellular oncogenes are genes that are essential for life. They control normal cell growth and differentiation, and it is thought carcinomas may develop if they have an altered or enhanced expression. Oncogenes may be classified by the function of their gene products known as oncoproteins. For example:

- *myc* - involved in cell proliferation
- *ras* - involved in cyclic nucleotide binding and hence intracellular signalling
- *bcl-2* – involved with apoptosis.

Abnormalities in oncogene expression, therefore, may account for an increased risk of carcinogenesis by:

- Production of abnormally functioning oncoproteins
- Production of an excessive amount of oncoprotein
- Loss of usual growth inhibition (tumour suppressor genes).

It is thought that abnormal or large amounts of oncoprotein encourage cells to grow of their own accord, to have an increased motility and to have reduced cell-to-cell adhesion. All of these properties enable the affected cells to develop into a malignant tumour.

TUMOUR MARKERS

Q. What is a tumour marker?

A. A tumour marker is a substance produced by a tumour which is present in the circulation. It may be measured in the serum and can aid diagnosis, it can be used to monitor the response to treatment, and rising levels can indicate recurrence. There are several types of tumour markers, including:

- Hormones – may be produced from tumours affecting endocrine organs e.g. cortisol from an adrenal tumour
- Ectopic hormones – may be produced aberrantly from tumours e.g. oat cell lung tumours may produce ACTH and ADH
- Isoenzymes – e.g. prostate cancer produces prostate acid phosphatase
- Oncofetal antigens – e.g. carcinoembryonic antigen (CEA) in colorectal tumours
- Growth factors – used by the tumour to aid autocrine growth and invasion.

Q. Can you give some examples of commonly used tumour markers in clinical practice?

A. Some examples of tumour markers used clinically include:

- α-fetoprotein (AFP) – produced by primary liver tumours and testicular teratomas
- Placental alkaline phosphatase (PLAP) – produced by testicular seminomas and tumours of the pancreas and lung
- Human chorionic gonadotrophin (hCG) – produced by choriocarcinoma
- Vanillyl mandelic acid (VMA) – produced by phaeochromocytomas and can be detected in the urine
- 5-hydroxyindole-acetic acid (5-HIAA) – produced by carcinoid tumours and is also detected in the urine.

Q. Give an example of one tumour marker that is used in the surveillance of tumour progression.

A. Commonly, the measurement of serum levels of α-fetoprotein is used to monitor the progress of testicular teratomas. Usually a sample is taken preoperatively. As with most tumour markers, the initial level is not indicative of the size of the tumour. It is simply used as a guide with which the response to treatment may be monitored. After an orchidectomy has been performed, serum levels must then be measured frequently until they return to normal. Samples can then be taken less frequently and a rise may indicate tumour recurrence, prompting further investigations.

TUMOUR CLASSIFICATION

Q. Tell me about any classifications of malignant tumours that you know. (This question is specific to malignant tumours. You will not be penalized for initially defining the difference between benign and malignant tumours, but the examiner will expect you to concentrate on malignant tumours.)

A. Malignant tumours may be broadly classified into epithelial tumours, known as carcinomas, and connective tissue tumours, known as sarcomas. However, some malignancies do not fit into this classification. These include lymphoma, myeloma and haematological malignancies such as leukaemia.

Q. Can you give me any examples of epithelial and connective tissue malignant tumours?

A. Malignant epithelial tumours may be categorized into:

- Squamous cell – squamous cell carcinoma
- Transitional cell – transitional cell carcinoma
- Basal cell – basal cell carcinoma
- Glandular – adenocarcinoma.

Malignant connective tissue tumours may be categorized into:

- Smooth muscle – leiomyosarcoma
- Striated muscle – rhabdomyosarcoma
- Adipose tissue – liposarcoma
- Blood vessels – angiosarcoma
- Bone – osteosarcoma
- Cartilage – chondrosarcoma
- Mesothelium – malignant mesothelioma
- Synovium – synovial sarcoma.

Q. **Tell me about the significance of the histological grade of the malignant tumour.**

A. Grading of tumours is used by histologists in order to classify the degree of differentiation of the tumour. The degree of differentiation of the tumour cell reflects how closely it resembles its cell of origin. If it closely resembles its cell of origin it is well differentiated and therefore low grade. Low-grade tumours are less aggressive than those with poorly differentiated cells which bear little or no resemblance to their cell of origin.

Q. **What is carcinogenesis?**

A. Carcinogenesis is the process which results in the formation of malignant tumours.

Q. **What is oncogenesis?**

A. Oncogenesis is the process which results in the formation of benign and malignant tumours.

Q. **How is this thought to occur?**

A. It may be congenital or acquired. Acquired or environmental factors are more common, but sometimes the formation of a tumour may result from a combination of both.

Q. **Can you give me examples of these?**

A. Yes, examples of congenital tumours include retinoblastoma, which involves a genetic mutation on chromosome 13, and familial adenomatous polyposis which involves a genetic mutation on chromosome 5. Examples of acquired tumours include skin cancer, associated with UV light, and lung cancer, associated with smoking.

TUMOUR METASTASES

Q. **What are metastases?**

A. Metastases develop when malignant tumours are able to spread from their original site and form secondary tumours elsewhere in the body.

Q. **What determines whether a tumour metastasizes or not?**

A. By definition, it is only malignant tumours that are able to metastasize. In order to do so, the tumour has to develop certain properties that will help it spread from the primary site and survive elsewhere. These include:

- Increased cellular mobility
- Reduced cellular adhesion (loss of contact inhibition that usually inhibits the cell from moving)
- Production of enzymes locally to aid spread.

Histologically, this is easy to detect in epithelial tumours where the basement membrane has been invaded. In other tumours it may not be as easy to detect. In these cases, the lymphovasculature is assessed for evidence of spread and other histological features are looked at in order to work out the likelihood that metastases have developed. These include:

- Increased number of mitoses/abnormal mitoses
- Increased nuclear/cytoplasm ratio
- Widespread nuclear hyperchromatism (aneuploidy/polyploidy are associated with aggressiveness)
- Cellular pleomorphism.

Other factors that may be taken into consideration include excessive necrosis and haemorrhage due to fragile new vasculature and obvious/excessive infiltrative borders.

Q. Where do tumours tend to metastasize to?

A. Primary tumours may metastasize via:

- Blood – they will then be carried to other organs to form secondary tumours (common in sarcomas).
- Lymphatics – from here they will travel to local lymph nodes (common in carcinomas).
- Transcoelomic – generally affects tumours of the stomach, ovary or colon where spread occurs across the peritoneal cavity. May also affect pleural and pericardial cavities in lung and breast cancer.
- CSF – affects CNS tumours.
- Perineural – tumours tend to favour the path of least resistance.
- Implantation – accidental contamination as a result of manual handling at the time of surgery or inappropriate biopsy.

Q. Which tumours classically metastasize to bone?

A. Primary tumours reach bone via haematogenous spread. Classically they include:

- *Breast*
- *Bronchus*
- *Kidney*
- *Prostate*
- *Thyroid.*

(Surgical mnemonics are often alliterative ('all the F's' for abdominal distension, 'all the P's' for vascular occlusion). I remember this using the mnemonic 'all the B's: *Breast, Bronchus, Bidney, Brostate* and *Byroid*'!)

Q. What clinical features may suggest to you that a patient is presenting with metastases?

A. Clinically, the patient may present with symptoms or signs from the affected area. For example, they may have palpable axillary lymph nodes in breast cancer, bone pain or pathological fractures with bony metastases or right upper quadrant pain from an enlarged liver. If metastases have developed in several places, the patient is said to have 'carcinomatosis' and may present with multiple problems such as ascites, cachexia, liver failure and respiratory difficulties.

Q. What are paraneoplastic syndromes?

A. Paraneoplastic syndromes are features that are associated with a malignant tumour that are not due to direct involvement or development of metastases. For example:

- Haematological – thrombocytopenia, thrombophlebitis, disseminated intravascular coagulation (DIC)
- Neuromuscular – myopathy, polymyositis
- Endocrine – hypercalcaemia, carcinoid syndrome (secretion of serotonin), ADH secretion
- Dermatological – clubbing, dermatomyositis, acanthosis nigricans.

Q. Which tumours are associated with the development of paraneoplastic syndromes?

A. Tumours associated with paraneoplastic syndromes include lung, pancreas, kidney and breast cancer.

PNEUMONIA

Q. How would you classify pneumonia?

A. There are several different ways to classify pneumonia. It may be primary, in someone who is otherwise well, or secondary due to local causes such as aspiration or systemic defects such as immunodeficiency.

Another method of classification is by aetiological agent. Most commonly the aetiological agent is a bacterium. Common bacterial agents include:

- *Streptococcus pneumonia*
- *Haemophilus influenzae*
- *Staphylococcus aureus.*

Viruses can also cause pneumonia: influenza and measles both cause pneumonia in a small proportion of patients who contract the virus. Fungal causes, such as *Aspergillus* and *Cryptococcus*, are also seen, particularly in immunosuppressed patients. Other causes include *Pneumocystis carinii* and *Mycoplasma*.

Grouping by anatomical site is another widely used classification of pneumonia:

- Bronchopneumonia is seen more commonly in the elderly, often secondary to pre-existing disease. One or both lungs show patchy consolidation centred on the bronchioles and bronchi, and surrounding alveoli. The causative organisms typically include staphylococci, streptococci, *haemophilis influenzae*, coliforms and fungi.

- Lobar pneumonia is more often seen in previously healthy individuals. Part or all of a lobe may be affected. By far the most common organism responsible for causing lobar pneumonia is *streptococcus pneumoniae*.

Q. Can you tell me the pathological changes seen in lobar pneumonia?

A. The changes seen in lobar pneumonia closely follow those of acute inflammation.

The first stage of the process is *congestion*, which lasts for about 24 hours. A protein-rich exudate pours into the alveolar spaces resulting in venous congestion and oedema.

The next stage is known as *red hepatization* and lasts for several days. Polymorphs, with lymphocytes and macrophages, accumulate in the alveolar spaces. The venous congestion leads to extravasation of red blood cells from the capillaries. The lung is red and airless, resembling liver, which is responsible for the name of this stage of the process.

The next stage is *grey hepatization*, again lasting for a few days. There is further accumulation of fibrin, particularly over the surrounding pleura. There is continued destruction of red and white blood cells. The lung remains solid but the colour is now grey-brown.

The final stage is *resolution* which is seen after about 8–10 days in untreated cases. The inflammatory debris is reabsorbed, preserving the underlying architecture of the lung.

Q. What do you know about nosocomial pneumonias?

A. A nosocomial infection is one which is acquired in hospital. It is estimated that up to 10% of all hospital inpatients develop an infection acquired while in hospital. Pneumonia is one of many infections that can be acquired in hospital; urinary tract infections and wound infections are also common problems on surgical wards. The source of infection may be from people as incidental carriers or via fomites (inanimate objects which come into contact with a patient such as surgical instruments and anaesthetic equipment). The routes of infection are similar to those for any infection: person-to-person contact, air-borne transmission or ingestion (food poisoning has been reported many times in British hospitals).

Simple hand washing between each patient can greatly reduce the amount of spread from person to person contact and its importance cannot be over-estimated.

Certain patients are more prone to acquiring nosocomial pneumonias than others. The very young or very elderly, patients with any form of immunosuppression, patients on intensive care wards and those receiving long-term antibiotics are all more likely to contract hospital-acquired infection. The organisms responsible for nosocomial infections are the same as those typically seen for community-acquired infections and the treatment is the same.

INFLAMMATORY BOWEL DISEASE

Q. Tell me what you know about Crohn's disease.

A. Crohn's disease is a chronic non-caseating granulomatous condition that affects the bowel. It has an approximately equal incidence in men and women, is commonly diagnosed between the ages of 20 and 30 years and has an increased incidence in Western societies. The aetiology is unknown; various theories have implicated *Mycobacterium paratuberculosis*, the MMR vaccine, microparticles (e.g. toothpaste) and diet.

The condition is characterized by chronic inflammation and granuloma formation. It may affect the gastrointestinal tract anywhere from the mouth to the anus, but most commonly affects the terminal ileum. Perianal disease, particularly fissures and fistulae, is also common.

The condition typically follows a relapsing and remitting course. Management is principally medical using steroids, sulphasalazine and azothiaprine. Occasionally surgical resection is required for complications. Crohn's disease is associated with long term amyloid deposition and an increased risk of small bowel lymphoma.

 TIP

This is a gift question provided you know enough information to pull it off! Even if you don't, there is a standard way to approach any question that starts off 'What is the condition?'. It follows this well known mnemonic: *Dressed In a Surgeon's Gown A Physician May Make Progress:*

Definition, Incidence, Age, Sex, Geography, Aetiology, Pathogenesis, Macropathology, Micropathology, Prognosis.

Q. You mentioned that there is granuloma formation; what other pathological features are associated with the disease?

A. The granulomas are composed of epitheloid macrophages and giant cells, and typically affect the bowel in a patchy manner. The affected areas are known as skip lesions. The inflammation also affects the entire bowel wall as opposed to just the mucosa, as is the case in ulcerative colitis.

Macroscopically, longitudinal ulcers result in deep fissures within the bowel. These cross transverse oedematous folds resulting in a 'cobblestone' appearance. There may also be some reactive lymphadenopathy.

Q. How does this differ from the pathological features of ulcerative colitis?

A. Ulcerative colitis is a non-specific inflammatory disorder, which primarily affects the large bowel. It usually begins in the rectum and progresses proximally, causing a proctitis or distal colitis. It usually results in superficial ulceration involving the mucosa but may sometimes extend into the muscle.

Microscopically there is an acute and chronic inflammatory infiltrate with formation of crypt abscesses and eventual distortion of the crypt lining. Macroscopically there is hyperaemia of the intact mucosa and haemorrhage from the ulcers. In the long term, there is an increased risk of colonic malignancy.

Q. What are the clinical features of ulcerative colitis?

A. Ulcerative colitis manifests itself as frequent, bloody stools. If there is a long history, the patient may become extremely unwell and present with dehydration and malnutrition. It may be complicated by toxic megacolon leading to haemorrhage and perforation. It is also associated with disorders of the skin, such as erythema nodosum and pyoderma gangrenosum, disorders of the liver, such as primary biliary cirrhosis and also eye disorders such as iritis and uveitis.

Q. What are the indications for surgery in an attack of severe colitis?

A. An attack of colitis is usually managed medically. This includes rehydration and symptom control using steroids, salicylic acids and anti-diarrhoeals. It is also important to improve nutrition levels using enteral or parenteral nutrition.

If the severe attack doesn't respond despite 4–5 days' high-dose steroids then an urgent colectomy must be considered. Other factors to be considered include eight or more bloody stools a day, persistent tachycardia, fever >38.5°C, dilatation of the colon >5 cm or increasing diameter on serial films and a falling serum albumin.

Q. Do you know of any markers thought to be indicative of severe colitis?

A. Yes, the ESR and CRP.

INTESTINAL POLYPS

Q. What is a polyp?

A. A polyp is an abnormal protuberance from an epithelial surface. It may be benign or malignant. Polyps are more common in the large intestine than the small intestine.

Q. What types of benign polyps do you know about?

A. Benign polyps may be categorized into epithelial and soft tissue. Epithelial polyps include:

- Adenoma (neoplastic)
- Inflammatory (e.g. pseudopolyps in ulcerative colitis)
- Hamartoma (e.g. Peutz–Jeghers syndrome)
- Hyperplastic (metaplastic).

The commonest type of benign polyp is the adenoma or 'neoplastic' polyp. They may be subdivided into tubular, villous or tubulo-villous. The tubular type is by far the most common. Adenomas are thought to be highly likely to develop into carcinomas.

Soft tissue polyps include:

- Lipoma
- Haemangioma
- Fibroma
- Leiomyoma.

These types of polyps are far less likely to progress into a carcinoma.

Q. Why is it that adenomatous polyps are at an increased risk of becoming malignant?

A. Adenomas, particularly the villous type, are lined with columnar epithelial cells which become dysplastic. The dysplasia is graded as mild, moderate or severe according to the number of mitoses present, nuclear pleomorphism and loss of nuclear polarity. It is thought that a series of mutations causes an adenoma to develop into a carcinoma. This process is known as the 'adenoma-carcinoma' sequence.

Q. What clinical features are associated with intestinal polyps?

A. Mostly, adenomatous polyps are picked up as incidental findings on sigmoidoscopy or colonoscopy. Symptoms of polyps depend on the site of the polyp, their size, number and histological type. Rectal polyps may present with rectal bleeding or even prolapse of the polyp itself. Villous adenomas are associated with mucus production; hence the patient may present with passage of mucus per rectum.

Alternatively, the patient may present with complications, e.g. development of colorectal cancer, anaemia secondary to blood loss from the surface of the polyp, electrolyte imbalance (protein and potassium loss) from copious mucus production in villous adenomas or intussusception.

Q. If a patient is found to have a polyp, what is the best management?

A. It should always be recommended that a polyp is removed unless the patient is not fit enough to withstand the procedure. Most polyps can be removed at the time of colonoscopy or sigmoidoscopy using biopsy forceps or a diathermy snare. Occasionally, it may be necessary to perform a laparotomy if the polyp is large.

Q. What is familial adenomatous polyposis?

A. Familial adenomatous polyposis is a rare genetic condition that results in the development of multiple adenomatous polyps, mostly affecting the large bowel. The genetic mutation affects chromosome 5. It affects males and females equally. The condition results in almost certain progression to carcinoma within one or more polyps by the age of 20–30 years.

Q. How is the condition diagnosed?

A. The diagnosis is usually made as a result of screening affected families. Sporadic cases may present in the teens/early twenties with alterations of bowel habit and passage of mucus PR. Alternatively, the undiagnosed patient may present later on when the cancer has developed. The diagnosis of familial adenomatous polyposis is then made if more than 100 adenomatous polyps are found in the colon and rectum.

Q. How is the condition treated?

A. This depends on when the condition is diagnosed and the extent of the disease. If the condition is detected early as a result of screening, the patient should undergo a total colectomy as a preventative measure with an ileorectal anastomosis or formation of an ileoanal pouch. Patients undergoing ileorectal anastomosis require yearly sigmoidoscopic surveillance of the rectal remnant.

The patient may already have developed a rectal carcinoma, in which case a total proctocolectomy may be necessary, depending on the site of the lesion.

Q. What other clinical features are associated with familial adenomatous polyposis?

A. Other features of this condition include:

- Abdominal desmoid tumours
- Dental cysts
- Jaw osteomata
- Epidermoid cysts
- Retinal pigmentation
- Hamartomatous polyps in the stomach.

COLORECTAL CARCINOMA

Q. A 69-year-old man presents to Accident and Emergency with a 3 day history of worsening abdominal pain and constipation. On examination, you find that he has a distended abdomen, generalized tenderness and high-pitched bowel sounds. What conclusions do you draw?

A. These findings suggest the presence of bowel obstruction which is more likely to be large bowel than small due to the absence of nausea and vomiting. I would like to perform a plain abdominal radiograph in order to confirm the diagnosis.

Q. What is the most likely cause of large bowel obstruction in a 69-year-old man?

A. The most likely cause is a colorectal carcinoma. It may also be caused by diverticulitis, sigmoid volvulus and, more rarely, strictures, hernias and ischaemia.

Q. How else does a colorectal carcinoma present?

A. A colorectal carcinoma may present differently according to its position. Left sided lesions may present acutely as large bowel obstruction. Right-sided lesions are associated with chronic blood loss and so patients may present with pallor and lethargy. Other presenting features include:

- PR bleeding – more common in rectal carcinoma
- PR mucus – more common in left-sided lesions
- Change of bowel habit with increased frequency and urgency
- Tenesmus – the painful, repeated desire to open the bowels
- Symptoms and signs of local spread – coccygeal or anal pain, colovesical or colovaginal fistulae
- Symptoms and signs of generalized spread i.e. ascites, weight loss, hepatomegaly.

Q. How would you treat this gentleman if you suspected a diagnosis of large bowel obstruction secondary to colorectal carcinoma?

A. First, I would take a full history and examine the patient, including carrying out a rectal examination. I would then review the imaging available to me and confirm the diagnosis of large bowel obstruction. Then I would resuscitate the patient using intravenous fluids and administer analgesia as appropriate. I would then place the patient NBM (nil by mouth), insert a nasogastric tube and arrange to take him to theatre in order to perform a laparotomy.

Q. What type of operation would you perform?

A. There are several options available. Firstly, I would like to assess the situation, looking specifically at the size of the tumour, the position and its involvement with surrounding structures. Then I would assess the bowel and look for the presence of sepsis. I would also feel the liver for the presence of metastases. Then I would consider the following options:

- Defunctioning colostomy, radiotherapy to downstage the tumour, then resection of the tumour at a later stage (fixed rectal tumours)
- Resection of the tumour, temporary end colostomy and closure of the distal bowel (Hartmann's procedure)
- Resection of the tumour and primary anastomosis (tumours of the right colon).

It is sensible to delay primary anastomoses in the presence of an obstructed or faecally loaded bowel, sepsis or locally advanced disease.

Q. What is the commonest histological type of colorectal carcinoma?

A. The commonest histological type of colorectal carcinoma is an adenocarcinoma with mucin production. Other types include APUD (amine precursor uptake and decarboxylation), cell tumours and lymphomas.

Q. What is Dukes' staging?

A. Dukes' staging is a pathological classification of colorectal carcinoma. It includes the following stages:

- A – tumour limited to the bowel wall (not breaching the muscularis propria)
- B – tumour invades through the bowel wall but does not involve the lymph nodes
- C – tumour has spread to the lymph nodes.

A recent addition to the staging classification is 'D' signifying distant metastases.

Q. How does the Dukes' stage correlate with survival?

A. Dukes' staging has an important correlation with survival.

- Dukes's A + B – 70–80% at 5 years
- Dukes' C – approximately 30%.

There are other factors that influence survival, for example:

- Histological grade – poorly differentiated tumours have a poorer prognosis
- Resection margins of the surgical specimen (most importantly the circumferential margin) – poorer outlook if involved
- Young age at presentation and short history of onset of symptoms are associated with a worse prognosis
- Complications associated with emergency presentation, e.g. perforation, sepsis, adversely affect survival.

BREAST DISEASE

Q. What do you know about Paget's disease of the nipple?

A. Paget's disease of the nipple presents as a red, roughened area which may be ulcerated. It resembles eczema and is associated with an underlying ductal breast cancer. It is often associated with late presentation of breast cancer.

Q. Approximately what percentage of women who develop breast cancer present with this condition?

A. It affects approximately 1–2% of all women with breast cancer.

Q. How would you distinguish this lesion from a patch of eczema?

A. Paget's disease may present as a localized lesion or may be quite widespread and so size would not distinguish it from a patch of eczema. Paget's disease tends to begin from the nipple and spread outwards whereas eczema or any other skin conditions would tend to affect the areola first.

It may be difficult to distinguish both lesions from direct spread of a nearby locally invasive cancer as this may affect the nipple or the areola first depending on the location of the tumour.

Q. How would you manage a patient who you suspected may have Paget's disease of the nipple?

A. First, I would take a full history and carry out an examination, looking at any risk factors for breast cancer. Then I would instigate triple assessment which involves a mammogram, ultrasound and scrape cytology of the lesion. If the imaging were to detect any underlying lesion, I would want to perform a fine needle aspiration on this lesion. If all of these investigations were negative, I would proceed to an incisional biopsy of the lesion under local anaesthetic.

Q. What are the commonest histological types of invasive breast cancer that you know about?

A. The commonest types of invasive breast cancer include:

- Infiltrating ductal carcinoma
- Infiltrating lobular carcinoma.

These account for approximately 95% of all breast cancers in women. Other less common types include:

- Mucinous carcinoma
- Tubular carcinoma
- Medullary carcinoma
- Papillary carcinoma.

Q. What is the usual mode of spread of invasive breast cancer?

A. Breast cancer can spread:

- Locally – to surrounding skin, breast tissue and muscle
- Via the lymphatics – commonly to the axillary nodes but also to supra-clavicular, internal mammary and occasionally to tracheobronchial nodes
- Via the bloodstream – to the lung, pleura, liver, adrenals, brain and bone.

Q. What do you know about non-invasive tumours of the breast?

A. Non-invasive tumours of the breast are otherwise known as carcinoma in situ. Carcinoma in situ is the presence of malignant cells within the ducts or the lobules that have not penetrated the basement membrane. The two main types are known as ductal carcinoma in situ (DCIS) and lobular carcinoma in situ (LCIS).

Q. What are the differences between the two types?

A. DCIS tends to affect post-menopausal women whereas LCIS tends to occur in pre-menopausal women.

DCIS is characterized by ducts with large, irregular cells and irregular nuclei. It may present with a mass in the breast, nipple discharge or Paget's disease of the nipple. It is associated with the presence of microcalcification on mammography and tends to be unifocal. DCIS is a group of lesions which may be categorized into low grade, high grade or comedo type which is characterized by creamy necrosis.

LCIS is rare and is characterized by lobules with regular cells and rounded nuclei. It is less likely to present as a lump and more likely to be picked up as an incidental finding in a breast biopsy. It has no characteristic mammographic appearances. It is often multifocal, can be bilateral and is rarely associated with necrosis.

Q. How likely is it that a patient with DCIS will develop invasive cancer?

A. It is likely that up to 50% of patients with DCIS will develop invasive breast cancer within 15 years. This figure is dependent on the grade of the DCIS and is obviously higher for high-grade lesions.

Q. What do you know about phyllodes tumours of the breast?

A. Phyllodes tumours are rare fibroepithelial tumours which used to be called 'giant fibroadenomas'. They are commonly benign, but are occasionally malignant. The commonest affected age group is 45–50 years and the typical presentation is a lump in the breast. Microscopically the tumour involves characteristic epithelium which projects into cystic spaces and stroma that is more cellular than a fibroadenoma. It may grow to as large as 4–5 cm.

The major problem associated with phyllodes is recurrence after it has been excised. Features associated with recurrence include:

- Large initial size
- High mitotic rate
- Cellular atypia
- Infiltrating edge (as opposed to rounded).

If a phyllodes recurs, there is an increased risk of metastases to the lungs and bone via the bloodstream. It rarely metastasizes to the lymphatics.

Q. What is the treatment of a phyllodes tumour?

A. Treatment involves excision of the lump with a clear margin and regular follow up according to local policy. Chest X-rays are of more use than mammograms as the tumours metastasize via the bloodstream.

LYMPHOMA

Q. What is lymphoma?

A. Lymphoma is a primary malignancy of the immune system that is classified by its cell type. It is broadly categorized into Hodgkin's and non-Hodgkin's lymphoma.

Q. What is Hodgkin's disease?

A. Hodgkin's disease is a type of lymphoma that is characterized by the presence of Reed–Sternberg cells. It most commonly occurs in young people in their early 20s and presents with painless lymphadenopathy, particularly in the neck and axilla. In approximately a third of cases there will also be systemic symptoms such as night sweats, weight loss and fever.

Q. Do you know of any classifications for Hodgkin's disease?

A. Yes, two exist. The first is the Ann Arbor staging system which classifies the disease anatomically. It consists of stages I to IV:

- Stage I – single lymph node region affected or single organ affected
- Stage II – more than one lymph node region affected, but only on one side of the diaphragm
- Stage III – both sides of the diaphragm affected
- Stage IV – disease spread to bone marrow, spleen, lung and bone.

The second is called the Rye pathological classification system:

- Lymphocyte predominant – this type is uncommon and consists of lymphocytes and histiocytes.
- Nodular sclerosing – lacunar cells predominate. These are variants of Reed–Sternberg cells. Clinically there is a thickening of the lymph node capsule.
- Mixed cellularity – more aggressive than lymphocyte predominant. Consists of a mixture of lymphocytes, histiocytes, Hodgkin's cells and Reed–Sternberg cells. Tends to present late.
- Lymphocyte depleted – rarest form, poorest outlook due to late presentation and may be subdivided into reticular and diffuse fibrosis.

The presence of 'B' affixed to any of the classifications denotes systemic symptoms such as fever or weight loss.

Q. How would you investigate a 19-year-old man who presents with a painless, enlarged node in his neck?

A. I would first take a full history and carry out an examination. I would pay particular attention to a history of night sweats, weight loss and fever persisting over several months. Then I would perform a thorough examination of cervical, axillary and inguinal nodes. I would also examine the abdomen for splenomegaly.

Then I would proceed to a full blood count (FBC), erythrocyte sediment rate (ESR) and liver function tests (LFTs). If the patient has systemic symptoms, anaemia and abnormal LFTs it is likely that they have bone marrow involvement. I would therefore proceed to a bone marrow trephine biopsy. I would then arrange imaging, ideally a CT scan of the chest and abdomen, to assess hilar, coeliac, para-aortic and pelvic lymph node involvement. Lymphography is also thought to be a reliable tool in investigating affected lymph nodes that may appear normally sized on imaging.

I would then proceed to a lymph node biopsy of the affected node for a definitive diagnosis.

Q. Why is it necessary to perform a lymph node biopsy if you have already performed a bone marrow trephine?

A. A bone marrow trephine would only be of use if the patient actually had marrow involvement. This only occurs in approximately 10% of cases of Hodgkin's disease. Therefore, it is unlikely to be of any use diagnostically if used in all presentations of enlarged painless lymph nodes. Similarly, a bone marrow aspiration, if positive, would only give cytological information.

A lymph node biopsy provides the tissue architecture to give an accurate histological diagnosis, whereas FNA cytology does not. With the results of this and any staging investigations, it would be possible to gain prognostic information prior to instigation of treatment.

Q. What is the role of a 'staging laparotomy' in Hodgkin's disease?

A. The staging laparotomy was introduced in the 1960s in order to assess the intra-abdominal extent of Hodgkin's disease. It commonly involved a splenectomy. It was based on the notion that the abdomen may be affected despite clear staging investigations. There has been no proven survival advantage in patients undergoing such laparotomies in comparison to controls, and it is now thought that the risks of abdominal surgery and the infection risk associated with splenectomy far outweigh the value of any information that may be gleaned from the surgery.

SKIN TUMOURS

Q. What skin tumours do you know of?

A. Skin tumours may be benign or malignant. Benign skin tumours include:

- Basal cell papilloma (seborrhoeic wart)
- Squamous cell papilloma
- Keratoacanthoma.

Malignant skin tumours include:

- Basal cell carcinoma (BCC)
- Squamous cell carcinoma (SCC)
- Malignant melanoma
- Kaposi's sarcoma.

Q. What causes skin cancer?

A. Skin cancer is classically associated with sun damage i.e. UV radiation. It is also caused by radiation from other sources i.e. X-rays. It may also be associated with topical carcinogens such as tar and rubber.

Q. Who is most at risk?

A. BCC and SCC tend to occur in the older patient and melanoma affects younger people. People who have fair skin and burn easily are more at risk of developing skin cancer. People who have an increased amount of melanin in their skin (e.g. Africans/South Americans) are protected against UV radiation.

Q. What is a malignant melanoma?

A. Malignant melanoma is a cancer of the melanocytes and is the commonest cancer affecting 20–40-year-olds. In the UK it is more prevalent in women; however, elsewhere in the world men are more commonly affected. It tends to occur in the fair skinned and is commonest on the legs in women and the trunk in men.

It presents as an irregular, pigmented skin lesion that may arise de novo or in a previously benign naevus. It is associated with a rapid increase in size, itchiness, ulceration and the development of satellite nodules. It may also arise elsewhere in the body such as the anus, nasal cavities, retina and the central nervous system.

Q. What determines the prognosis of malignant melanoma?

A. There are several factors involved in the prognosis. These include:

- Increasing age (associated with a poorer prognosis)
- Female sex (better prognosis)
- Site of lesion – trunk associated with a poorer outcome
- Presence of ulceration or satellite lesions
- Tumour grade and stage
- Tumour type – nodular, superficial spreading, acral lentiginous and lentigo maligna (progressively better prognosis)
- Tumour thickness – vertical spread.

The most important indicators of outcome are the Breslow thickness and Clarke's levels. Percentage survival at 10 years according to the Breslow thickness (tumour thickness from the most superficial point to the deepest) is:

- < 0.75 mm – 92%
- 0.76 – 3 mm – 50%
- > 4 mm – <30%.

Clarke's levels predict the survival at 5 years according to the involvement of the underlying tissue:

- I (intra-epidermal) – 98%
- II (papillary dermis) – 96%
- III (papillary/reticular junction) – 94%
- IV (reticular dermis) – 78%
- V (subcutaneous fat) – 74%.

Q. Which is the more reliable indicator of prognosis?

A. It is thought that the Breslow thickness is the more reliable indicator of outcome as the thickness of the papillary and reticular dermis can vary at different sites around the body and also from person to person. Other factors such as site and age of patient should be taken into account as up to 20% of 'thin' melanomas metastasize.

INTRACRANIAL SPACE OCCUPYING LESIONS

Q. Tell me about any central nervous system (CNS) tumours that you know of:

A. CNS tumours are uncommon. Most brain tumours tend to be metastases from primary tumours elsewhere. Classically tumours from the breast, lung, kidney, colon and melanomas from skin spread to the brain via the bloodstream.

Primary CNS tumours are relatively more frequent in children than in adults. In children, they are the second commonest tumours after leukaemia. Mostly they are astrocytomas which tend to occur in the posterior fossa. In adults, the most frequently occurring primary CNS tumour is a glioblastoma which tends to occur in the supratentorial region.

Q. How may CNS tumours be classified?

A. CNS tumours may be classified according to their cell of origin:

- Glial cells (neuroepithelial cells) – astrocytoma, glioblastoma, ependyoma, oligodendroglioma
- Neuroectodermal cells – medulloblastoma, neuroblastoma
- Nerve sheath cells – schwannoma, neurofibroma
- Arachnoid cell – meningioma
- Lymphoma
- Haemangioblastoma.

Q. What are the risk factors for developing CNS tumours?

A. Risk factors include a positive family history, inherited conditions such as neurofibromatosis, radiation as a child, immunosuppression, trauma and virally induced in HIV infection.

Q. How do CNS tumours tend to present?

A. CNS tumours may present as:

- Raised intracranial pressure
- Local/mass effects.

Q. What are the clinical features of a raised intracranial pressure?

A. The classic symptoms include headache, drowsiness and vomiting. The headache is present on waking and is usually progressive throughout the day. With increasing intracranial pressure, the patient becomes increasingly drowsy and eventually loses consciousness.

Signs of a raised intracranial pressure tend to occur late and include 'Cushing's reflex' which is a raised blood pressure and a low pulse. A sixth nerve palsy may also occur and is a false localizing sign. Visual disturbances are also a presenting feature and papilloedema may be visualized as blurring of the margins of the optic disc. Disturbances of eye movement such as nystagmus are far more common in children due to an increased incidence of brainstem involvement. Late features of a raised intracranial pressure include pulmonary oedema, pancreatitis and gastrointestinal tract haemorrhage and ulceration.

Features specific to the tumour are dependent on the size and site of the tumour. For example, focal lesions may result in:

- Frontal lobe – a change in personality, incontinence
- Temporal region – epilepsy and dysphasia
- Parietal lobe – hemiparesis, sensory abnormalities
- Pituitary gland – visual disturbances, classically bitemporal hemianopia
- Cerebellum – truncal ataxia, disturbances of coordination.

Q. What is the result of untreated raised intracranial pressure?

A. If a focal CNS tumour enlarges, a mass effect occurs due to the tumour itself and to the surrounding oedema. In infants the fontanelles allow some room for expansion in hydrocephalus due to a posterior fossa tumour or a rise in intracranial pressure. In adults, however, the skull is a rigid structure. In untreated raised intracranial pressure there is an initial compensation by a reduction in CSF around the brain, less blood within the brain and a reactive atrophy that occurs with slow-growing lesions. Eventually, intracranial herniation may occur at several sites including:

- Any weak spot in the dura or skull
- Cerebellar tonsil through the foramen magnum
- Hippocampal uncus or parahippocampal gyrus across the tentorium cerebelli
- Lateral shift of the cingulated gyrus beneath the falx cerebri.

The outcome is usually fatal.

Q. What is hydrocephalus?

A. Hydrocephalus is an increase in cerebrospinal fluid (CSF) within the intracranial cavity.

Q. How is CSF regulated?

A. CSF is produced by the choroid plexus in the lateral, third and fourth ventricles at a rate of approximately 400 ml per 24 hours in adults. From the lateral ventricles, CSF travels through the foramen of Munro to the third ventricle and then through the aqueduct of Sylvius to the fourth ventricle. From the fourth ventricle it then passes through the foramina of Magendie and Luschka to the subarachnoid space.

Most CSF is then reabsorbed through the arachnoid villi within the sagittal venous sinuses. Hydrocephalus occurs when the flow is obstructed or there is reduced absorption at the villi.

Q. How is hydrocephalus classified and what is the most common cause?

A. Hydrocephalus may be classified into communicating and obstructive. Obstructive is by far the commonest type. This is mostly as a result of congenital structural abnormalities in children and CNS tumours in adults.

PRINCIPLES OF SURGERY

CONSENT FOR TREATMENT

Q. How would you go about obtaining informed consent?

A. Informed consent for a surgical procedure involves discussion of:

- The main treatment options available
- The individual benefits of each treatment option
- Accurate information regarding this particular surgical option
- The risks associated with each option, including risks involved with other aspects of the procedure i.e. as a result of the anaesthetic, catheter etc.
- Whether the operation is entirely necessary and the effects of possibly not having the procedure at all
- The success rates of each option.

All of the above should be discussed in a calm, non-pressurized environment and in a manner that is understandable to the patient. It is a good idea to have such a discussion in the presence of a close friend or relative and to answer any questions they may have about the treatment itself or its possible implications for the patient's social circumstances.

It is also well known that patients don't always take in all of what is discussed. It is therefore a good idea to provide leaflet information and arrange a time for the patient to return once they've had a chance to think about the options.

Once they've come to an informed decision, I would then ask the patient to sign a consent form and assure them that they are entitled to change their mind at a later date.

Q. Are you obliged to inform all of your patients about all of the possible risks?

A. It is always a good idea to be as honest and informative as possible these days as patients tend to be better informed as a result of accessing information from the internet. However, as the surgeon obtaining informed consent, it is up to you how much information you wish to divulge.

Generally, you tend to give as much information as you feel the patient is able to understand. Sometimes, complications may have a greater impact on a person's life according to their profession i.e. an opera singer unable to reach the high notes after thyroid surgery.

Q. If you thought that some risks may upset your patient, for example the chance of death whilst undergoing a heart bypass procedure, is it acceptable not to mention it?

A. No, it is not acceptable to withhold vital information, no matter how distressing it may be to the patient. It is their right to make the decision about what's best for them.

Q. Who signs the consent form?

A. The patient and the surgeon obtaining the informed consent.

Q. What is the age limit?

A. Sixteen years of age is the cut-off limit; for children under 16 years of age the parent or carer must act on their behalf. Consent for a child under 16 may be obtained from the child if the child is deemed competent to understand the information and make an informed decision.

Q. Is a child allowed to refuse treatment?

A. A child's wishes should always be taken into consideration, however, if a child refuses treatment that will save their life, their decision may be overridden up to the age of 18.

Exceptions to this rule occur when a child has a terminal illness and has already undergone surgical treatment and understands the implications.

Q. If you have a patient with learning difficulties or mental illness, is it acceptable to obtain consent from their carer?

A. If a patient has learning difficulties, their competence and understanding may be assessed prior to any decision making. It may be that they are unable to make a decision regarding emergency or elective surgery, in which case, no other adult is allowed to sign the consent form for them. The surgeon must then take responsibility for the patient and come to a decision with the carer as to what is in the patient's best interests.

In the case of mental illness, a similar level of competence must be assessed. A person may be placed under a mental health act and given treatment for their mental illness without consent. However, consent must be obtained for treatment/ procedures that are not related to their mental illness i.e. appendicitis. The only circumstances in which consent may be overridden are when a procedure is required to save the person's life and where the person is delusional and is unable to give informed consent. In these circumstances, the surgeon must take responsibility for the decision and the patient's carer must be in full agreement.

Q. Is the consent form legal proof that informed consent was obtained?

A. No, it is documentation that provides some evidence that informed consent was obtained. However, it does not prove that the information given was comprehensive and satisfactory under the circumstances.

Q. What is battery?

A. Battery is the violation of a civil law which forbids intentionally touching another person without consent.

Q. When is confidentiality legally allowed to be breached?

A. It may be breached in the public interest when:

- A patient is suspected to be involved with terrorism
- A patient is known to have a notifiable disease
- When a judge demands it
- When evidence is required in an NHS tribunal.

It may also be breached in the patient's interests:

- If a patient is unable to communicate their medical history due to psychological or physical effects of illness, relatives may be consulted
- In the case of a surgeon sharing the information with colleagues who will be helping with the procedure, as the success of the operation will depend on all of those involved being well informed.

ANTIBIOTIC PROPHYLAXIS

Q. What is the point of antibiotic prophylaxis?

A. Antibiotic prophylaxis is used to:

- Prevent postoperative wound infection
- Prevent sepsis in sites where instrumentation may introduce colonization of bacteria.

It is also used in surgery where there is a high risk of infection i.e. bowel surgery, and where the consequences of infection would be disastrous i.e. cardiac valve/joint replacement surgery.

Q. What regimes do you know of?

A. The choice of antibiotic is dependent on the likely microorgansims i.e. cefuroxime and metronidazole in bowel surgery, gentamicin in urological procedures.

It has been shown that short courses are the most effective. Anything longer is deemed unnecessary. It is therefore given as a single intravenous dose on induction so that tissue levels are maximal when surgery occurs. A second dose may be given if the surgery proves to be lengthy. In high-risk cases, a short course comprising two further postoperative doses, at 8 and 16 hours, may be given.

SURGICAL INFECTION

Q. In what sorts of surgery is infection a serious problem?

- Surgery with a high risk of contamination and thus a high incidence of infection.
- Surgery with a low risk of infection but where the consequences are catastrophic (e.g. prosthetic heart valves, ventriculo-peritoneal shunts, joint replacement).

Q. What are the sources of surgical infection?

A. They may be endogenous and exogenous.

Endogenous

This means it is found within the patient. It may be normal flora or organisms that have colonized after antibiotic therapy:

- Respiratory tract – *Haemophilus*, *Streptococcus viridans*, diphtheriods
- Gastrointestinal tract – *E. coli*, anaerobes, *Pseudomonas*
- Genitourinary tract – anaerobes, lactobacilli.

Exogenous

The source may come from other patients, hospital staff, visitors, hospital equipment.

Q. Different types of surgery pose different risks of endogenous infection. How may these types of surgery be classified? What are the approximate rates of deep infection for each category?

Clean	No non-sterile viscus breached	1.5%
	No inflammation encountered	
Clean contaminated	Non-sterile viscus breached	6%
	No significant spillage	
Contaminated	Inflammation without pus encountered or	13%
	Gross spillage from viscus	
Dirty	Frank pus or perforation encountered	40%

National Research Council Division of Medical Sciences (1964).

Q. How are exogenous risks minimized?

A.
- Hand scrub (chlorhexidene or povidone iodine)
- Sterile gown and gloves
- *Not* shaving the area (if absolutely necessary, use clippers immediately preoperatively)
  Clean wound infection rates (CWIR):
  - Shaved > 2 hours preoperatively   2.3%
  - Clipped   1.7%
  - Neither   0.9%.

- Skin preparation:
  - 1% iodine in 70% alcohol (antibacterial action as skin prep dries)
  - 0.5% chlorhexidine in 70% alcohol
  - Aqueous povidone iodine (non-flammable/may be used on open wounds).

- Drapes:
  - Cotton or disposable equally good
  - Plastic adhesive drapes *increase* infection rates.

- Duration of surgery – CWIR doubles every hour.
- Surgical technique:
  - Respect for tissue
  - Minimize foreign material

- Haemostasis
- Care in closure (CWIR: sutures > clips > steristrips).

Q. What other techniques are of proven benefit in ultra-clean prosthetic surgery?

A.
- Ultra-clean air with laminar flow (halves major joint infection rate from 3.4% to 1.6%)
- Exhaust ventilated suits (major joint infection rate is 0.9%).

Q. What is the role of perioperative antibiotic prophylaxis?

A. Antibiotic prophylaxis is only ever an adjunct to good surgical practice.

Antibiotic prophylaxis is mandatory for prosthetic surgery and when the risk of contamination is significant.

There is some evidence that antibiotic prophylaxis may reduce the infection rate even in clean surgery (Platt et al NEJM 1989).

Q. What are the risks associated with antibiotic therapy?

A.
- Allergy/anaphylaxis
- Toxicity (e.g. oto/nephrotoxicity of aminoglycosides)
- Gastrointestinal upset
- Resistance
- Superinfection from resistant organisms (e.g. pseudomembranous colitis secondary to *Clostridium difficile*).

References

National Research Council Division of Medical Sciences, Ad hoc committee of the Committee of Trauma. Post-operative wound infections: the influence of ultra-violet irradiation of the operating room and various other factors. Ann Surg (1964) 160 (suppl 2) p. 1.
Platt R, Zaleznik DF, Hopkins CC et al. Perioperative antibiotic prophylaxis for herniorrhaphy and breast surgery. N Engl J Med (1989) 322 pp 153–60.

DVT PROPHYLAXIS

Q. You are called to see a 65-year old lady on the ward who is day 5, post left total knee replacement. She is complaining of pain in her left calf and on examination you find that she has a swollen lower limb. What is the most likely diagnosis?

A. A deep vein thrombosis.

Q. What else may the diagnosis be?

A. The differential diagnosis includes:

- Cellulitis
- Peripheral oedema – as a result of congestive cardiac failure
- Calf haematoma
- Achilles tendonitis
- Torn gastrocnemius
- Ruptured Baker's cyst
- Knee haemarthrosis
- Thrombophlebitis.

Q. Where do deep vein thromboses commonly occur?

A. They can occur in any limb; however, they are commonest in the pelvis and lower limbs.

Q. What are the risk factors associated with deep vein thromboses?

A. The risk factors include:

- Increasing age
- Sex
- Immobilization/bed rest/long-haul flights
- Operations especially orthopaedic/anaesthetic
- Pregnancy
- Malignancy
- Obesity
- Injury
- Cardiac failure
- Myocardial infarction
- Varicose veins
- Previous history of DVT/PE
- Occupation
- Arterial ischaemia
- Drugs especially the combined oral contraceptive pill
- Vasculitis i.e. Buerger's disease
- Congenital disorders i.e. Hippel–Trenaunay syndrome.

Q. How would you investigate a patient who you felt clinically had a DVT?

A. I would take a full history and examine the patient. I would look for any relevant risk factors such as recent long flights or operations. I would then commence empirical treatment for a DVT and arrange for an urgent duplex scan to be performed of the affected limb.

Q. Is there any other way of confirming a diagnosis of a DVT?

A. Phlebography.

Q. What is the treatment of DVT?

A. The usual treatment involves heparinization until the diagnosis is confirmed and then warfarinization for 6 months for above-knee DVTs. Below-knee DVTs don't require formal warfarinization.

Q. How would you go about reducing the risk of a DVT developing in a patient coming in for surgery?

A. Firstly, I would identify any patients at high risk of developing a DVT such as the elderly and anyone who has previously been diagnosed with a DVT. Then I would ensure that all patients were given TED stockings preoperatively and given advice on mobilizing and perhaps not smoking, if appropriate. Intraoperatively there are several devices available to help reduce the risk of developing a DVT. These include:

- Intermittent pneumatic compression devices
- Electrical calf-stimulation devices.

Postoperatively, I would prescribe daily subcutaneous injections of low molecular weight heparin and encourage early mobilization.

Q. What are the risks associated with an untreated DVT?

A. The risks include the formation of a pulmonary embolism which is a potentially life-threatening condition.

FITNESS FOR ANAESTHESIA

Q. What do you know about the Confidential Enquiry into Perioperative Deaths (CEPOD)?

A. CEPOD was a report conducted in 1987 looking specifically at factors that may have contributed to perioperative deaths. The essential message from the report was that patients undergoing surgery, particularly emergency surgery, after 9 p.m. seemed to be at increased risk of perioperative mortality.

Q. Why do you think that this is the case?

A. The main contributing factors were:

- Poor surgical pre-assessment
- Poor preparation for anaesthesia
- Emergency surgery
- Lack of supervision for junior anaesthetists and surgeons late at night.

Q. Do you know of any classification systems that quantify the risk of death while under an anaesthetic?

A. The American Society of Anaesthesiologists have produced a grading system used by anaesthetists that quantifies mortality risk with physical status. It is called the ASA classification system (American Association of Anesthesiologists, 1963):

- ASA 1 – normal patient
- ASA 2 – mild systemic disease i.e. diabetes mellitus
- ASA 3 – severe disease that limits activity i.e. stable angina
- ASA 4 – severe systemic disease that is a constant threat to life i.e. heart failure
- ASA 5 – moribund, not expected to survive more than 24 hours i.e. ruptured aortic aneurysm.
- E – emergency

Q. How would you go about assessing a patient's fitness for anaesthesia?

A. First, I would confirm that the planned operation was appropriate for the patient in question. Then I would take a full history and carry out an examination in order to exclude any significant medical problems.

I would also pay particular attention to the patient's drug history as they may have allergies, for example to penicillin. Similarly, special care needs to be taken with patients on warfarin and oral steroids.

Q. What investigations would you consider performing?

A. Depending on the age and medical condition of the patient and type of operation, I would consider the following:

- Blood tests – FBC, U+E, LFT, G+S and cross-match if necessary
- Chest X-ray – anyone over 50 years of age or with a history of smoking or respiratory problems
- ECG – anyone over 40 years of age or with a history of cardiac disease.

Q. Is it always necessary to perform these investigations?

A. No, in a young and fit patient no investigations need be performed. They are usually performed for patients over 40 years of age or with underlying medical problems.

Q. What other issues are there for you to consider preoperatively as a surgical SHO?

A. Other preoperative considerations include:

- Obtaining informed consent
- Preparation of the operation site – hair removal
- Marking of the operation site – using an indelible marker pen
- Writing up antibiotic prophylaxis if necessary
- Bowel preparation – if necessary
- DVT prophylaxis – a consideration for all patients undergoing surgery.

Q. **You are a surgical SHO called to see a patient in Accident and Emergency (A&E) who needs a laparotomy for bowel obstruction. The patient is a 79-year-old man who has smoked all of his life and also has diabetes. How would you go about preparing him for theatre?**

A. First, I would take a full history and do an examination, and check that the planned operation was appropriate for the patient. Then I would contact the duty anaesthetist and inform him/her about the patient, the need for surgery and the patient's medical problems.

I would then assess the patient for hypovolaemia, electrolyte imbalance and hypothermia. I would insert a urinary catheter, ensure that the patient was adequately resuscitated and treat any underlying hypothermia. I would like to take blood for FBC, U+Es, LFTs and cross-match four units of blood. I would also obtain a chest X-ray and an ECG.

Since the patient was a lifelong smoker, I would be concerned about his respiratory function. Out of hours it is difficult to obtain respiratory function tests which would be my ideal investigation of choice. Given the circumstances, I would obtain a chest X-ray and peak flow in A&E and then perform an arterial blood gas analysis. This would give me some indication of the patient's lung function and would also detect an acidosis which may need correcting preoperatively.

If I detected severe underlying chronic obstructive airway disease, I would also be concerned about the cardiac function of this gentleman. The diabetes would also be a contributing factor to this. Unfortunately, only an ECG and chest X-ray would aid me in assessing this patient's cardiac function at this stage. However, if I was very concerned I would arrange an urgent assessment by a cardiology registrar in A&E.

I would also like to obtain more information regarding the type of diabetes this gentleman has, the treatment he has for it, and whether it generally is under control. I would obtain a bedside BM glucose measurement and send a blood sample to the laboratory for a serum glucose measurement. If there was any doubt regarding the control of the diabetes, I would place the patient on a sliding scale.

I would like to discuss intravenous access with the anaesthetist. Given the patient's age, underlying medical problems and the risks of surgery, I would consider the need for a central line and an arterial line. I would also inform ITU of the need for a bed postoperatively.

Before surgery, I would ensure that informed consent was obtained. I would specifically consent this gentleman for:

- Operative mortality
- ITU admission postoperatively
- Possibility of a stoma
- Chest infection
- Poor wound healing/infection.

I would also like to discuss the treatment plan with any relatives, if available.

I would commence prophylactic antibiotics, DVT prophylaxis and inform my registrar before proceeding to theatre.

Q. What antibiotics would you commence?

A. I would commence intravenous cefuroxime and metronidazole.

Reference

American Society of Anesthesiologists. Anesthesiology (1963) 24 p. 111

DISINFECTION AND STERILIZATION

Q. What is the difference between sterilization and disinfection?

A. Sterilization is the eradication of *all* microorganisms including bacterial spores and viruses.

Disinfection is the eradication of most microorganisms (bacterial spores and slow viruses may survive). Note: prions survive many modern 'sterilization' procedures.)

Q. How may surgical instruments be sterilized?

A. • Wet heat (wrapped instrument sets are sterilized in a porous load autoclave; 'Little Sister' type autoclaves may be used for unwrapped instruments):
  – 134°C at 30 lbs/square inch for 3–10 min
  – 121°C at 15 lbs/square inch for 15–30 min

(Note: brown stripes appear on Bowie–Dick tape after a sterilizing period of wet heat.)

- Dry heat (less corrosive but poorer results) – 160°C for 2 hours
- Ethylene oxide gas (e.g. for sutures)
- Gamma irradiation (e.g. for catheters and syringes)
- Glutaraldehyde (e.g. 'Cidex' for gastroscopes):
  – 4 min immersion for disinfection
  – Up to 3 hours for sterilization.

Q. What disinfection agents are used on skin?

A. There are several commercially available skin disinfectants:

- Alcohol – effective against gram positive and negative bacteria but not fungi and spores
- Chlorhexidine – non-toxic and effective against *Staphylococcus aureus*
- Iodine – effective against bacteria, fungi, viruses and spores; can stain.

Q. What does the term 'cleaning' mean?

A. Cleaning entails the removal of obvious dirt/contamination without eradication of any organisms.

METHICILLIN-RESISTANT STAPHYLOCOCCUS AUREUS

Q. What is *Staphylococcus aureus*?

A. *Staphylococcus aureus* is a bacterium which is prevalent within the community and hospital populations. It is aerobic and gram-stain positive, appearing in clusters on the gram stain. It can colonize up to 30% of the healthy population, and is usually found in the nose or skin. It leads to localized, superficial, self-limiting abscesses when the skin is disrupted.

Q. Tell me about the different antibiotics that are available for treating *S. aureus*.

A. The antibiotic treatment of *S. aureus* infections was transformed by the introduction of penicillin. Penicillin and semi-synthetic penicillins act by interfering with the synthesis of the bacterial cell wall peptidoglycan.

Since the initial introduction of penicillin in the 1940s, resistant strains of *S. aureus* have become increasingly isolated. It is now estimated that over 80% of *S. aureus* strains are resistant to penicillin alone. Through plasmid transmission, a gene responsible for the formation of the enzyme β-lactamase has enabled the bacterium to become resistant. The enzyme cleaves the β-lactam ring, an integral part of the antibiotic structure. Cephalosporins are also degraded by β-lactamases, which makes them equally as ineffective.

Some semi-synthetic penicillins, such as methicillin and flucloxacillin, are relatively resistant to the effects of β-lactamases. This enables them to still be an effective treatment against the majority of strains of *S. aureus*.

Other penicillins have been combined with clavulanic acid, a natural inhibitor of β-lactamase. Clavulanic acid binds covalently to the enzyme. The resulting complex is cleaved very slowly, protecting the penicillin from the enzyme.

Since the 1960s, strains of resistance have been found even to methicillin and flucloxacillin. By the production of a penicillin-binding protein, the bacterium is able to gain resistance. It is estimated that 50% of nosocomial infections are now methicillin-resistant *S. aureus*.

Vancomycin and teicoplanin, both glycopeptide antibiotics inhibiting cell wall synthesis, or the anti-tuberculosis drug rifampicin are now the treatment for cases of methicillin-resistant *S. aureus*.

There are now reported cases of methicillin-resistant *S. aureus* which are resistant to even these antibiotics. Newer antibiotics, such as linezolid, an oxazolidione, are however still effective.

Q. Who is susceptible to methicillin-resistant *S. aureus*?

A. The majority of carriers will not be susceptible to infection. Methicillin-resistant *S. aureus* seems to be more virile than methicillin-sensitive *S. aureus*, although the vast majority of healthy individuals who are colonized with it will remain disease free. In vulnerable populations, it can lead to clinical infection, particularly wound and skin infections, osteomyelitis, endocarditis, pneumonia, urinary tract infections and septicaemia.

It tends to colonize institutions, such as nursing homes and hospitals. Factors associated with the acquisition of methicillin-resistant *S. aureus* in the acute care setting include the use of broad-spectrum antibiotics, the longer duration of use and the greater number of antibiotics, surgery, chronic illness, ITU or burns unit admissions or proximity to another methicillin-resistant *S. aureus* infected patient.

Transmission between hospitals is common, presumably from movement of infected health care workers. These strains are known as endemic methicillin-resistant *S. aureus*. Worryingly, these strains are the most likely to be responsible for clinical infection.

Q. What can be done to control the spread of methicillin-resistant *S. aureus*?

A. The single most important measure in controlling the spread of methicillin-resistant *S. aureus* is thorough hand washing of health workers and patients. This is by far the most important strategy for the prevention of transmission. Gloves and aprons should be worn, by staff and visitors. Patients should be in an isolated room, which is cleaned after they have left.

Colonized patients and staff should be treated with mupirocin, to the skin and nose, in addition to washing the rest of the body and hair with disinfectants, such as chlorhexidine. This eliminates the bacteria and limits the spread to other parts of the body.

Strict adherence to microbial guidelines for the use of all antibiotics is also essential. This will help to prevent the potentially devastating growth of resistance to all antimicrobials.

PRINCIPLES OF SKIN COVER

Q. In what circumstances may it be difficult or inappropriate to close a surgical incision?

A. It may be difficult to close wounds in the following circumstances:

- Loss of skin – excision of cutaneous lesion; traumatic skin loss (with or without further debridement); secondary defect (harvest site for graft or flap)
- Subcutaneous swelling – post fasciotomy
- Infection – incision and drainage of abscess.

Q. What options are available to the surgeon if the skin cannot be closed directly?

A. • Leave it open – either pending further surgery or for it to heal spontaneously ('secondary intent')
• Skin graft
• Flap.

Q. What is a skin graft?

A. A graft is organic material harvested from one site on an individual and transferred to another site or another individual. Nutrition at the recipient site depends on diffusion over short distances or rapid neovascularization:

• Autograft – from one site to another in the same individual (Gr Autos – self)
• Allograft – from one individual to another of the same species (Gr Allos – other)
• Xenograft – from one individual to another of a different species (Gr Xenos – stranger).

Q. What tissues may be used as graft material?

A. Skin, bone, cornea, vein and artery.

Q. What difference does the thickness of a skin graft make?

A. The difference is as follows:

Full thickness skin graft (epidermis and full dermis)	Split thick skin graft (epidermis and variable depth of dermis)
Donor site must be closed or grafted	Donor site healing from dermal islands
More likely to fail	Less likely to fail (the thinner the better)
Better cosmesis	Less good cosmesis
Less cicatricial contracture	More contracture (the thicker the better)

Q. What tissues will not accept skin grafts?

A. Tendon, bone and cartilage. Note: paratenon, periosteum and perichondrium *will* accept a graft, but poorly.)

Q. What is a flap?

A. A flap is a vascularized single tissue type or combination of tissue types transferred from one site to another on the same individual. The vascular pedicle for the flap either remains intact or is divided and then re-anastomosed at the recipient site. (Note: vascularized tissues transferred between different individuals are not alloflaps but transplants.)

Q. What tissue types may be transferred as flaps?

A. Cutaneous/fasciocutaneous/myocutaneous/osteomyocutaneous/muscle.

Q. How else might flaps be classified?

A. According to the treatment of the vascular pedicle:

- Local flaps – transposition, rotation
- Pedicled flaps – latissimus dorsi (LD)
- Free flaps – transverse rectus abdominis muscle (TRAM), deep inferior epigastric perforator (DIEP).

SCARS

Q. What factors affect the appearance of a scar following the excision of a simple skin lesion?

A. The patient, the lesion and the surgery all affect the appearance of the scar.

Patient

- Age (more prominent in young/keloids and hypertrophy more common)
- Skin type (more prominent in oily and coarse skin types)
- Skin colour (affects keloid risk, see below).

Lesion

- Size
- Shape
- Site (keloids most common overlying the sternum).

Surgery

- Planning – orientation of incision (Langer's lines/lines of election); 'hiding' incision in natural junctions (e.g. nasolabial fold on face); local flaps
- Technique – tissue handling; asepsis; haemostasis; accurate suture technique (accurate apposition, no inversion or tension).

Q. What is the difference between a keloid and a hypertrophic scar?

A. A hypertrophic scar is raised above the surrounding skin but is restricted to the area of the scar.

A keloid scar encroaches into the skin beyond the original scar.

Q. What factors make keloids more likely?

A. The factors predisposing to keloids include:

- Skin colour – most prevalent in black skin, followed by Asian then Caucasian
- Age – more common in the young
- Site – order of prevalence is pre-sternal > deltoid > chest.

Q. What treatments are available for keloid scars?

A. Intralesional triamcinolone and silicon gel pads.

WOUND DEHISCENCE

Q. What is wound dehiscence?

A. Wound dehiscence is the breakdown of a wound, which occurs around 5–10 days after surgery. It is rare and has an incidence of 1%. There may be a warning discharge of serosanguinous fluid known as the 'pink fluid' sign. This is followed by protrusion of the omentum with or without intestine through the wound margins and can be seen beneath the skin sutures. It most commonly occurs in abdominal wounds.

Q. Can you tell me the risk factors associated with this condition?

A. The commonest cause is inadequate abdominal wall repair. This may be due to poor surgical technique involving suture technique and choice of suture material. It is more common in emergency procedures. The same risk factors for incisional hernia apply to wound dehiscence. These include:

General

- Nutritional – deficiencies of zinc and vitamin C
- Systemic disease – diabetes, malignancy, jaundice and respiratory disease
- Drug-related – steroid therapy, smoking
- Obesity
- Emergency procedures.

Local

- Skin conditions – local infection, previous irradiation
- Poor blood supply
- Foreign body in the wound
- Site of wound – anterior tibial, scaphoid, neck of femur and talus
- Surgeon-related.

Maximizing these preoperatively reduces the risk of a dehiscence occurring.

Q. How might you avoid wound dehiscence?

A. Wound dehiscence may be avoided by identifying those most at risk preoperatively, correcting the risk factors if possible, and then using good surgical technique at all times. Good surgical technique involves choosing the right type of suture. Generally it is acceptable to close the abdomen on mass with non-absorbable nylon or a slowly absorbable synthetic suture such as polydioxanone, which retains its tensile strength. Sutures must be placed approximately 1 cm apart, taking large bites, and the suture length must be at least four times as long as the length of the wound.

Q. Who described this rule?

A. Jenkins.

Q. How would you manage a case of abdominal wound dehiscence?

A. In cases of wound dehiscence it is important to recognize the problem early, as the condition is associated with a mortality of up to 40%. As I mentioned earlier, there may be an initial discharge of pink watery fluid, a low-grade pyrexia and abdominal pain. It is important at this stage to adequately resuscitate the patient by obtaining intravenous access, giving fluid therapy and possibly using antibiotics. If the omentum and intestines were visible I would cover them with warm, betadine soaked towels. I would then proceed quickly to re-explore the abdomen under general anaesthetic followed by peritoneal lavage. I would then re-suture the abdominal wall by mass closure using interrupted deep tension suture.

RADIOTHERAPY

Q. What is the purpose of tumour staging?

A. The purpose of tumour staging is:

- To plan treatment
- To gain an indication of prognosis
- To evaluate results
- To exchange information between centres
- To contribute to the investigation/research into cancer.

Q. What do you understand by the terms 'adjuvant' and 'neoadjuvant therapy?'

A. Adjuvant therapy is cancer treatment that occurs after surgery and neoadjuvant therapy is treatment that occurs prior to surgery. It may include radiotherapy, chemotherapy or hormonal therapy. The aim of neoadjuvant therapy is to shrink or downstage an inoperable tumour thereby making it operable. The patient is treated with radiotherapy, for example, and is later re-imaged to assess response prior to surgery.

Q. How does this differ from primary treatment?

A. Primary treatment is the use of radiotherapy, chemotherapy or hormonal therapy in the first instance. The clinical response is monitored; however, surgery may or may not occur in the future. This is usually reserved for patients with advanced disease whose outcome will not be affected by surgery, and elderly patients not fit for an anaesthetic or not willing to undergo surgery.

Q. What is radiotherapy?

A. Radiotherapy involves the therapeutic use of photons (X-rays, γ-rays) or subatomic particles (electrons, neutrons) in cancer management.

The definition of ionizing radiation is the amount of energy absorbed per unit mass of tissue. It is measured in grays (Gy). 1 Gy = the absorption of 1 joule per kilogram of tissue.

Q. What is a linear accelerator?

A. A linear accelerator is a machine used to deliver accelerated electrons at the speed of light. The depth of tissue penetration can be altered for each individual tumour and, once delivered, the radiation decays rapidly in the tissues targeted.

Q. What is the mechanism by which radiotherapy damages cancer cells?

A. Radiotherapy damages nuclear DNA. It does this indirectly by producing highly reactive radicals which then damage the cell's DNA. The unstable radicals cause chromosomal damage and, if left unrepaired, result in cell death. The cellular damage that results may also cause the cell to undergo apoptosis.

The amount of damage is proportional to the dose of radiation administered.

Q. Which tumours are sensitive to radiotherapy and which are resistant?

A. They may be classified into the following groups:

- Highly sensitive – lymphoma, myeloma, seminoma, Ewing's sarcoma, Wilm's tumour
- Moderately sensitive – breast cancer, ovarian cancer, teratoma, basal cell carcinoma, small cell lung cancer
- Moderately resistant – cervical carcinoma, bladder carcinoma, rectal carcinoma, sarcomas, squamous cell lung cancer
- Highly resistant – melanoma, osteosarcoma, carcinoma of the pancreas.

Q. What determines whether a tumour will be sensitive to radiotherapy?

A. Cells are thought to be less affected by radiation-induced damage if they are hypoxic. Therefore a tumour will only be sensitive to radiotherapy if it is well vascularized.

Generally, the most effective way of administering the doses is by small daily doses as opposed to fewer larger ones. This is because the tumour is allowed to shrink, and it becomes less hypoxic; also the surrounding normal tissues have time to recover.

Q. What factors does the radiotherapist have to take into account when planning treatment?

A. There are several factors to take into consideration:

- The extent of the tumour (assessed by CT or MRI scan)
- Tolerance of normal tissues to the radiation i.e. bowel
- Radiosensitivity of the tumour
- Possible inclusion of nearby lymph nodes.

Q. How is damage to surrounding structures minimized?

A. Careful planning using three-dimensional imaging is undertaken to ensure that the maximum radiation dose is delivered to the tumour itself and not to the normal surrounding tissues. This is achieved by creating moulds as in head and neck cancers or tattooing the chest wall as in breast cancer. This ensures that the same position is achieved each time the patient returns for their next radiation dose.

Radiotherapists may also use 'wedged' fields. This technique is used when multiple fields are necessary; it is a process by which fields are wedged to alter the distribution of the dose and so don't cause excess damage at the sites where they overlap.

A 'shrinking technique' is also employed these days to allow the margins of treatment to be reduced in the last few weeks of treatment.

Q. What are the possible complications associated with radiotherapy?

A. These may be separated into acute and late onset. Acute side effects usually occur within the first 2–3 months and include:

- Fatigue
- Anorexia and nausea
- Erythema/desquamation (skin irradiation)
- Mucosal irradiation (oral cavity irradiation)
- Dysphagia (thoracic irradiation)
- Temporary alopecia (mantle irradiation)
- Diarrhoea (abdominal irradiation)
- Sterility (gonadal irradiation).

Late-onset side effects tend to occur months to years after treatment and are usually as a result of damage to the surrounding normal structures. They include:

- Telangiectasia, SCC (skin irradiation)
- Loss of saliva production (oral cavity irradiation)
- Pulmonary damage (thoracic irradiation)
- Bowel strictures (abdominal irradiation)
- Lhermitte's syndrome – numbness and shooting pains in the lumbar spine (associated with mantle irradiation)
- Permanent azoospermia and amenorrhoea (gonadal irradiation).

CHEMOTHERAPY

Q. Why would you consider giving a patient chemotherapy?

A. Chemotherapy is used in the treatment of cancer: for cure, for the prevention of recurrence, to shrink tumours and so prolong life. There are several treatment regimes:

- Primary chemotherapy – chemotherapy is given as the mainstay of treatment.
- Neoadjuvant chemotherapy – chemotherapy is given as the initial treatment with the aim of future surgery (for example, in a young woman with a large, high-grade breast cancer neoadjuvant therapy is given in order to downsize it and potentially avoid a mastectomy).

- Adjuvant chemotherapy – given after surgery in order to gain control of the primary disease.
- Palliative chemotherapy.

Q. What factors are there to consider when planning to administer chemotherapy?

A. There are several factors:

- Type of cancer
- Stage of cancer and extent of spread
- Patient's age
- State of health including other medical conditions i.e. diabetes
- Previous treatments for cancer i.e. radiotherapy, hormonal therapy.

Q. Do all patients receive the same dose?

A. No, it is adjusted according to weight and height. Each patient's body surface area (BSA) is estimated and cycles are given at intervals so as to allow the body's normal tissues to recover.

Q. What cancers do you know of that are chemosensitive?

A. Chemosensitive tumours include:

- Breast cancer
- Lymphomas
- Leukaemia
- Small cell lung cancer
- Testicular – teratoma and seminoma
- Ewing's sarcoma
- Ovarian
- Head and neck cancers.

Q. Can you name any that don't respond to chemotherapy?

A. Melanoma, cervical and pancreatic cancers don't respond to chemotherapy.

Q. What determines whether or not a tumour is chemosensitive?

A. Cytotoxic agents interfere with cellular proliferation and growth in different ways. Tumours, however, often develop resistance to the drugs. Once a tumour has become very large, the efficacy of cytotoxics is reduced, however, generally there is a dose–response relationship with most cytotoxics. But since cytotoxics also interfere with normal cellular proliferation, the dosage is limited by the toxic effects on normal tissues.

Q. When is it appropriate to give high dose chemotherapy?

A. High dose chemotherapy is indicated in otherwise fit patients where a cure may be achieved e.g. leukaemia.

Q. What are the drawbacks of this?

A. The drawback of this regime is the possible profound toxic effects on the bone marrow. It is now possible to use stem cell support in order to protect the body from overwhelming sepsis during treatment. This may be harvested from the patient (autologous transplant) or from a matched donor (allogenic transplant).

Q. How would you categorize cytotoxics?

A. Cytotoxics may be categorized according to their mechanism of action:

- Alkylating agents – impair the function of enzymes which form DNA strands, thereby inhibiting mitosis. Examples chlorambucil/cyclophosphamide.
- Anti-metabolites – irreversibly interrupt DNA. Examples methotrexate/5-FU.
- Vinca alkaloids – inhibit microtubule function. Examples vincristine/vinblastine.
- Anti-mitotic agents – cause damage by the production of free radicals. Examples adriamycin/doxorubicin.

Q. Can you name any side effects of chemotherapy?

A. Side effects of chemotherapy may be categorized into early and late:

Early

- Nausea and vomiting
- Diarrhoea/constipation
- Ulcers/mucositis
- Alopecia
- Local thrombophlebitis
- Bone marrow suppression – neutropenia, thrombocytopenia, leucopenia.

Late

- Infertility
- Risk of developing a second cancer.

Q. What do you know about the use of hormonal therapy in oncology?

A. Hormonal therapy has a well recognized use in the treatment of oestrogen (ER) and progesterone (PR) receptor-positive breast tumours. Approximately 70% of breast tumours are ER/PR positive. As a result, these tumours are amenable to hormonal manipulation using various agents:

- Tamoxifen – longstanding, effective oestrogen receptor antagonist.
- Anastrazole – newer, highly effective aromatase inhibitor (prevents the conversion of androgens into oestrogen in peripheral fatty tissues). Currently it is only licensed in the treatment of advanced breast cancer. Trials are underway to assess its use as adjuvant therapy in place of tamoxifen.

- Exemestane – aromatase inhibitor. As with anastrazole, aromatase inhibitors are associated with fewer side effects than tamoxifen (vaginal bleeding, discharge, hot flushes, endometrial cancer, ischaemic heart disease, deep vein thrombosis and pulmonary embolus).

Patients who are ER/PR positive and receive hormonal therapy tend to have an overall improved prognosis.

Q. Do you know of any recent advances in chemotherapy?

A. Liposomal therapy

This involves the use of synthetic fat globules ('liposomes') in order to administer cytotoxics. This method of administration leads to a more selective penetration of cancer cells and thereby causes fewer adverse effects.

- An example of a cytotoxic administered by liposomes is DOXIL – encapsulated doxorubicin.

Chemoprotective agents

Several agents have been developed in order to prevent adverse effects associated with specific cytotoxic agents:

- Dexrazoxane – prevents cardiac effects
- Amifostine – protects the kidney
- Mesna – protects the bladder.

PALLIATIVE CARE

Q. What do you understand by the term palliative care?

A. Palliative care is the branch of medicine that deals with dying. It involves all aspects of a patient's care, including social, psychological and medical needs.

Q. One of your patients has deteriorated overnight. They have been thoroughly reviewed and after discussion with the patient's family it is decided that the patient should be allowed to die. How would you proceed?

A. It is important that the patient is allowed to die without symptoms and with dignity.

I would make sure that the patient was not in any pain. If necessary, adequate analgesia should be given. This can be given orally, intravenously or by using a subcutaneous pump.

Problems such as constipation should be treated with laxatives. Sickness should be treated with anti-emetics.

Ideally the patient should be moved to a quiet side room; their family might wish to be present. Any religious wishes should be respected.

Most hospitals employ palliative care nurses. They should be contacted for specific advice regarding symptoms. Family members may also wish to speak with them, and their advice in these situations is usually extremely helpful (see Tip).

Any investigations or blood tests which may have been previously requested should be cancelled. Potentially degrading objects, such as nasogastric tubes, should be removed, unless they are obviously benefiting the patient.

Q. Could you tell me more about the use of subcutaneous pumps?

A. They can be used to relieve a range of symptoms. They are small, automated pumps which deliver regular amounts of drugs. They are usually changed every 24 hours and the amount of drugs to be used in the next 24-hour period is reviewed. It is important to ensure symptom relief without overdosing the patient; an example is the use of diamorphine to relieve pain without causing increased nausea.

Q. Do you know of any other drugs that can be used in a subcutaneous pump?

A. Many combinations of drugs can be used in a subcutaneous pump. Unfortunately many drugs can interact within the pump and great caution should always be used when combining them.

The combination of drugs used will reflect the clinical needs of the patient. They can include anti-emetics, such as cyclizine, and anti-cholinergic drugs, such as hyoscine, to decrease secretions.

Q. What is the place of surgery in palliative care?

A. Surgery has many roles in palliative care. It is often done to relieve specific symptoms. There are many examples, including a defunctioning colostomy if an inoperable bowel tumour is causing obstruction; ERCP and insertion of a stent to relieve jaundice in a patient with pancreatic or gallbladder malignancy; pathological fractures caused by metastatic bone deposits are often nailed to provide stability, restoration of function and pain relief; stents can be inserted into the bronchus or oesophagus to relieve obstruction and improve symptoms.

 TIP

Any opportunity to mention other health care professionals should be taken. They provide both expert advice and time, both of which improve patient satisfaction and care. This may include physiotherapists, occupational therapists, breast, bowel or palliative care nurses; these are just some examples.

Mentioning other disciplines improves viva technique and shows a level of clinical experience in the candidate, earned from hard hours on the wards.

SCREENING

Q. What do you understand by the term screening?

A. Screening is population testing in order to identify asymptomatic individuals with a particular disease or pre-disease states. It can be directed towards the whole population, for example mammography, or groups considered to be at high risk of developing disease e.g. familial polyposis coli.

Q. What factors are considered necessary for a good screening program?

A. Screening offers a test to previously asymptomatic individuals, which leads to many ethical considerations and false-positive results. In addition, the high financial cost of screening programs means that the benefits have to be clearly and undeniably established.

These reasons have led the WHO to draw up guidelines in order to judge whether a screening program is likely to be effective:

1. The condition being screened for should be an important health problem.
2. The natural history of the disease should be well understood.
3. There should be a detectable early stage.
4. Treatment at an early stage should be of more benefit than at a later stage.
5. There should be a suitable test for the early stage.
6. The test should be acceptable.
7. Intervals for repeating the test should be determined.
8. There should be adequate health service provision for the extra clinical workload resulting from the screening.
9. The risks, both physical and psychological, should be less than the benefits.
10. The costs should be balanced against the benefits.

Q. What do you understand by the terms specificity and sensitivity?

A. A screening test is measured by its ability to do what it is supposed to do; this is the ability to correctly categorize persons who have pre-clinical disease as test positive and those who do not as test negative. In order to do this, the screening test needs to have high specificity and sensitivity. Sensitivity is the probability of testing positive if the disease is truly present. Specificity is defined as the probability of screening negative if the disease is truly absent.

Q. Do you know of any criticisms of screening programs?

A. There are several problems associated with screening programs, which lead to difficulty in evaluating screening programs. These include the type of patients who participate in screening programs. They tend to be more health conscious than those who do not, for example, women who have regular mammography will also tend to self-examine their breasts at other times.

Apparent improvements in the length of survival may be due to adding extra months or years as a result of earlier diagnosis. Screening is also more likely to detect slow-growing tumours with a better prognosis. Pre-invasive conditions, such as cervical neoplasia in situ, are treated as 'cases'. Not all of these conditions would have led to invasive or fatal disease.

All of these factors can lead to overestimation of the benefits of screening programs.

Q. Do you know of any screening programs, directly related to surgery, which are performed in the NHS?

A. At the moment the only national screening program available is for breast screening.

This screening program offers all women aged between 50 and 64 years the opportunity to attend for a mammography every 3 years. This screening service is expanding and by 2004 all women up to the age of 70 will be offered screening. Also by 2004 all women will have two views taken at every visit rather than just the first, as it is estimated that this will further increase the specificity of the test.

There has been debate about the effectiveness of this program, with some of the decreasing mortality attributed to improvements in health awareness and treatments such as tamoxifen. As the screening program continues and the amount of reliable data increases, it appears that screening does have additional benefits to the other recent advances in care. Research published in the British Medical Journal (September 2000) has estimated that the NHS breast-screening program is saving at least 300 lives per year. With the continued expansion and uptake of the service, this figure is set to rise to 1250 by 2010.

Sadly, screening programs for prostate cancer, using prostate specific antigen, have proved to be unacceptable for the male population as a whole, although individuals may still request testing.

The screening test does not satisfy many of the criteria outlined above, which are needed for a successful screening program. There are several reasons for this. Firstly, prostate specific antigen is not very sensitive, leading to large numbers of false-positive results. The resulting prostate biopsy then exposes far too many healthy individuals to the risk of impotence and incontinence. Secondly, there is no consensus of medical opinion as to what is the correct treatment for early-stage disease. Finally, prostatic cancer can often run an indolent course, with many men never likely to suffer any ill effects of it. The subsequent detection of the condition causes unnecessary anxiety and treatment to many of these men.

Reference

Blanks RG, Moss SM, McGahan CE, Quinn MJ, Babb PJ. Effect of NHS breast screening programme on mortality from breast cancer in England and Wales, 1990–8: comparison of observed with predicted mortality. BMJ (2000) 321 (7262) pp. 665–9

AUDIT

Q. Why is clinical audit used in the National Health Service?

A. Clinical audit is used in the NHS to monitor the care received by patients and the use of interventions within the NHS. By comparing service provision against either local or nationally agreed guidelines, deviation from 'best practice' can be highlighted and clinical standards maintained and improved.

Audit allows for improvements to be made within a system, in a non-threatening or non-judgemental environment. The audit cycle allows for continued assessment of that system, once improvements have been implemented.

Q. What are the benefits of clinical audit?

A. Audit is important for health professionals, health-care managers and patients alike.

Health professionals are supported in making sure that their patients are receiving the best possible care.

Health-care managers can be informed of areas that require organizational change and additional investment.

Both patients and the general public gain confidence in the service provided knowing that best practice has been ensured.

Q. What is the audit cycle?

A. For audit to be successful and complete, several steps should be implemented in a specified order. For an audit to ensure maximum benefit, all these steps should be conducted in a process known as the audit cycle.

First, a suitable topic should be selected, which is appropriate to the experience and time constraints of the lead person conducting the audit. A small and simple, but complete, audit is far more useful than anything that remains unfinished.

Standards to be compared should be agreed and the audit planned. Next the initial data are collected and analysed.

The next steps are crucial to the audit cycle – these are highlighting areas for change, allowing those changes to be implemented and then collecting the data again.

It is essential that data are collected again; this is the key to the audit cycle. It ensures that improvements have been put in place and implemented. The cycle can be repeated again and again, to continue to improve standards of care. Repeat data collections can be made after several years to confirm high standards are still the norm.

Q. Are you aware of any surgical audits which are carried out at national level?

A. The Royal College of Surgeons of England has been actively involved in audit for many years and is integral in running national surgical audits through its clinical effectiveness unit. This is supported financially by the National Institute of Clinical Effectiveness and academically by the locally based London School of Hygiene and Tropical Medicine. Current audits include the national liver transplant audit, the national audit on intrathoracic transplantation and the national audit on the outcome of subarachnoid haemorrhage.

In Scotland, both the Royal Colleges and the Royal College of Anaesthetists run the Scottish audit of surgical mortality. This is an audit of all surgical deaths in Scotland. All surgical deaths are peer reviewed and, although voluntary, it has nearly 100% compliance. This enables the system to reflect a sense of ownership by the profession. It serves as a testament to the clinicians involved and improves public confidence in Scottish surgery.

Q. What are your own experiences of clinical audit?

A. While this question would normally be asked in an interview setting, audit is such an important part of modern surgery, that a prospective member of the Royal College of Surgeons should be expected to have completed at least one.

I suggest that you familiarize yourself with an old audit that you (or a friend) have completed prior to the viva. The examiner will not be interested in the exact details of your audit, just the fact that you have done one.

A common failing in audit by junior members of staff is a lack of time and follow-up, due to rotating through different surgical specialties, departments and hospitals, usually at 6-monthly intervals.

If you really haven't experienced clinical audit for yourself, you must. It will hinder your future career progress. Most people find audit tedious and dull; however, it is less tedious and dull than not getting short-listed for a registrar job.

STATISTICS

Q. What is the difference between the mean and the median?

A. The mean is the arithmetical average of a series of measurements. The median is an alternative measure of the central value. It is the value, not necessarily a whole number, which halves the measurements, with 50% above the median and 50% below.

Q What do you understand by a normal distribution?

A. A normal distribution is a frequency distribution which is symmetrical and unimodal (it has a single peak). It is called a 'bell-shaped' or Gaussian distribution. When a variable is normally distributed, half the results will lie below the mean and the other half lies above the mean.

Normal distributions measure continuous variables, such as height or weight. Theoretically, normal distributions have no upper or lower limits, they extend from minus infinity ($-\infty$) to plus infinity ($+\infty$).

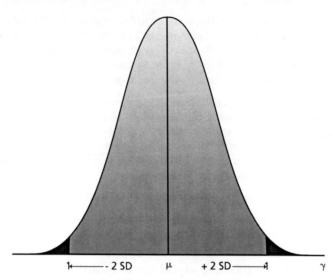

Fig. 8 A normal distribution. SD = standard deviation, μ = mean

A normal distribution can be completely described by two parameters; these are the mean (μ) and the standard deviation. The standard deviation can be thought of as approximately the average distance of the observations from the mean. Mathematically, it can be shown that the probability of being within two standard deviations of the mean is just over 95%. In other words, 95% of observations will lie between two standard deviations above and below the mean.

The majority of a population, e.g. adult men and women, will have a height roughly the same as the mean height. Just over 95% of the population's height will lie within two standard deviations either side of the mean height, but there will still be a few very tall people and a few very short people at either end of the distribution.

Q. What is a significance test?

A. When comparing means or associations, for example height, we want to be sure that the differences measured are real and not just a chance finding. A significance test is a method of accurately gauging this. There are a huge number of significance tests which can be used depending on what you are comparing. If you are comparing means, you can use a Z test for large samples and a T test for smaller sample sizes. Associations between different variables are often tested using the Chi-squared test (χ^2).

Q. When is a Chi-squared (χ^2) test used?

A. Chi-squared (χ^2) testing is another form of significance testing. A Chi-squared (χ^2) test is used to test for an association between two variables. An example would be whether rectal bleeding is associated with cancer of the bowel. A Chi-squared (χ^2) test could be used to confirm that rectal bleeding is associated with cancer.

Chi-squared (χ^2) testing works by using proportions. In this example, it will compare the proportion of people with rectal bleeding and bowel cancer against the proportion of people with rectal bleeding and no bowel cancer.

Q. What is statistical significance?

A. The statistical significance of a result is the probability that the observed relationship or difference occurred by chance alone, when no such relationship or differences exist. In other words, the statistical significance of a result tells us something about the degree to which the result is true.

The strength of the difference is often represented by a 'p' value. The p value represents an index of the reliability of the result. The higher the p value, the less we can believe the observed relation between variables. Specifically, the p value represents the probability of error that is involved in accepting our observed result as valid, that is, as 'representative of the population.' For example, a p value of 0.05 (i.e. 1/20) indicates that there is a 5% probability that the relation between the variables found in our sample occurred by chance alone. In other words, assuming that in the population there was no relation between those variables whatsoever, and we were repeating experiments like ours one after another, we could expect that in every 20 replications of the experiment there would be one in which the relation between the variables in question would be equal or stronger than in ours. In many areas of research, the p value of 0.05 is customarily treated as a 'border-line acceptable' error level, although this is an arbitrary figure.

Q. What is a confidence interval?

A. Confidence intervals give us a range of values where we expect the 'true' value to be located, with a given level of certainty. For example, if the mean in a sample is 23, and the lower and upper limits of the 95% confidence interval are 19 and 27 respectively, then you can conclude that there is a 95% probability that the true population mean is greater than 19 and lower than 27.

Q. What is the null hypothesis?

A. When using statistical tests, it is usual to have a position of truth which is constantly being refuted. The null hypothesis is the position of truth. It states that there is no difference between two results. It is the job of the investigators to challenge this statement and refute it. If a statistical test rejects the null hypothesis, on the basis of the p value generated, we can conclude that there is evidence to reject the null hypothesis.

Q. What is the power of a study?

A. When planning a clinical trial, it is important to have some idea of the number of participants that need to be involved in order that we can be reasonably sure that the result is not due to chance.

If the null hypothesis is rejected when it is true, this is known as a type 1 error (often denoted by α). Likewise, if the null hypothesis is rejected when it is not true, this is known as a type 2 error (denoted by β).

The power of a study is defined as $1-\beta$. It is the probability of rejecting the null hypothesis when it is false. The commonest reason for type 2 errors is that the study was too small.

PAPER CRITIQUE

Q. How would you structure a paper critique?

A. When reviewing a paper I would concentrate on three broad areas. These are:

- The aims of the paper
- The methods used to generate the results
- The discussion.

When looking at the aims of the paper, the first question to be considered is the central research question. Exactly what is this paper trying to achieve and what will this piece of work add to the established knowledge about this subject? The research question should be stated in a concise and unambiguous form. It should be up to date and based on a thorough review of the literature.

After establishing an appropriate research question, the methods used to answer that question should then be examined.

It is important to note that ethical considerations are an integral part of modern research. Laboratory techniques should be checked to ensure that they conform to recognized standards and that normal laboratory methods have been adhered to.

The study design also needs close inspection. What study design was used and which population selected for study? What was used as a comparative group and was it an appropriate comparative group?

How were the data analysed – what methods were used? What is the significance of the statistical findings? Is the evidence weak from a small sample or very strong based on an analysis of tens of thousands of patients? P values of greater than 0.05 are not normally considered to be of significance.

Finally, the presentation of the data should be considered. The data should be clearly presented in an understandable manner. Graphs should be correctly labelled and simple to comprehend.

The final area for consideration involves the interpretation of the data. Are the inferences in accordance with the data? Any conclusions stated by the authors need to be backed up by their findings. Has the influence of the study's limitations or flaws been considered? Could any of the effects obtained be explained by chance, bias or confounding? The findings presented need to be assessed in relation to those of other studies. Are the inferences supported by plausible biological theories?

Q. What is the peer review process which occurs before publication in scientific journals?

A. This is the process that reviews scientific papers before they are accepted for publication in a journal. As the name suggests, it is conducted by 'peers'. The scientific journal will have a panel of suitable reviewers who have a breadth of knowledge of the field covered by the journal. For medical journals, these include clinicians, clinical scientists, epidemiologists and statisticians. The number of reviews which each paper is subjected to will vary according to the size and financial position of the journal.

Initially the journal will internally review the paper using the resident editorial staff to ensure that it is an appropriate paper for that journal. It is then sent to external reviewers for their opinions. The journal will take the decision on whether to publish based on those reviews. It is an important function of those reviewers to suggest any improvements that they feel will add to the publication, even if it is rejected by that journal.

Q. Do you know of any problems associated with the peer-review system?

A. It is a slow and expensive process. It is biased and open to abuse. It is poor at detecting errors and fraud. It is largely an unpaid job and is time consuming, which makes it hard for journals to find suitable reviewers.

Q. What biases do you know of concerning peer review?

A. Research has shown that a prestigious author or institution is more likely to be given a favourable review. The geographical location of the results influences the outcome, as do positive findings and research published in the English language.

Q. What is the impact factor of a research journal?

A. All research publications are graded according to their impact factor. It is calculated by the number of citations a journal receives compared to the number of articles that it publishes. It is not simply a count; it also reflects the size and frequency of publication.

The impact factor has importance for British academia because funding is based in part on the standard of research. The impact factor of the journals in which a department publishes is used to help gauge the standard of research.

CLINICAL TRIALS

Q. What do you understand by the term a clinical trial?

A. They are a scientific method of detecting differences between treatments. They detect the merits of specific treatments for patients with specific diseases. They aim to provide reliable evidence of efficacy and safety.

Q. What do you understand by the term randomized clinical trial?

A. Randomization is the most important aspect of a clinical trial. It ensures that each patient has an equal chance of receiving either treatment. It is essential that the randomization is fair and unbiased. This process allows for a fair and accurate comparison between the treatment options.

Treatment options will usually include the standard treatment, which could be a placebo treatment. Trials also need to be large to allow for small but significant differences to be detected.

Q. What do you know about blinding within clinical trials? Why is this such a problem for surgery?

A. In order to limit bias in the results obtained, it is preferable to keep both doctors and patients unaware of which treatment the patients are receiving. This is known as a 'double blind' trial. These are most easily carried out with drug treatments e.g. tamoxifen versus placebo following mastectomy.

Double blind trials are difficult to carry out in a surgical setting because surgery usually involves a physical procedure being carried out on a patient. Both surgeon and patient are aware of what treatment has been carried out. To improve the reliability of a surgical study 'single blinding' may occur. The surgeon is aware of which procedure was carried out but the patient is unaware. The major disadvantage is that single blind studies are much more prone to bias.

Q. What are the ethics behind a clinical trial?

A. There has been huge international debate about the ethics of clinical trials. These issues were addressed by the Declaration of Helsinki. This was initially written by the World Medical Association in Finland in 1964 and most recently revised in Edinburgh in 2000. It describes the ethical principles for medical research involving human subjects. All clinical trials should abide by the principles which it describes.

Patients should not be denied effective treatments; therefore, when true doubt exists about the effectiveness of a treatment or when no effective treatment exists, it is possible to conduct a clinical trial.

It is essential that any new treatment is also safe; no patient should suffer as a result of a clinical trial.

Within the UK, each hospital has an ethics committee designed to regulate clinical trials. All clinical trials must pass through this committee for research to be conducted within a hospital. If a clinical trial involves several centres, this process would be conducted at a regional level, often with a central coordinating hospital heading the clinical trial.

For a trial which involves a drug company, then governmental regulatory authorities should be involved. In the UK, this is the Medicines Control Agency and in the USA, the Food and Drug Administration (FDA).

It is also ideal, but not always possible, for informed patient consent to be obtained before a patient is enrolled in a clinical trial. If it is not possible for informed consent to be obtained, e.g. in an unconscious patient, the principles described above allow for a clinical trial to proceed.

Q. Do you know about the different phases of clinical trials?

A. Clinical trials are divided into four different phases, each of which requires ethical approval. The first three are conducted before a treatment is fully licensed and the fourth takes place after a treatment is available for use.

Phase one clinical trials are the first to be carried out on patients, usually not more than 20. Their role is to assess toxicology, clinical pharmacology and appropriate dosage. Different routes of drug administration will be assessed and the methodology refined.

Phase two clinical trials involve more patients, up to 100 or so. The initial efficacy will be evaluated. It is not ethical for unhelpful treatments to proceed for further evaluation. In addition, clinical trials are often extremely expensive to organize and it would be a waste of resources to continue if the new treatment did not seem effective.

This phase of the trial process acts as a pilot study for the next large phase of the trial. Organizational issues and the management of the trial should be perfected during this stage of a trial.

Phase three clinical trials involve many more patients, often several thousand. They assess both efficacy and safety. If, after finishing phase three of a clinical trial, a treatment is found to be both safe and effective it can be licensed for use.

Phase four clinical trials are used as a form of post-marketing surveillance. They serve as a means of continued safety monitoring and assessing new clinical applications of a treatment.

EPIDEMIOLOGY

Q. How would you define epidemiology?

A. The word epidemiology is derived from the Greek word '*epidemos*', *epi* meaning upon and *demos* meaning people. Hippocrates used the word '*epidemeion*' over 2400 years ago to refer to diseases that *visit* the community.

A modern definition is given in Lasts' dictionary of epidemiology – 'Epidemiology is the study of the distribution and determinants of health-related states or events in specified populations, and the application of this study to control of health problems'.

Q. What do you understand by the terms incidence and prevalence?

A. These are both measures of disease frequency. Incidence measures the frequency of new cases in a specified time period in a specified population. Prevalence is the measure of all cases in a population at a given point in time. If we use ulcerative colitis as an example, there are approximately eight new cases per 100 000 people per year (this is the incidence) and 116 cases per 100 000 people (the prevalence). Diseases with a rapid onset and a short duration, such as appendicitis, have a high incidence and a low prevalence. Diseases which are chronic, such as ulcerative colitis, have a low incidence and a high prevalence.

Q. What is the relationship between incidence and prevalence?

A. Prevalence depends on the duration of the disease and on the incidence of the disease. Prevalence can be approximated to the product of the mean duration and the incidence of a disease. For example, a disease with ten incidence cases per year per 1 000 000, with a mean duration of 10 years, will have a prevalence of 100 per 1 000 000 within that population.

Q. What different types of study design do you know about?

A. There are several different types of study used in epidemiology. Each study is useful for different questions and each provides different information. The most common studies include ecological studies, cross-sectional studies, case-control studies, cohort studies and intervention studies (clinical trials).

An ecological study is one that is conducted at a population level on the basis of place and time. For example, a study of the rate of cirrhosis of the liver and alcohol intake shows a clear increase in rate the more alcohol is consumed, when compared across different countries.

Ecological studies are good at generating hypotheses. A major disadvantage is that not all findings at the population level can be extrapolated to the individual level.

Cross-sectional studies are studies which collect information to measure prevalence at any point in time; for example, 'What proportion of abscesses is caused by intravenous drug abuse?'. They have the advantage of being simple, cheap and quick. They are widely used to assess the burden of disease. They are good for hypothesis generation; for example, is there a high rate of abscesses in intravenous drug abusers – yes or no? However, they are not always representative e.g. different rates of abscess formation, in intravenous drug abusers, would be obtained in rural and in urban settings, as intravenous drug abusers tend to live in deprived urban areas.

Case-control studies are useful for studying rare diseases, for example primary bile duct carcinoma. Also, many risk factors can be assessed for that rare disease. Each case of a disease can be compared to a control selected at random to assess for different risk factors, for example, 'Do cases drink alcohol more than controls?' 'Do cases have a history of gallbladder disease?'. A major disadvantage of case-control studies is bias in the selection of controls. It can be difficult to select controls that truly represent the general population. For example, a subject who volunteers to be a control subject is unlikely to be truly 'normal'. They are likely to have different characteristics from those of the whole population; to volunteer in the first place shows a high level of health awareness.

Cohort studies are another type of study. A cohort of patients with a specified condition or exposure are followed up over a period of time: 'Does a cohort of patients with an enlarged aortic aneurysm have an increased rate of death compared to the general population of a similar age?'. Cohort studies are good for establishing a temporal sequence i.e. the aneurysm was diagnosed before death and so an increased rate in these patients can be assumed to be due to the aneurysm.

Cohort studies are also useful in studying rare risk factors but not rare diseases. For example, a whole factory which is exposed to a rare chemical (risk factor) can be followed for a very rare cancer, potentially linked to the chemical. To find enough cases of a very rare cancer in the population would require following millions of people. Cohort studies are also time consuming, expensive and participants are easily lost to follow-up.

Intervention studies usually take the form of clinical trials and have several advantages. They can measure the effect of intervention: 'Does hepatitis B vaccine prevent hepatitis infection?'. They can also test causal hypotheses e.g. hepatitis B is widely thought to cause hepatocellular cancer. If a vaccine prevents hepatitis infection and leads to a subsequent drop in the rate of hepatocellular cancer, then this is evidence for a causal link between the two.

Intervention studies are also very epidemiologically robust. High-quality randomization in sufficiently large studies means that confounding factors are likely to be approximately balanced between the different groups.

Q. **What do you understand by the term bias?**

A. In epidemiology the term is used to describe methods and results which are not representative of the truth.

There are many types of bias; some are listed below:

- Selection bias. This was discussed with reference to case-control studies. Is the control group from the same population that the cases came from? We know, for example, that controls drawn from a hospital population are more likely to smoke, drink and have other chronic diseases than those out of hospital. Should these patients then be used as a representative control group?
- Recall bias. A subject's ability to recall an event depends on whether or not they are a case or a control. Women recently diagnosed with breast cancer may be more likely to recall their use of oral contraception more accurately than those who have not been diagnosed.

- Observer bias. A bias common to all studies. This is a bias introduced by personnel involved in the study. For example, a pathologist who is aware that a patient has been exposed to asbestos may be more likely to diagnose mesothelioma than in a patient they know has not been exposed. Blinding of all staff as much as possible will help prevent this problem.
- Publication bias. Positive results are generally deemed more interesting than negative ones. Hence, positive results are more likely to be published than negative ones. This leads to an over-representation of any, usually positive, effect in the medical literature.

Q. What do you understand by the term confounding?

A. Confounding is another source of error seen in epidemiology. It is about alternative explanations. It can occur when two risk factors have not been separated and it is incorrectly concluded that an effect is due to one, rather than the other, variable. For example, pancreatic cancer is more likely to occur in smokers. Smokers also drink more coffee than non smokers. It could, therefore, wrongly be concluded that coffee is a risk factor for pancreatic cancer. Coffee is said to confound the relationship between smoking and pancreatic cancer.

Q. What is causality in the epidemiological setting?

A. In order to conclude that something is caused by something else, several questions need to be answered. In 1965, the famous epidemiologist Austin Bradford-Hill devised a set of criteria which need to be established before something can be said to be causal. There were nine original points:

1. Temporal sequence. Does the exposure precede the outcome e.g. smoking precedes lung cancer.
2. Strength of association. Strong associations, as measured by risk or odds ratios, are less likely to be due to chance, bias or undetected bias.
3. Consistency of association. Do different studies agree?
4. Dose–response gradient. An observed increase in risk with an increase in exposure. For example, heavy smokers suffer more lung cancer than light smokers.
5. Specificity of association. A single factor is associated with a single outcome. This is no longer so useful now that the majority of diseases are believed to be multifactorial.
6. Biological plausibility of association. For example, carcinogens isolated from tobacco smoke.
7. Coherence of association. Reported associations do not conflict with current knowledge.
8. Reversibility. Removal of an exposure leads to a reduction in the risk of the outcome. For example, ex-smokers have a lower rate of lung cancer than current smokers.
9. Analogy. Are there other demonstrated associations? For example, kuru and scrapie show similar pathology to BSE and nCJD.

Recently two further criteria have been added. The first is prediction; for example, the current increasing rates of smoking in women will lead to a higher rate of lung cancer in the future. The second is to generate and if possible reject alternative hypotheses i.e. 'Could this be due to anything else?'.

Reference

Last JM. A dictionary of epidemiology. 4th edn. Oxford University Press, 2001

DEATH CERTIFICATES AND THE CORONER

Q. What is the purpose of the death certificate?

A. Since 1837 births, deaths and marriages have been registered in the United Kingdom. A death certificate is a formal document that is issued by a medical practitioner after death, which allows a death to be registered. If a death has not been registered it is illegal for a funeral director to conduct a funeral service.

The national registration system also provides an excellent resource for the NHS, allowing for rates and trends of death to be monitored. All deaths in the UK are collected by the NHS Central Register. It is possible to alert research groups to the death of an individual if they have been previously flagged up to the register. For example, a participant in a trial involving different types of treatment for prostate cancer would be registered when they die, including the cause of death. It is then possible to see how long they survived and what they died of.

Q. Which deaths should be reported to the Coroner?

A. Only a small number of deaths are reported to the Coroner before a death certificate can be issued and a funeral take place. These include:

1. Where there is no doctor who can issue a medical certificate of the cause of death.
2. Where the deceased was not seen by the doctor issuing the medical certificate after death nor within 14 days prior to death.
3. Where the cause of death is unknown.
4. Where the cause of death is believed to be unnatural or suspicious.
5. Where the death occurred during an operation or before recovery from anaesthetic.
6. Where death is due to industrial disease or industrial poisoning.

The vast majority of cases which are reported to the Coroner will have a medical certificate of death issued without any further investigation. It is up to the Coroner to decide whether any further action, such as a post-mortem, is required.

Q. What is an inquest?

A. When a patient's identity or cause of death cannot be established, the Coroner will sometimes arrange for an inquest into the death. An inquest is a legal body, designed to hear evidence from parties concerned with the death, such as the police, the surgeon attending the patient or the pathologist who conducted the post-mortem.

At the discretion of the Coroner, relatives and friends can ask questions. It can be very cathartic for the families involved to hear the facts surrounding the death of their loved one and ask questions relating to the death which were not aired at the time of death.

At the end of the inquest the Coroner will record their verdict, according to what he or she feels was the reason for the death, which is often natural causes. If there is doubt involved in the cause of death or the possibility of foul play, the verdict given by the Coroner will reflect this. It is then dependent on the individual case as to what further legal proceedings take place.

TOURNIQUET

Q. When would you use a tourniquet in surgery?

A. I would use a tourniquet for operating on the upper or lower limb. The tourniquet would allow me to operate in a bloodless field and so decrease my chances of injuring any nearby vessels, nerves or tendons.

Q. When would you not use a tourniquet?

A. I would not use a tourniquet in an elderly patient or one who had a compromised circulation.

Q. What are the potential problems associated with tourniquet use? How would you avoid them?

A. Tourniquet use is associated with ischaemia and possible nerve damage. Nerve injury is most likely to occur with direct as opposed to prolonged pressure. The acceptable length of time for tourniquet use is 90 min; damage begins to occur after 3 hours. The pressure should be set to no more than 100–125 mmHg above the systolic blood pressure. Injury is also most likely to occur with narrow cuffs and non-pneumatic tourniquets.

Q. How else may nerves be injured intraoperatively?

A. Nerves may be injured intraoperatively by:

- Direct scalpel/diathermy injury
- Compression/traction
- Accidental injection i.e. epidural/during venepuncture
- Irradiation.

Q. Which nerves are particularly at risk?

A. These include:

- Head and neck surgery – accessory nerve and brachial plexus
- Shoulder – axillary and musculocutaneous nerves
- Proximal radius – posterior interosseous branch of the radial nerve
- Wrist – median nerve
- Dupuytren's disease – digital nerves
- Hip – sciatic nerve
- Knee – common peroneal nerve
- Calcaneum – sural nerve.

Q. How would you prevent these injuries from occurring?

A. A good knowledge of anatomy and adequate preparation are required in order to prevent such injuries occurring. Care should be taken with exposure, gentle handling and retraction of tissues. If a nerve is inadvertently divided, it should be repaired immediately; however, if it is discovered postoperatively, the level of function should be carefully assessed. If only a minor disability is observed, the injury may be treated conservatively. If severe, the wound must be explored and the injury repaired or grafted.

> *'Keep away from nerves or see them clearly,*
> *For if you cut them it may cost you dearly;*
> *But if you have, you must confess –*
> *In the long run it will cost you less'*

(From Apley G Solomon L. Peripheral nerve lesions. Concise system of orthopaedics and fractures. Butterworth-Heinemann 1988, pp. 80–86).

POSTOPERATIVE MONITORING

Q. You have just performed an emergency appendicectomy on a 16-year-old girl. The surgery was uncomplicated and the anaesthetist is now waking her up. How would you go about monitoring her progress?

A. Firstly, I would liaise with the anaesthetist regarding any specific difficulties encountered during the anaesthetic. In particular, I would be concerned about laryngospasm, nausea or vomiting. Assuming the anaesthetic was uneventful, I would arrange for the patient to be taken to recovery where she will be monitored by a designated recovery nurse. Specific tasks include:

- Adequate pain relief.
- Gentle reassurance as the patient comes round from the anaesthetic to reduce fears.
- Mouthwash/glass of water available for dry mouth.
- Care of pressure areas.

- **A** – ensuring a patent airway; nasopharyngeal, guedel airway and oxygen mask if necessary. Nursing upright if the patient is drowsy and there is a risk of aspiration.
- **B** – suctioning the airway until the patient is able to maintain their own airway. Monitoring oxygen saturation using pulse oximetry.
- **C** – regular blood pressure measurements, continuous pulse measurement by the pulse oximeter and regular recordings of blood/fluid loss from the drains and catheter.
- Hypothermia needs to be checked for and corrected prior to the patient leaving recovery.
- Encouraging deep breathing and early mobilization to prevent basal atelectasis and DVT.

Q. What are the commonest causes of hypoxia in the early postoperative period?

A. The commonest causes of hypoxia at this stage include:

- Laryngospasm/airway obstruction
- Respiratory depression secondary to opiate use
- Residual effects of inhalational agents.

Some patients may have a previous history of respiratory problems whilst under anaesthetic.

Q. Would you give this girl intravenous fluids postoperatively?

A. Presuming that this was an otherwise fit and healthy young girl who had undergone an uncomplicated procedure, I would not instigate intravenous fluids. I would encourage her to drink oral fluids as early as possible.

If I was concerned that she had a significant fluid loss, I would work out her fluid balance and correct any deficit using normal saline or Hartman's solution. I would then monitor her urinary output and encourage her to drink oral fluids as early as possible.

Q. What analgesia would you give to this patient?

A. I would prescribe a non-steroidal anti-inflammatory suppository to be given to the patient at the end of the operation, providing she wasn't asthmatic. I would then prescribe a combination of regular paracetamol and either a non-steroidal anti-inflammatory or codeine phosphate. I would also prescribe a stronger analgesic such as pethidine to be given intramuscularly and as required.

NUTRITION

Q. Why would you assess a patient's nutritional status preoperatively and how would you go about doing so?

A. Preoperative malnutrition and obesity can result in an increased morbidity and mortality postoperatively.

It is possible to assess nutrition preoperatively by:

- Taking a history and assessing recent weight gain or weight loss
- Anthropomorphic measurements – skin fold thickness (assesses subcutaneous fat) and mid-arm circumference
- Dynamometric assessment i.e. hand-grip strength
- Blood tests – serum albumin, transferrin
- Immunology i.e. lymphocyte count
- Measurement of body mass index (BMI)

$$\frac{\text{Weight (kg)}}{\text{Height (m}^2)}$$

To be forewarned is to be forearmed. Obese patients are specifically at risk of:

- Operative mortality – ischaemic heart disease and CVA
- Wound sepsis
- DVT and PE.

Prior knowledge allows adequate optimization of conditions i.e. preoperative attempts to lose weight, DVT prophylaxis and early mobilization.

Unfortunately, early detection of malnutrition by a low serum albumin is not easily correctable. Use of human albumin is expensive and ineffective. Attempts should be made to improve nutrition preoperatively; however, if this is not possible postoperative enteral or parenteral nutrition should be considered early. Otherwise, malnourished patients are particularly at risk of:

- Infection, for example, chest and wound
- Poor wound healing
- Wound breakdown/dehiscence.

Q. What clinical signs of malnutrition could you look for?

A. On examination, I would first look at the patient's general habitus. I would assess body fat stores by pinching the biceps and triceps skin fold; if the dermis can be felt the patient is composed of <10% fat (Hill et al. 1977, positive 'finger-thumb' test; Forsel et al. 1981). Then, I would check if the patient's bones were prominent, specifically the rib cage and scapula.

Other clinical features include:

- Reduced muscle power
- Angular stomatitis
- Glossitis

- Peripheral oedema
- Generalized loss of muscle power
- Neuropathies.

Q. Do you know what the usual energy requirements are for a patient undergoing surgery?

A. 2200–2500 kcal per 24 hours.

Q. What do you know about the different kinds of postoperative nutritional support?

A. Nutritional support may be enteral, meaning oral, or parenteral, meaning intravenous. Enteral nutrition is regarded as the gold standard as it helps reduce the overall metabolic insult associated with surgery and trauma.

Q. How does it do that?

A. Early enteral nutrition allows the gut to function as normally as possible under the circumstances. It maintains the barrier and mucosal function of the gut and as a result the gut bacteria are not disrupted. In the absence of enteral nutrition, translocation of the bacteria occurs across the gut wall and the presence of such endotoxins in the circulation is thought to contribute to the development of GIT and multiorgan failure in the critically ill.

Q. Why can't all patients have enteral nutrition postoperatively?

A. It is contraindicated in some patients, for example:

- Bowel obstruction
- Bowel dysfunction i.e. excessive vomiting
- Bowel anastomoses (although enteral feeding may be commenced after approximately 5 days providing there has been no complication).

Enteral feeding may be administered by the patient themselves i.e sips of water or maybe via a nasogastric tube. Some patients may be at risk of aspiration or regurgitation via this method:

- Major abdominal surgery
- Ventilated/critically ill
- Head injuries
- Neuropatholgical conditions i.e. diabetes
- Deglutition disorders.

In such cases, a feeding tube may be placed beyond the pylorus. This may be done through the nose i.e. naso-jejunal tube or percutaneously:

- Percutaneous endoscopic gastrostomy (PEG)
- Percutaneous endoscopic jejunostomy (PEJ).

These two options are usually reserved for long term nutritional care.

Q. What are the complications associated with enteral nutrition?

A. Complications include:

- Feeding tube blockage (occurs commonly and may be prevented by regular flushing with water), also wrongly positioned feeding tube
- Bloating, abdominal distension and pain (may be helped by slowing down the infusion)
- Nausea, vomiting and diarrhoea
- Regurgitation and aspiration into lungs
- Metabolic – vitamin and mineral deficiencies, biochemical derangements, interactions with other administered drugs
- Infection – feeding tubes, giving sets.

Q. How do these complications compare with parenteral nutrition?

A. Parenteral nutrition or TPN is intravenous and therefore more invasive. Complications include:

- Line insertion – wrong position, haematoma, arterial puncture, air embolism, pneumothorax, cardiac arrhythmias, haemopericardium, chylothorax, infection, thrombophlebitis
- Metabolic – hyper/hypoglycaemia, hyper/hypokalaemia, hyper/hyponatraemia, hypercalcaemia, hypophosphataemia, zinc, magnesium and folate deficiencies
- Liver dysfunction – elevated liver enzymes, cholestasis, fatty infiltration of the liver
- Late – venous thrombosis, line occlusion, sepsis.

References

Hill GL, Blackett RL, Pickford et al. Lancet (1977) i, 689–92.
Forsel et al. Reliability of skin testing as a measure of nutritional state. Archives of Surgery (1981) 116, 1284–8.

BLOOD TRANSFUSION

Q. Prior to blood transfusion, what viruses are tested for?

A. Donated blood is tested for:

- Hepatitis B surface antigen
- Hepatitis C antibodies
- Syphilis antibodies
- HIV types 1 and 2 (antibodies).

Q. Can you donate blood if you've had malaria?

A. You are allowed to donate blood if you no longer have malarial antibodies.

Q. Apart from microbiological screening, what else is blood tested for?

A. All donated blood is tested for blood group antigens. In particular:

- ABO blood grouping system
- Rh CDE phenotype
- Red cell antibodies.

Q. What are the frequencies of the various common blood groups?

A. O is the commonest blood group, accounting for approximately 50% of all blood groups. The next is A which is marginally less frequent. B and AB are the least frequent, accounting for approximately 10% of blood groups in total.

It is genetically determined which blood group a person is; two genes are located on each of the paired chromosomes. It is therefore possible to be OO, OA, OB, AA, AB or AO.

Q. What is the significance of the Rhesus D antigen?

A. Rhesus D antigen is prevalent within the population and is considered to be the most antigenic of all the Rhesus antigens – C, D, E, c, d and e. Patients are grouped as Rh positive or negative according to the presence of the D antigen.

Q. What happens if you were to transfuse a Rhesus negative person with Rhesus positive blood?

A. There would be no immediate 'transfusion reaction'. Anti-Rhesus antibodies would develop over a period of approximately 2–4 weeks and may occasionally be sufficient to result in agglutination of transfused cells within the circulation. This is known as a delayed transfusion reaction. The next time that person encounters Rhesus positive blood, the transfusion reaction is a lot worse and has a quicker onset. It is then called an immediate transfusion reaction.

Q. What other types of transfusion reactions do you know of?

A. Transfusion reactions occur as a result of blood incompatibilities. This may be a result of:

- ABO agglutinin incompatibility (usually results in a severe, immediate transfusion reaction)
- Rhesus incompatibility
- HLA antigens as a result of multiple transfusions
- Haemolytic disease of the newborn – occurs as a result of a Rhesus negative mother carrying a Rhesus positive baby (inherited from the father). The result is that the mother may develop antibodies which may cause agglutination of fetal blood in future pregnancies.

Q. What would lead you to suspect a diagnosis of a transfusion reaction?

A. Transfusion reactions as a result of incompatibility are rare due to the fact that rigorous testing now occurs on all donated blood. If it does occur, usually as a result of a clerical error, the patient may become extremely unwell very quickly. They may complain of gastrointestinal symptoms, dizziness and palpitations. Clinically they may develop anaphylaxis and become haemodynamically unstable. This may lead to renal failure.

In delayed transfusion reactions, the patient may become jaundiced or suffer renal abnormalities a few days after the blood transfusion.

Q. What other side effects are associated with blood transfusions?

A. The incidence of side effects from blood transfusions increases if the blood has not been stored at the right temperature of 4°C. The side effects that may be seen include:

- Viral transmission, particularly HIV (this has decreased in incidence due to better screening).
- Bacterial infection i.e. skin contaminants can result in a profound clinical reaction such as hypotension, DIC and renal failure.
- Immunological reactions i.e. reactions to transfused plasma proteins/immunoglobulins in patients who have had multiple transfusions. This may present as rigors, low-grade temperature and urticaria. Also, antibodies within the donated blood may react with the patient's white blood cells causing lung oedema that may require treatment.
- Thrombocytopenic purpura may develop after a blood transfusion as a result of antibodies in the donor blood to the patient's antibodies.

Q. What other products are obtained when blood is donated?

A. Other blood products include:

- Platelets (stored at −22°C)
- Plasma and cryoprecipitate (FFP stored at −30°C)
- Clotting factors i.e. factor VIII
- Albumin.

APPLIED PHYSIOLOGY

MUSCLE MECHANICS

Q. What different types of muscle are there?

A. Skeletal muscle, smooth muscle and cardiac muscle.

Q. Tell me the general principles involved in muscle contraction.

A. The initial stimulus is an action potential, which travels along the nerve ending at the muscle fibre. In the case of skeletal muscle, acetylcholine is released at the neuromuscular junction causing a large influx of sodium ions into the muscle fibre. This produces an action potential within the muscle, causing depolarization. This results in the release of large quantities of stored calcium, which initiates the actin and myosin fibres to slide over each other and produce a contraction. The whole process ends by the calcium ions being pumped back into the sarcoplasmic reticulum for storage until the next action potential comes along.

Q. How does this differ in smooth and cardiac muscle?

A. Skeletal muscle contraction has a very rapid onset and brief duration. Cardiac and smooth muscle, however, have a more prolonged action. They also don't contain motor end plates like skeletal muscle.

In the case of smooth muscle, the contraction is similarly initiated by an influx of calcium ions. This may be produced by nerve stimulation, hormonal stimulation or stretching of the fibres. It is the autonomic nervous system which supplies smooth muscle via the release of acetylcholine and norepinephrine, which may be excitatory or inhibitory. Smooth muscle contraction requires far less energy to produce the same tension as skeletal muscle. This is because in the case of organs such as the intestines and gallbladder, tonic muscular contraction is sustained most of the time. The onset of contraction followed by relaxation is also approximately 30 times as long. Despite all this, however, the force of contraction is often greater than skeletal muscle.

Cardiac muscle differs from both smooth and skeletal muscle in that it acts as a syncytium. This is an 'all or nothing' phenomenon. The heart is composed of an atrial syncytium and a ventricular syncytium separated by specialized conductive fibres. This allows the atria to contract before the ventricles thereby allowing the heart to pump effectively. As with skeletal muscle, the action potential is caused by the opening of fast sodium channels; however, this is also accompanied by the opening of slow calcium channels resulting in a more prolonged period of depolarization. Cardiac muscle also differs from skeletal muscle in that immediately after the onset of the action potential, the permeability of the muscle to potassium ions decreases significantly. This refractory period prevents premature repolarization of the muscle membrane (see Tip).

Q. What is the Frank–Starling law of the heart?

A. The Frank–Starling law describes the ability of the heart to cope with changes in volumes of inflowing blood. It states that the force of myocardial contraction is directly proportional to the initial muscle fibre length. Therefore, as the fibre length increases with the end diastolic volume, the stroke volume increases. This is a characteristic of all striated muscle.

Q. What happens with excessive ventricular filling?

A. As the ventricle becomes overstretched, the myocardium is unable to function efficiently and the stroke volume decreases, with a risk of pulmonary oedema.

 TIP

A comprehensive assessment of the differences between contraction of skeletal, smooth and cardiac muscle has been given. In the viva, you may be asked to simply state the differences between the three types of muscle, so it is a good idea to learn a few basic differences off by heart:

Skeletal	Cardiac	Smooth
Motor end plates	No motor end plates	No motor end plates
Cylindrical fibres	Branched fibres	Fusiform fibres
Sarcomeres	Sarcomeres	No sarcomeres
Few mitochondria	Many mitochondria	Gap junctions
Lots of ATPase	Average ATPase	Little ATPase
Graded response	All or nothing	Graded response
Tetany	No tetany	Tetany
No pacemaker activity	Pacemaker potential	Slow pacemaker potential

ATPase is the enzyme which splits ATP (adenosine triphosphate) to form ADP (adenosine diphosphate) and inorganic phosphate. This reaction provides the energy required for muscular contraction.

AUTONOMIC NERVOUS SYSTEM

Q. What is the autonomic nervous system? (This is an open-ended question. The examiner is trying to test your depth of knowledge in a specialized area. In these situations, if you know the answer it is best to keep it simple; this is your opportunity to shine. If not, don't panic, admit you don't know and move on, rather than trying to make it up.)

A. The autonomic nervous system regulates the involuntary control of internal organs including cardiac muscle, smooth muscle, blood vessel tone and gut via afferent and efferent pathways.

Q. What is the somatic nervous system?

A. The somatic nervous system innervates skeletal muscle and is under voluntary control.

Q. Tell me what you know about the neuromuscular junction.

A. The neuromuscular junction consists of a single motor neuron and the muscle fibres it innervates. The junction between them is similar to a synapse and is called the motor end plate. When a presynaptic action potential arrives, there is an influx of calcium resulting in the release of the neurotransmitter acetylcholine into the synaptic cleft. Acetylcholine is released from stored vesicles and reacts with the nicotinic receptors on the muscle membrane. This results in an influx of sodium. An action potential is fired into the muscle, which results in contraction.

Q. What happens to the acetylcholine after this has occurred?

A. Acetylcholinesterases, which are enzymes in the synaptic cleft, rapidly hydrolyse acetylcholine. Choline is then taken back up by the presynaptic membrane in order for more acetylcholine to be produced.

Q. Can you give me any examples of substances that block neuromuscular transmission?

A. Yes, botulinum toxin inhibits acetylcholine release from vesicles. There are various anaesthetic agents which prevent the action of acetylcholine on acetylcholine receptor sites and they form the basis of neuromuscular blocking agents i.e. atracurium, vecuronium. This prevents the formation of an action potential in the muscle membrane.

Q. What is myasthenia gravis?

A. Myasthenia gravis is a condition where antibodies are formed against acetylcholine receptors. Paralysis occurs due to the inability to transmit action potentials from the nerve to the muscle through the motor end plate.

BLOOD

Q. Can you estimate the total blood volume in human beings for me?

A. The estimated blood volume for an average male is roughly 75 ml per kg and for females roughly 65 ml per kg (it is 80 ml/kg in children).

Q. What is the division of total body water in a normal 70 kg man?

A. Total body water in a 70 kg man is roughly 60% of total body mass or around 45 litres.

- Intracellular compartment – 30 l
- Extracellular compartment – interstitial 10 l, vascular 5 l, transcellular 1 l.

Q. What are the normal physiological compensatory mechanisms for volume loss?

A. You will see an increase in cardiac output, redistribution of blood flow to oxygen-supply-dependent tissue such as heart and brain, and an increase in oxygen extraction.

Q. What would you regard as an acceptable haematocrit in a healthy individual compared to someone with respiratory disease?

A. The haematocrit is the percentage of the blood that is cells (the remainder is plasma). The haematocrit of an average man is 0.42 and of an average women is 0.38. It is much higher in a patient with respiratory disease.

Q. What is a normal haemoglobin?

A. A normal haemoglobin for a man is 13–16 g/dl and 11–14 g/dl for a woman.

Q. How is oxygen transported in the blood?

A. Approximately 97–98% of oxygen is transported in combination with haemoglobin in red blood cells. The rest is dissolved in water.

Q. What is haemoglobin made up of?

A. Haemoglobin is made up of:

- Haem component – iron and protoporphyrin
- Globin chain.

They combine together to form a haemoglobin chain. In humans this mostly consists of two alpha and two beta chains. Each haemoglobin molecule carries four molecules of oxygen.

Q. What do you know about the oxygen dissociation curve?

A. The oxygen dissociation curve is a graph with percentage saturation of haemoglobin on the y-axis and Po_2 (mmHg) of blood on the x-axis. It is a sigmoid curve, demonstrating that there is a steady increase in the percentage of haemoglobin bound with oxygen as the blood Po_2 rises.

Q. Can you explain the differences seen in arterial and venous blood?

A. Yes, arterial blood has a Po_2 of 95 mmHg and therefore an oxygen saturation of approximately 97%. Venous blood, however, has a Po_2 of 45 mmHg and so has an oxygen saturation of 75%.

Q. Why does the oxygen dissociation curve have a sigmoid shape?

A. This is because of the nature of oxygen binding to the haemoglobin molecule. As one molecule of oxygen binds to haemoglobin, the binding of the next is easier and so forth. It is known as 'cooperative' binding.

Q. What happens to oxygen saturation in the steep portion of the curve?

A. A small decrease in Po_2 on the steep portion of the curve can result in a large decrease in oxygen saturation. Similarly, increasing the Po_2 by small amounts can lead to a significant increase in the oxygen saturation.

Q. Can you name any factors that may shift the oxygen dissociation curve?

A. Factors shifting the curve to the right include:

- Increasing [H⁺]
- Increasing CO_2
- Increasing temperature
- Increasing DPG (2,3-diphosphoglycerate).

Factors shifting the curve to the left include:
- Increasing pH
- Decreasing CO_2.

Q. Do you know what the Bohr effect is?

A. The Bohr effect occurs when the oxygen dissociation curve is shifted to the right. This occurs when there is an increase in carbon dioxide and hydrogen ions, and results in an increase in oxygenation of blood in the lungs and an increase in oxygen release into the tissues.

Q. What are the effects on the circulation of a low haemoglobin?

A. In patients who are anaemic:

- Blood viscosity decreases
- Blood flow resistance also decreases and so cardiac output increases
- A reduction in the transport of oxygen to the tissues causing hypoxia
- Dilatation of the peripheral blood vessels (as a result of the hypoxia) which further increases cardiac output.

Q. What haemoglobin would you accept pre- and postoperatively, and when would you consider a blood transfusion?

A. The ideal haemoglobin for oxygen carriage is 8–10 g/dl. Ideally I would only consider a transfusion below this level. However, if a patient had a haemoglobin of 8 g/dl preoperatively, I would consider a transfusion as, depending on the nature of the surgery, some volume loss would be expected intraoperatively. Therefore they may become significantly hypoxic and cardiovascularly compromised.

Q. What blood products are available that you know of?

A. These include:

- Packed red cells
- Fresh frozen plasma (FFP)
- Albumin

- Immunoglobulins
- Cryoprecipitate
- Individual factors i.e. factor VIII, IX, X etc.
- Platelets.

Leucocyte-depleted blood may be given to reduce the risk of Creutzfeld–Jacob disease transmission.

Q. When would you consider giving fresh frozen plasma?

A. I would consider giving FFP in the following situations:

- To control bleeding in surgery associated with significant blood loss
- To treat the effects of warfarinization
- Post-massive blood transfusion i.e. trauma
- In the management of DIC.

Q. What is the average volume in a unit of blood?

A. The average volume is approximately 300–350 ml.

Q. How is blood stored and how long does it last for?

A. It is stored in a fridge at 4°C and lasts approximately 35 days.

Q. What changes occur to the blood as it ages?

A. The following changes occur:

- Increase in potassium and phosphate
- Decrease in pH
- Haemolysis
- Loss of certain clotting factors i.e. factor VIII
- Aggregates of dead cells/'clumping'.

Q. What is blood screened for?

A. Blood is screened for:

- Hepatitis B and C
- CMV
- HIV1 and 2
- Syphilis.

Q. Are there any other infections that may be transmitted?

A. Yes, other organisms include:

- Bacteria – *Pseudomonas, Yersinia enterocolitica*, staphylococci
- Parasites – malaria, Chaga's disease
- Prion disease.

Q. Who might require a transfusion of factor VIII?

A. Patients with haemophilia A or von Willebrand's disease.

Q. How would you know if a patient was experiencing immediate haemolysis post-transfusion?

A. They would exhibit the following clinical features:

- Rapid onset of symptoms i.e. as soon as the transfusion is commenced
- Rigors
- Chest pain
- Pyrexia
- Hypotension
- Oliguria/haemoglobinuria
- Jaundice
- Bleeding.

Q. What is the cause of this?

A. If severe, it is usually caused by an ABO incompatibility. Less severe reactions are caused by Rhesus incompatibility.

COAGULATION

Q. What is haemostasis?

A. Haemostasis is the mechanism by which blood is kept in a fluid state within blood vessels.

Q. What stimulates the haemostatic response?

A. It is usually stimulated by a ruptured/damaged vessel. The clotting cascade may also be activated in the rare condition adult respiratory distress syndrome (ARDS) where disseminated intravascular coagulation (DIC) occurs.

Q. When a blood vessel is severed, what are the main components that make up the haemostatic response?

A. The haemostatic response stimulated by a cut vessel involves an initial spasm of the vessel followed by a platelet plug over the site of the injury. The coagulation cascade is then activated resulting in the formation of a blood clot. The blood clot then organizes and is replaced by fibrin which permanently closes the defect.

Q. What factors may alert you preoperatively to a patient at risk of bleeding intraoperatively?

A.
- Past history of spontaneous bleeding
- Previous bleeding problems during operations/injury
- Drug history i.e. aspirin, anticoagulants, NSAIDS.

Q. Could you describe the intrinsic and extrinsic coagulation cascades for me?

A. The extrinsic system is classically stimulated by traumatized tissues which release thromboplastin. Thromboplastin is mostly made up of phospholipid from tissue membranes and lipoprotein. Factor X is activated and, with the help of calcium, prothrombin is split into thrombin.

The intrinsic system is stimulated by trauma to vessel walls, thereby exposing blood to collagen, or by trauma to blood itself. Factor XII becomes activated and platelets release phospholipids. Through a series of complex reactions involving phospholipids and factor VIII, factor X is activated. Factor X then acts to split prothrombin into thrombin as in the extrinsic pathway. Calcium is also required in several steps in the pathway.

Traditionally, the extrinsic and intrinsic pathways have been considered as separate pathways that merge after activation of factor X; in reality, however, these are linked pathways.

Q. What part does the liver play?

A. The liver produces many clotting factors; therefore, diseases such as hepatitis and cirrhosis may cause a reduced production of clotting factors, causing a bleeding tendency.

Patients with obstructed bile ducts may also bleed as bile is essential for the absorption of vitamin K.

Q. Tell me about the effect of heparin on coagulation.

A. Heparin is a strong anticoagulant. It is used widely in medicine to prevent the formation of thromboses.

Q. Is it normally present in blood?

A. Yes, it is produced by mast cells and basophils and is present in very low concentrations in the blood. Its purpose is to enhance the actions of anti-thrombin III which is a protein that protects the body from excessive thrombosis. It also aids the removal of other activated clotting factors i.e. XII, XI, IX and X thereby adding to the anticoagulant effect.

Q. What coagulation tests do you know of and how do they reflect the pathways?

A. There is the partial thromboplastin time (PTT) which reflects the intrinsic and common pathways, and which is normally around 40–100 seconds in duration. Calcium and a substitute for platelet phospholipid are used in order to reduce the effects of platelet variability. If kaolin is added, this becomes the activated PTT (APTT) which has a normal range of 25–30 seconds. This is a good marker of heparin activity, expressed as a ratio 2–4 × normal, and is considered therapeutic for treatment of DVT or PE.

Then there is the activated clotting time (ACT), which involves taking fresh whole blood plus an activator. This is a good bedside monitor of heparin activity (used commonly in cardiac surgery); its normal range is 90–120 seconds.

The prothrombin time (PT) is where plasma and calcium are added to tissue thromboplastin; this has a normal range of 10–12 seconds and can be expressed as a ratio (INR). This reflects the extrinsic and common pathways. It is a good monitor of warfarin activity.

Q. What is DIC?

A. DIC stands for disseminated intravascular coagulopathy, which is the manifestation of a disease process whereby pathways are activated by circulating phospholipid. There is formation of thrombus, platelet and clotting factor (I, II and XIII) consumption and activation of fibrinolysis. The consequence is a reduction in platelet number and function, deficiency in clotting factors and the production of FDPs (fibrin degradation products). FDPs may themselves impair platelet function, compete with fibrin and affect thrombin. Thus, excess fibrinolysis has a 'knock-on' effect on coagulation.

Q. Can you name some of the causes of DIC?

A. The causes of DIC include:

- Obstetric causes, for example amniotic fluid embolus, placental abruption, eclampsia and fetal retention
- Sepsis
- Viraemia
- Disseminated malignancy
- Burns
- Trauma
- Severe liver disease.

Q. How would you diagnose DIC?

A. I would expect to see a raised INR and a raised APTT. I may also expect to find a reduced platelet count, reduced fibrinogen level, raised FDP and raised D-dimers. The absence of D-dimers (normally <10 mg/l) excludes the presence of thrombosis and fibrinolysis.

Q. How would you manage DIC?

A. Treat the cause, where possible, and replace clotting factors and blood products according to clinical need. Close and early liaison with a senior haematologist is vital.

MECHANICS OF RESPIRATION

Q. Define 'respiration'.

A. The term 'respiration' includes both 'internal' respiration (the cellular utilization of oxygen) and 'external' respiration. The latter is defined as the periodic exchange of alveolar gas with fresh gas from the upper airways to reoxygenate desaturated blood and eliminate carbon dioxide.

Q. What mechanisms are involved in 'external' respiration?

A. Three basic mechanisms are involved:

- Ventilatory drive via central control
- Mechanics of ventilation resulting in gas flow in and out of lung units
- Gas exchange occurring across the alveolar–capillary membrane along partial pressure gradients.

Q. What muscles aid inspiration and expiration?

A. Inspiration

- Diaphragm.
- External intercostal muscles.
- Accessory muscles – scalene muscles (elevate the first two ribs) and sternocleidomastoids (raise the sternum). These muscles are mostly active during laboured breathing.
- Other contributions from small muscles in the head and neck; alae nasi (flares the nostrils).

During inspiration the diaphragm contracts and moves downwards approximately 1 cm. The abdominal contents are forced forwards and downwards. The thorax is increased vertically by the diaphragmatic movements and transversely by the lifting of the ribs ('bucket handle' movements by the external intercostals).

Expiration

- Usually occurs passively during normal breathing as a result of elastic recoil of the lungs and chest wall.
- Active expiration (exercise, hyperventilation etc.) involves the abdominal musculature – rectus abdominis, internal/external oblique muscles, transverse abdominis. The muscles contract and force the diaphragm upwards.
- Internal intercostal muscles play a part in active expiration as they have the opposite action to the external intercostals.

Q. Can you explain how the cough reflex works?

A. The cough reflex is stimulated by an irritation to the highly sensitive larynx, trachea or bronchi. The autonomic nervous system is stimulated via the vagus nerves and the cough reflex is triggered. Firstly, approximately 2.5 l of air is inspired. The epiglottis and vocal cords then close tightly and there is a sudden forceful contraction of the abdominal musculature against the diaphragm. As a result, there is a rise in intrathoracic pressure. The epiglottis and vocal cords then open and the intrathoracic high-pressure air bursts out (sometimes up to 100 mph). The purpose of this explosion of air is to carry the irritant out of the airways.

Q. What do you understand by the term 'lung compliance'?

A. Lung compliance is the change in lung volume by a given change in pressure. The lungs are extremely compliant – normal compliance is approximately 200 ml/cm water. Normal expanding pressure is approximately –5 to –10 cm water.

Q. What causes a reduced compliance?

A. Reduced lung compliance may be caused by:

- Pulmonary fibrosis
- Alveolar oedema
- Atelectasis i.e. postoperatively
- Pulmonary hypertension.

An increase in compliance may be seen in emphysema, acute asthma and ageing lungs.

Q. What is the role of surfactant?

A. Surfactant is a phospholipid produced by type II alveolar cells. It dramatically reduces the surface tension of the lining of the alveoli. It contains a hydrophobic and a hydrophilic end which line up on the surface of the alveolus and oppose the normal attracting forces between liquid molecules that are responsible for surface tension.

The consequence of this is to reduce the surface tension within the alveoli, thereby increasing lung compliance and reducing the overall work of breathing. Surfactant also enhances alveoli stability by reducing the incidence of small alveoli collapsing into larger ones and also helps to keep the alveoli dry.

Q. What controls the respiratory system?

A. The respiratory system is controlled by:

- Respiratory sensors – sense information.
- Respiratory control centres – medullary and pontine respiratory centres in the brainstem (may be overridden by the cortex). Process and coordinate information.
- Respiratory effectors – intercostals, accessory muscles, diaphragm, abdominal muscles. Muscles that produce the ventilation.

Q. Tell me about the respiratory sensors.

A. The respiratory sensors are responsible for detecting a change in blood gas tension or acid/base status. They may be categorized into central and peripheral chemoreceptors and mechanoreceptors.

Central chemoreceptors

These can be found on the surface of the medulla oblongata, near the exit of the ninth and tenth cranial nerves. They respond to a rise in H^+ concentration in the CSF. The H^+ concentration rises in the CSF as P_{CO_2} increases and CO_2 diffuses into the CSF from cerebral vessels (the blood–brain barrier is impermeable to H^+ ions). This results in an increase in H^+ ion production within the CSF which stimulates the central chemoreceptors.

Peripheral chemoreceptors

These may be found in *carotid bodies* at the bifurcation of the common carotid arteries and in the *aortic bodies* along the aortic arch. They are sensitive to changes in arterial P_{O_2}, P_{CO_2} and pH (carotids only) and are mainly responsible for the increase in ventilation seen with arterial hypoxia.

Mechanoreceptors

These include chest wall and pulmonary receptors. Chest wall receptors are stimulated by stretch and inhibit excessive forces of contraction. Pulmonary receptors are located within the smooth muscle of the airways. They are stimulated by stretching of the lung and slow the respiratory rate by increasing expiration. Irritant receptors also lie within the airways' epithelial cells. They are stimulated by cold air, cigarette smoke etc. and cause bronchoconstriction.

Pain and hyperthermia are also known to cause an increase in ventilation.

Q. What is Cheyne–Stokes breathing?

A. Cheyne–Stokes breathing is an abnormal pattern of breathing characterized by periodic episodes of apnoea associated with hypoxia. There are episodes of apnoea followed by episodes of hyperventilation as respiration is said to 'wax and wane'. It is thought that the hyperventilation causes a sudden increase in blood oxygen concentration, a short delay occurs whilst the patient is over-breathing and the respiratory centre detects this and acts to depress it by causing apnoea. Carbon dioxide then builds up and the cycle continues.

This condition occurs in patients with heart failure (when there is a delay in blood travelling from the lung to the brain) and in cerebral dysfunction where an exaggerated response may occur (premorbid condition).

Q. What principles underlie ventilatory gas flow and how is ventilation normally distributed?

A. Inspiration is an active process whereby respiratory muscle contraction increases the intrathoracic volume. The pressure in the 'space' between the lungs and the chest wall (the 'intrapleural' pressure) is subatmospheric and reduces further on inspiration, effectively 'pulling' the lungs into a more expanded position and resulting in a negative airway pressure which allows air flow into the lungs along a pressure gradient generated between the mouth and alveoli. This air flow is also influenced by the resistant forces to flow (Hagen–Poiseulle law) and the pattern of flow (laminar or turbulent).

In the upright position, ventilation is greater at the base of the lungs than at the apex. This is because the basal lung intrapleural pressure is greater (less negative) than that at the apex at the start of inspiration; thus the apical alveoli are already partially expanded compared to those at the base before inspiration begins as the intrapulmonary–intrapleural pressure difference is greater. In lung disease where the natural lung tissue elastic recoil is reduced, intrapleural pressures become 'less negative' and during normal expiration this can cause airway/alveolar collapse in the lung bases.

Q. What are 'respiratory compliance' and 'FRC'? What is their relevance in ventilation?

A. Lung tissue elastic recoil is usually measured in terms of compliance, which is defined as the change in lung volume per unit change in distending lung inflation pressure. Normal human lung compliance is approximately 200 ml/cmH$_2$0 and determines gas flow through its influence on lung/airway volume and pressures. A reduced thoracic compliance, such as in fibrotic lung disease and pulmonary oedema, will reduce inspiratory flow and tidal volumes.

The FRC is the 'functional residual capacity'; it reflects the lung volume at the end of a normal exhalation and constitutes an oxygen reserve. It is important because hypoxaemia may result if it is reduced, as well as lung compliance and increased pulmonary vascular resistance (limiting pulmonary blood flow for gas exchange). A lung volume exists below which airway collapse will occur in the dependent basal regions of the lungs – this is called the closing capacity. This volume is normally well below the FRC but with advancing age and conditions reducing FRC it can encroach on and even exceed FRC with subsequent collapse.

Q. What are the determinants of pulmonary blood flow?

A. The major determinants are gravity and hypoxic pulmonary vasoconstriction (HPV). The actual perfusion to an alveolus depends on multiple factors. West (2000) described zones of perfusion in an upright lung with Zone 1 at the apex where alveolar pressure exceeds pulmonary artery pressure and effectively prevents alveolar perfusion despite ventilation (Starling resistor effect). As you descend the lung pulmonary artery pressure increases due to gravitational effects and eventually exceeds alveolar pressure with resulting increasing flow. Hypotension will 'push' further lung units into Zone 1 due to reduced pulmonary artery pressure, leading to hypoxaemia from impaired gas exchange.

Q. What is 'V/Q' mismatch and how does HPV help to prevent it?

A. Ventilation (V) and perfusion (Q) increase toward the gravity-dependent portion of the lungs at different rates. Therefore V/Q is >1 at the apex and <1 at the base. V/Q mismatch exists where there is ventilation without perfusion or vice versa and can result in hypoxaemia. HPV is a reflex vasoconstriction of pulmonary arterioles in response to low PO$_2$ in nearby alveoli. It results in flow of blood away from poorly ventilated areas of the lung, helping to limit V/Q mismatch.

Q. How do surgery and anaesthesia affect respiratory mechanics?

A.   Uncomplicated anaesthesia alters pulmonary function through effects on ventilatory control (responses to hypoxia and hypercapnia are depressed – can persist into early postoperative period), lung volumes and gas exchange. V/Q mismatch increases due to (1) reduced FRC (additive effect of both supine posture and anaesthesia) and lung compliance (leading to airway collapse), (2) inhibition of HPV, (3) decreased pulmonary artery pressures and (4) increased alveolar pressures with mechanical positive pressure ventilation (IPPV). The overall effects on gas exchange are exacerbated in patients with pre-existing lung disease.

Operative sites in close proximity to the diaphragm cause diaphragmatic dysfunction and a restrictive ventilatory defect. Upper abdominal and thoracic incisions are associated with a 60% decrease in FRC – this is at a maximum on day 1 postoperatively and lasts up to 14 days (vertical incisions are worse than horizontal ones).The result is a tendency towards a rapid, shallow breathing pattern in the postoperative period with ineffective cough and microatelectasis.

Reference

West JB. Respiratory physiology. 6th edn. Lippincott Williams & Wilkins, 2000, pp. 36–38

GAS EXCHANGE

Q. What is the concentration of oxygen in atmospheric air?

A.   21%.

Q. Is it the same concentration as oxygen in the alveolus?

A.   No, the concentration of oxygen in the alveolus is approximately 104 mmHg (13.6%). This is because:

- Inspired air mixes with alveolar gas
- O_2 is continually absorbed
- CO_2 content rises
- The moisture content also rises through the respiratory passages.

Q. What determines the rate at which gases diffuse across the respiratory membrane?

A.   There are several factors:

- Membrane thickness – composed of a layer of surfactant, alveolar epithelium, epithelial basement membrane, interstitial space, capillary basement membrane and capillary endothelial membrane
- Surface area of membrane

- Gas diffusion coefficient (based on solubility and molecular weight)
- The pressure of the gas on either side of the membrane.

Q. Can you think of any factors that may impair gas diffusion across the respiratory membrane?

A. Any change in thickness of the respiratory membrane will affect gas exchange, for example as a result of:

- Oedema
- Pulmonary fibrosis.

The surface area of the respiratory membrane may be reduced in emphysema, thereby affecting gas exchange.

Q. Tell me some of the main causes of hypoxaemia.

A. These include:

- Poor oxygenation due to extrinsic causes – low inspired oxygen concentration, hypoventilation as a result of neuromuscular disease
- Respiratory disease – high airway resistance, decreased lung compliance, ventilation-perfusion mismatch, diffusion abnormalities
- Shunts – 'right to left' cardiac shunts
- Abnormal oxygen carriage to tissues – anaemia, haemoglobinopathies, hypovolaemia, oedema, vascular disorders (i.e. peripheral vascular disease)
- Abnormal utilization of oxygen at tissue level – i.e. cyanide poisoning, vitamin B deficiency.

Q. What is a common cause of postoperative hypoxaemia and describe how you would help prevent it?

A. A common cause of postoperative hypoxaemia is basal atelectasis leading to chest infection. Treatment should involve:

- Non sedative analgesia
- Early mobilization
- Chest physiotherapy
- Humidified O_2 supplementation.

Other relatively common problems include:

- Decreased level of consciousness secondary to opioids or sedatives
- Pulmonary embolism.

Q. What is V/Q mismatch?

A. Ventilation/perfusion mismatch occurs in the lung where there is either:

- No ventilation, but adequate perfusion, or
- No perfusion, but adequate ventilation.

Both ventilation and perfusion increase towards the base of the lungs, but perfusion increases to a greater extent than ventilation (Q > V). This creates a physiological dead space at the top of the lung where there is more ventilation than perfusion (see Fig. 9).

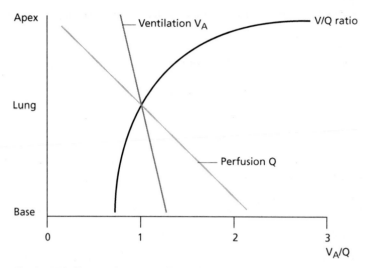

Fig. 9 V/Q diagram in a normal upright individual (V_A = alveolar ventilation)

Q. Why does surgery plus anaesthesia worsen V/Q mismatch?

A. Surgery can worsen the mismatch as a result of:

- Reduced functional residual capacity (FRC) secondary to a reduction in intra-thoracic volume secondary to supine positioning
- Reduced hypoxic pulmonary vasoconstriction (HPV)
- Further reduction in FRC is seen with pregnancy and obesity.

Q. What is PEEP?

A. PEEP is positive end expiratory pressure – it is used as an adjunct to IPPV for prevention or improvement of small airway and alveolar collapse. It increases compliance and FRC, thereby improving oxygenation.

It is used at levels of 5 – 20 cm H_2O (or higher in extreme cases). Problems include the risk of barotrauma and it may increase the dead space. Cardiac output may be reduced especially in hypovolaemia. Intracranial pressure is also increased, thus caution is required for patients with head injuries or neuro-surgical patients.

Q. Define absolute shunt.

A. Absolute shunt is defined as a V/Q = 0, i.e. blood entering the arterial circulation having not taken part in gas exchange. This blood is known as 'shunted blood'.

Q. Can you give me any examples of 'shunted blood?'

A. These include:

- Bronchial arterial blood

- Coronary venous blood (drains directly into the left ventricle via Thebesian veins)
- Aterovenous fistulae.

Q. What is the effect of increased Fio_2?

A. It has little impact on the absolute shunt, because shunted blood has bypassed the alveoli and so has not been exposed to a high alveolar Po_2 (however, this is rarely ever the case).

Q. Define dead space.

A. Dead space is defined as the proportion of tidal volume that does not participate in gas exchange (i.e. V/Q = ∞).

- Anatomical dead space = conducting airways
- Physiological dead space = anatomical plus alveolar.

Q. What happens when the dead space is large?

A. This can interfere with breathing, as the body works to ventilate the lungs, and the ventilated air doesn't reach the alveoli.

ARTERIAL BLOOD GASES

Q. You are handed the following arterial blood gas results and asked to interpret them:

- pH = 7.20
- Pco_2 = 3.1
- Po_2 = 12.5
- HCO_3^- = 11.0
- BE = –15.4
- O_2 saturation = 98%

A. These results demonstrate an acidosis due to the low pH. It is most likely to be metabolic in cause due to the negative base excess. There is also evidence of hyperventilation to compensate as there is a low Pco_2.

Q. Is the Po_2 normal?

A. Yes, the Po_2 is normal; however, I would like to know if the patient was receiving any form of inspired oxygen (Fio_2), as this may affect the Po_2.

Q. Which values are directly measured in an arterial blood gas analyser?

A. pH, Pco_2, Po_2.

Q. Is there any other information that an arterial blood gas may give you?

A. Yes, bicarbonate and base excess, both of which are useful in determining acidosis.

Q. Can you define pH, and what is the normal range?

A. pH is the negative logarithm (to base 10) of the hydrogen ion concentration. It is normally maintained between 7.36 and 7.44. Hydrogen ions govern the pH of extracellular fluid. An acidosis develops below this level and an alkalosis above it.

Q. Can you categorize acid–base disturbances?

A. Yes, they may be categorized as:

Acidosis

Respiratory	Metabolic
Low pH due to an increase in P_{CO_2} (i.e. hypoventilation).	Low pH due to an increase in acid (not P_{CO_2}) or loss of bicarbonate i.e. diabetic ketoacidosis.

Alkalosis

Respiratory	Metabolic
Rise in pH as a result of a fall in P_{CO_2} i.e. hyperventilation.	Rise in pH due to an increase in bicarbonate or loss of acid (not P_{CO_2}) i.e. pyloric stenosis.

These may also be categorized as acute/chronic and compensated/decompensated as the body attempts to correct the disturbance.

Q. Can you define an acidosis?

A. Acidosis is the process which reduces the pH below 7.36, thus causing an acidaemia (the suffix 'aemia' refers to an alteration in blood pH, where 'osis' refers to the process). It is metabolic in origin if bicarbonate is affected, respiratory if $Paco_2$ is affected.

Q. Is it dangerous to be acidotic?

A. With increasing acidosis, normal cellular metabolism is inhibited and depression of cerebral and cardiac function develops.

Q. Take me through the compensatory mechanisms that you know of.

A. Responses to altered pH occur in three phases:

(1) Immediate chemical buffering (rapid):

- Bicarbonate (the most important ECF buffer)
- Hb (intracellular red cell buffer)
- Phosphate and ammonia (urinary system buffers)
- Plasma proteins.

(2) Respiratory compensation (rapid):

- – Increasing minute volume with increasing $PaCO_2$
- – Increasing minute volume with increasing hydrogen ion concentration in CSF, stimulating brainstem chemoreceptors.

(3) Chronic renal compensation (much slower):

- – Increased reabsorption of filtered bicarbonate
- – Increased excretion of excretable acids
- – Increased ammonia production (buffer).

Q. What is a buffer?

A. A buffer is a mixture of a weak acid and its conjugate base. Its purpose is to minimize the change in pH that may occur with sudden changes in acid/alkali concentration.

In solution it is therefore able to accept or donate hydrogen ions.

$$HA \rightleftharpoons H^+ + A^-$$
Weak acid   Conjugate base
Proton donator   Proton acceptor

Buffer systems are most effective when they are maximally dissociated i.e. when the pH is close to the pKa.

Q. Can you give me any examples of a buffer?

A. Buffers include:

- Proteins
- Phosphates
- Haemoglobin
- Bicarbonate.

Q. What is the base excess?

A. It is the amount of base that needs to be added or removed to return the pH of fluid to 7.4, at a $PaCO_2$ of 40 mm Hg and at 37°C. A normal value is 0, a positive value signifies a metabolic alkalosis and a negative value signifies a metabolic acidosis.

Q. Can you name any potential complications of arterial blood sampling?

A. There are several complications including:

- Haematoma/thrombosis
- Infection
- Damage to the vessel – intima/aneurysm formation
- Ischaemia.

These complications occur more frequently with the insertion of an arterial line as opposed to occasional arterial puncture.

Q. How might you assess the circulation in a patient's hand prior to the insertion of an arterial line?

A. I would assess the circulation using Allen's test. This involves occluding the ulnar and radial arteries at the wrist whilst the patient repeatedly makes a fist. This empties the vessels in the hand and so when the occlusion is released from one of the arteries, a flush should be seen within the palm.

Q. What is the significance of no flush?

A. This suggests that the arterial supply from whichever artery has been released is not sufficient to supply the hand. It may have implications in procedures such as radial artery harvest for a coronary artery bypass graft, where the risk of hand ischaemia may be too great.

ACID/BASE BUFFERS

Q. What is the anion gap?

A. It is traditionally defined as the difference between the major measured anions (negative) and cations (positive).

Anions include:

- Chloride
- Bicarbonate
- Albumin
- Phosphate
- Sulphate
- Lactate
- Ketones.

Cations include:

- Sodium
- Potassium
- Magnesium
- Calcium.

An attempt to calculate it may be made in the presence of a metabolic acidosis of unknown aetiology.

Q. Where do most of the body's hydrogen ions come from?

A. They are usually derived from the production of carbon dioxide.

$$H_2O + CO_2 \leftrightarrow H_2CO_3 \leftrightarrow H^+ + HCO_3^-$$

CO_2 dissolves in water to form carbonic acid which then produces hydrogen ions.

A small amount is produced as a result of anaerobic metabolism, metabolism of amino acids and also in the production of ketone bodies.

Q. Can you give an example of a metabolic acidosis with a raised anion gap?

A. Yes, aspirin overdose.

A good mnemonic for these conditions is Luke's Map:

- Lactic acidosis
- Uraemia
- Ketoacidosis
- Ethanol
- Methanol
- Aspirin
- Paraldehyde.

Q. Can you give a value for a normal Pa_{O_2}?

A. Yes, the normal value is 8–13 KPa or 60–100 mmHg. (A rough and basic rule of thumb is mmHg/7 = KPa = %.)

Q. Define hypoxia.

A. Hypoxia is an oxygen deficiency at tissue level. It may be classified as follows:

- Hypoxic hypoxia – too little oxygen in the blood
- Anaemic hypoxia – too little oxygen-carrying capacity
- Ischaemic hypoxia – reduced blood flow
- Histotoxic hypoxia – metabolic poison.

Q. What factors do a normal arterial partial pressure of oxygen depend upon?

A. • Temperature
- Atmospheric pressure
- Age
- Inspired oxygen content ($F_{I_{O_2}}$).

Note that a large rise in Pa_{CO_2} readily produces hypoxia in room air, but not at high $F_{I_{O_2}}$.

EXERCISE AND THE CIRCULATION

Q. What are the regional blood flows to the different organs during rest?

A.

	Blood flow (ml/min)	% Cardiac output
Brain	750	15
Heart	250	5
Muscle	1000	20
Skin	500	10
Kidneys	1250	25
Liver	1500	30
Total	5250	100

Q. How are these altered during moderate exercise?

A.

	Blood flow (ml/min)	Approximate change
Brain	750	Same
Heart	750	Increase × 3
Muscle	10 000	Increase ×10
Skin	2000	Increase × 4
Kidneys	700	Decrease × 2
Liver	800	Decrease × 2
Total	15 000	Increase × 3

The predominant change is seen in the muscle blood flow, which increases about ten-fold with moderate exercise. This comes about due to an increase in the total cardiac output, but there is also a slight increase due to blood being diverted from other organ systems, namely the abdominal viscera and the kidneys. Blood flow to the skin normally decreases initially, then increases along with rising body temperature, which aids heat loss. This cutaneous blood flow may alter again with maximal exertion to resting levels, as vasoconstriction occurs when oxygen consumption reaches maximum levels, to divert further blood to the muscles. Blood flow to the heart normally increases along with cardiac output, so as to maintain the metabolic demands of the myocardium.

Q. How is the increase in cardiac output achieved?

A. Cardiac output is the product of heart rate and stroke volume:

$$CO = HR \times SV$$

At rest, the average cardiac output is 5000 ml/min (70/min × 70 ml). Although there is an increase in stroke volume with exercise by about 20%, the predominant change comes about due to an increase in the heart rate. The heart rate is adjusted to pump the increase in venous return. This is also a result of increased sympathetic stimulation of the sino-atrial node and a decrease in parasympathetic drive. At moderate exercise levels, the heart rate increases in line with the cardiac output, and then is maintained at this new level.

Q. What occurs when maximal exercise levels are achieved?

A. As work rate increases, the heart rate increases until the maximal rate is achieved (approximately 180 – 200). At this level, maximum work has to be interrupted after a brief period since the heart rate cannot keep up the high performance required of it, i.e. fatigue occurs.

Q. What influences blood flow to the skeletal muscle during exercise?

A. Flow increases with increasing work rate of the muscle tissue. This is predominantly brought about by local chemical means, where vasodilatation occurs as a result of build-up of lactate, adenosine and potassium. There is also an increase in P_{CO_2} together with a decrease in P_{O_2} and pH. At near-maximal work, blood flow to muscle alone can amount to over 20 l/min, or four to five times the total resting cardiac output. Also, oxygen extraction can increase dramatically to over 50 times the resting value, which results therefore in greater arterio-venous oxygen differences. This increase is aided by a right shift in the oxy-haemoglobin dissociation curve.

Q. What happens to arterial pressures during exercise?

A. The systolic blood pressure (SBP) rises significantly during exercise, up to more than 180 mmHg, and although the diastolic pressure (DBP) also increases, it does so to a much lesser degree. The increase in pulse pressure (SBP–DBP) occurring in line with the vasodilatation of the muscle vasculature (i.e. decrease in systemic vascular resistance) reflects therefore the significant increases seen in cardiac output with exercise.

Q. What changes occur in athletes with training?

A. Athletes can achieve cardiac outputs of about 40% greater than untrained people (up to seven times the resting values). This occurs as a result of an increase in heart muscle mass as well as heart rate. The end-diastolic volume and the stroke volume both increase (stroke volume increases up to two times the resting value). Also their resting heart rate is lower. There is also improved blood supply during exercise, due to an increase in capillaries supplying the muscles, decreasing the intercapillary distance. A trained athlete also has more mitochondria in their muscles, enabling them to breakdown more glucose by oxidative pathways. Therefore blood lactate levels rise less and oxygen debt occurs later in exercise.

Q. What respiratory changes occur due to the increased oxygen demand?

A. Pulmonary ventilation increases from a resting value of 6 l/min to values of up to 100 l/min. Again, this predominantly occurs as a result of an increase in respiratory rate and, to a lesser degree, an increase in the tidal volume. Although there is an increase in blood volume in the thorax, as well as an increase in residual volume, the tidal volume rises predominantly as a result of a decrease in the inspiratory reserve volume. The respiratory rate increases from about 10–15/min to around 50/min.

ASSESSMENT OF RENAL FUNCTION

Q. Discuss the major causes of acute renal failure.

A. Acute renal failure is defined as a sudden and usually reversible failure of the kidneys to excrete the products of metabolism. It can be subdivided into pre-renal, renal or post-renal. Pre-renal causes account for 60% of acute renal failure.

Acute renal failure and acute tubular necrosis (ATN) are synonymous and account for approximately 30% of acute renal failure presentations. It is commonly secondary to underperfusion. It may also be caused by nephrotoxins:

- Contrast media
- Immunoglycosides – gentamicin
- Myoglobin from crush injuries
- Products of haemolysis (haemoglobin, urea).

Post-renal causes include:

- Obstructive nephropathy such as prostatism
- Raised intra-abdominal pressure
- Pelvic malignancies causing extrinsic compression
- Diabetic neuropathy (affecting bladder function)
- Ureteric obstruction
- Anticholinergic bladder dysfunction including agents of anaesthesia or antihistamines.

Q. Tell me about the methods you know of assessing renal function.

A. Urine output is the commonest and simplest method of assessing renal function and is an indicator of renal perfusion. Others include:

- Plasma levels of urea and creatinine (these may still be normal even in the face of some 75% reduction in nephron capacity)
- Urine to plasma ratios
- Urinary sodium and osmolality
- Specific gravity
- Plasma pH (metabolic acidosis)
- Creatinine clearance
- Clearance of other substances such as PAHA (para amino hippuric acid) and inulin as predictors of renal blood flow
- Radiology of the kidney.

Q. What would you consider to be the most sensitive measure of renal function?

A. Creatinine clearance is a sensitive measure of renal function, but is dependent on prolonged collection periods to allow averaging (up to 24 hours). As a perioperative measure, urine output is easily available; however, it is indirect and non-specific.

Q. How useful is urine specific gravity and osmolality?

A. They are both useful measures of renal concentrating ability. Pre-renal insult will manifest an osmolality of ≥ 500 mOsm/kg H_2O. In ATN there is likely to be an osmolality of <350 mOsm/kg H_2O.

Specific gravity is the comparison of 1 ml of urine to 1 ml of distilled water and has a normal range of 1.010 – 1.030 mOsm/l.

Pre-renal failure specific gravity > 1.030 is seen due to salt and water retention, as opposed to ATN (loss of concentrating ability) where the specific gravity will be less than 1.010.

Q. What other factors might affect the specific gravity and osmolality?

A. Clearly these figures will be altered by the use of diuretics. Other factors include:

- Dextrans
- Mannitol
- Contrast media
- Urinary protein and glucose
- Extremes of age.

RENIN–ANGIOTENSIN SYSTEM

Q. Briefly describe the components and significance of the whole renin–angiotensin system.

A. Renin is a hormone secreted by the juxtaglomerular apparatus of the renal tubule in response to hypotension, hypovolaemia, cardiac failure, cirrhosis and renal artery stenosis.

Renin stimulates the release of angiotensin I via antigiotensinogen. Angiotensin I is converted to angiotensin II in the lungs by angiotensin- converting enzyme.

Angiotensin II causes the release of norepinephrine from sympathetic nerves, and aldosterone from the renal cortex. This promotes sodium reabsorption by the kidney and increases plasma volume, and raises arterial blood pressure. It is also a potent vasoconstrictor by its actions on peripheral adrenergic neurones.

Angiotensin II also directly causes thirst and the release of ADH vasopressin which reduces the excretion of sodium and water from the kidneys. This therefore increases/preserves the circulating volume.

Feedback

In health, an increase in extracellular volume/salt intake or an increase in arterial blood pressure causes a reduction in renin and angiotensin, and therefore the extracellular volume and blood pressure return to normal.

In disease states this feedback mechanism may be inappropriate.

Significance

ACE inhibitors block the conversion of Agt I to Agt II and this increases the levels of natural vasodilator kinins. Vasodilatation may be profound at the first dose and the kinins may cause a metallic taste or persistent cough in some patients.

They are indicated in hypertension and heart failure and reduce mortality and morbidity post-myocardial infarction.

Angiotensin II receptor inhibitors are a new class of antihypertensive drug; they block the action of Agt II on the receptors of the arteriolar smooth muscle, and they have fewer kinin-related side effects.

GLYCOSURIA

Q. Can you explain how electrolytes are reabsorbed in the kidney?

A. Reabsorption in the kidney occurs via passive or active transport. Passive transport involves the movement of electrolytes according to a concentration gradient (osmosis). Active transport requires energy, usually adenosine triphosphate (ATP) and can move electrolytes against a concentration gradient i.e. sodium–potassium pump.

Q. How is glucose filtered in the kidney's tubules?

A. Glucose is freely filtered into the tubules with most other solutes except for plasma proteins. In normal people, nearly 100% of filtered glucose is reabsorbed in the proximal tubule.

Q. Does it appear in the urine?

A. No, usually it doesn't.

Q. When might it appear in the urine?

A. Glucose may appear in the urine when there is a large increase in the glomerular filtration rate or when there is a plasma increase in glucose concentration i.e. diabetes mellitus. There is a threshold within the kidney for the absorption of glucose; below this level, as in most normal patients, all glucose is reabsorbed. When plasma concentrations reach high levels, glucose spills over into the urine.

Q. How else does glycosuria affect the kidney?

A. Large amounts of glucose in the urine cause an osmotic diuresis. As a result, there is a significant reduction in the amount of fluid reabsorbed in the tubules causing a polyuria and dehydration.

Q. What then are the symptoms of diabetes?

A. Patients tend to complain of thirst and urinary frequency.

CARDIAC CYCLE

Q. What is ventricular systole?

A. Ventricular systole is the phase of the cardiac cycle when blood is ejected from the ventricles into the pulmonary and systemic circulations. It begins soon after ventricular excitation – this depolarizes by the start of the QRS complex. The ventricle undergoes isovolumetric contraction until intraventricular pressure supersedes intra-aortic pressure. At this point the aortic and pulmonary valves open and blood is ejected from the ventricle into the aorta and pulmonary artery. The first heart sound corresponds to the closure of the mitral and tricuspid valves at the beginning of isovolumetric contraction. Left ventricular systole ends on the beginning of the second heart sound at closure of the aortic valve (see Fig. 10).

Q. What does the P wave on the ECG correspond to?

A. The P wave signals atrial contraction, which occurs at the end of passive ventricle filling. Under normal circumstances this would account for 25% of ventricular filling; the other 75% of ventricular filling has occurred passively following opening of the mitral and tricuspid valves at the point at which intra-atrial pressure is greater than intraventricular pressure.

Q. What do the third and fourth heart sounds correspond to?

A. The third heart sound, if present, occurs shortly after the second sound. It may occur in normal subjects. It will also occur with reduced ventricular compliance or increased volume such as in cardiac failure. It may also occur with a VSD. It is thought to be due to ventricular filling.

The fourth heart sound occurs shortly before the first heart sound and may occur in hypertension, aortic and pulmonary stenosis. It is said to occur due to increased pressure of atrial contraction with forceful ventricular distension.

Q. What other signs and symptoms would you expect to see in somebody with left ventricular failure?

A. The symptoms of left-sided failure include dyspnoea, which will typically be worse on lying flat (orthopnoea). The patient may sometimes give a history of being woken at night with breathlessness (paroxysmal nocturnal dyspnoea). On examination, they may be peripherally shut down, with basal crepitations, ventricular hypertrophy and the gallop rhythm as previously mentioned. There may also be evidence of heart murmurs.

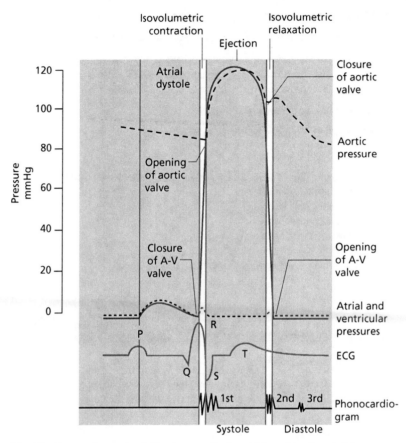

Fig. 10 The cardiac cycle. A-V valves = mitral and tricuspid valves ('atrio-ventricular')

Q. What murmurs may you expect to find?

A. You may find evidence of aortic regurgitation, which will increase pre-load and thus increase cardiac workload. Aortic stenosis may cause left ventricular failure due to an increase in after-load. Chest radiograph may reveal:

- Cardiomegaly
- Increased fluid in the pulmonary fissures
- Pleural effusions
- Evidence of pulmonary oedema.

There will also be evidence of ventricular hypertrophy/strain on the ECG.

Q. What are the mainstays of treatment for cardiac failure?

A. The main aim is to reduce after-load, thereby reducing the work of the heart.

- Diuretics reduce systemic vascular resistance, blood volume and oedema
- Vasodilator drugs reduce pre-load and after-load i.e. nitrates
- Inotropes improve left ventricular muscle contraction.

Arrhythmias are commonly associated.

Q. What are the causes of cardiogenic shock?

A. Causes of cardiogenic shock include:

- The commonest cause is an acute myocardial infarction (if >40 % of the left ventricle is damaged)
- Left ventricular aneurysm
- Aortic incompetence
- Acute mitral regurgitation
- Traumatic myocardial contusion
- Myocardial 'stunning' post prolonged cardiac surgery.

MAINTENANCE OF BLOOD PRESSURE

Q. What is blood pressure?

A. Blood pressure is the force exerted by blood onto a vessel wall. It is measured as a systolic and diastolic pressure in mmHg. It is affected by:

- Stroke volume
- Systemic vascular resistance (SVR).

Q. How is it controlled in normal subjects?

A. Blood pressure is controlled by a vasomotor centre in the medulla and pons. It has three essential components:

- Vasoconstrictor area – stimulates sympathetic nervous system
- Vasodilator area – inhibits vasoconstrictor area
- Sensory area (tractus solitarius) – via the vagus and glossopharyngeal nerves, this provides reflex control of vasodilator and vasoconstrictor effects.

The normal resting vasomotor tone is controlled by continual signals from the vasoconstrictor centre.

Other areas of the brain such as the hypothalamus, cerebral cortex and frontal lobe can play a part in the regulation of the vasomotor centre.

Q. What is the baroreceptor reflex?

A. Baroreceptors are stretch receptors located in the walls of large arteries, e.g. in the internal carotid artery (at bifurcation), known as the carotid sinus, and the arch of the aorta. They provide information on pulse rate, arterial and filling pressure via signals to the vasomotor centre in the medulla and minimize variations in blood pressure:

- Carotid sinus – transmits signals to the glossopharyngeal nerve and then to the tractus solitarius in the brainstem
- Aortic arch – transmits signals to the vagus nerves and then to the tractus solitarius in the brainstem.

A rise in blood pressure stimulates signals from the baroreceptors which travel to the brainstem. The vasoconstrictor area is inhibited and the parasympathetic area is stimulated. The result is a vasodilation of arterioles and veins in the peripheral system. There is also a drop in heart rate and strength of contraction.

Q. What happens when there is a drop in blood pressure?

A. When the blood pressure drops, the opposite effect occurs. The baroreceptors become inactive, there is a loss of the inhibition of the vasoconstrictor centre and the blood pressure rises.

Q. Can you explain the changes that occur in blood pressure in going from a lying to a standing position?

A. When a person stands up from the lying position, there is a drop in blood pressure in the head and upper part of the body and the person may feel faint. The baroreceptors feedback to the brainstem and there is a loss of the vasoconstrictor inhibition. As a result, there is a strong sympathetic drive to restore the blood pressure.

Q. Are there any other receptors involved in blood pressure control?

A. There are chemoreceptors and low-pressure receptors.

Chemoreceptors

Chemoreceptors are present within the carotid bodies (at the bifurcation) and aortic bodies. They are sensitive to changes in oxygen, carbon dioxide and hydrogen ion concentrations in blood. They are stimulated specifically by:

- Low oxygen
- High carbon dioxide
- Excess of H^+ ions.

Their signals are also transmitted through the glossopharyngeal and vagus nerves to the brainstem. Once stimulated, the vasomotor centre is also stimulated which causes a sympathetic drive to return the blood pressure to normal.

Low-pressure receptors

These are stretch receptors present in the walls of the atria and pulmonary arteries. An increasing volume in the atrium causes an increase in heart rate and the strength of contraction by stimulating a sympathetic drive.

Q. Tell me about hormonal control.

A. The release of catecholamines from the adrenal medulla is under hypothalamic control in response to physiological stress ('fight or flight'). Adrenaline and noradrenaline result in the following effects:

- Constriction of blood vessels
- Cardiac effects – increased rate and strength of contraction
- Dilated pupils
- Sweating
- Decreased GIT activity.

Q. What is cardiac output?

A. Cardiac output = stroke volume × heart rate.

Q. What are the determinants of stroke volume?

A. Stroke volume (SV) is determined by three factors:

- Pre-load (ventricular filling)
- After-load (total peripheral resistance)
- Myocardial contractility.

Pre-load reflects left ventricular end diastolic volume (LVEDV) and initial fibre length. Therefore an increase in pre-load will increase initial fibre length, thus increasing SV, according to the Frank–Starling relationship (the force of contraction being proportional to the initial fibre length).

After-load is the tension generated in the left ventricular muscle during systole.

Q. How is heart rate controlled?

There is a balance between parasympathetic (vagal) and sympathetic efferents. A relative dominance of sympathetic outflow will lead to an increase in chronotropism (rate) as well as inotropism (force of contraction), dromotropism (impulse conduction speed) and bathmotropism (increased excitability due to lowered threshold potential).

Q. Can you tell me about regional homeostatic mechanisms?

A. Vessel diameter is the principal determinant of regional blood flow (laminar flow in a tube is directly related to the pressure) and the 'radius to the power 4'. The arterioles are the main vessels involved in determining total and regional resistance to flow.

Neural control influences the vascular tone via the sympathetic system, post-ganglionic transmission via α-1 receptors causing vasoconstriction, and via β-2 receptors causing vasodilation.

Autoregulation also allows tissues to dictate blood flow independently of fluctuations in systemic blood pressure.

Q. Can you site some of the principal areas where autoregulation occurs?

A. Coronary and cerebral blood flow is virtually entirely locally controlled. A rise in such metabolites as H^+ ions, CO_2, ADP and AMP as well as potassium increase blood flow to facilitate their removal. There is a myogenic reflex, whereby vessels constrict in direct response to increases in blood pressure. This is of particular importance in brain and kidney homeostasis. Hypoxaemia causes all vascular beds, except lung, to vasodilate (hypoxic pulmonary vasoconstriction occurs in the lungs to alter V/Q mismatch).

There are also many locally produced vasoactive substances. Vasodilators include NO, histamine, kallikrein, bradykinin and prostacyclin. Vasoconstrictors include prostaglandin F2∞ and angiotensin II.

VALSALVA

Q. Tell me about the Valsalva manoeuvre.

A. The Valsalva manoeuvre is described as a forced expiration against a closed glottis after full inspiration. It was originally described by an Italian anatomist, Antonio Valsalva (1666–1723). It was used as a means of expelling pus from the middle ear.

It is effectively an increase in intrathoracic pressure of 40 mmHg for 10 seconds whilst direct arterial blood pressure tracing is undertaken.

Q. Can you describe the four cardiovascular phases of the Valsalva manoeuvre?

A. (1) There is an increase in blood pressure and also an increase in intrathoracic pressure expelling blood from the thorax.

(2) There is a reduction in cardiac output and blood pressure secondary to the reduced venous return. The subsequent baroreceptor reflex causes an increased heart rate and vasoconstriction that brings the blood pressure towards normal.

(3) Upon opening of the glottis, the venous return increases and there is an increase in cardiac output due to venous return.

(4) As the blood pressure increases, the baroreceptors respond and cause bradycardia.

Q. Can you give me an example of an abnormal response to the Valsalva manoeuvre?

A. In patients with an autonomic neuropathy, blood pressure falls and stays low until the increased intrathoracic pressure is released. Pulse changes are absent e.g. diabetics.

In hypovolaemic patients there will be an exaggerated response.

Q. Can you think of any other uses of the Valsalva manoeuvre?

A. Besides being a test for autonomic dysfunction, it may also be a useful manoeuvre for terminating SVT or evaluating heart murmurs.

THERMOREGULATION

Q. How would you go about measuring a patient's core temperature?

A. It may be measured orally, rectally and via the tympanic membrane.

Q. Describe the concept of thermoregulation in humans.

A. Humans are homeotherms and have a system to maintain a core temperature within close limits. Normally, it is 37°C plus or minus 0.4°C. Thermoreceptors are present in the hypothalamus, spinal cord and skin. These are heat sensitive and respond to changes in core temperature. In the normal subject, as body temperature rises, vasodilatation will occur followed by sweating. As the core temperature reduces, vasoconstriction will occur first of all, followed by non-shivering thermogenesis. This is closely followed by shivering and piloerection.

Q. What are the effects of anaesthesia on thermoregulation control?

A. There is a reduction in the thermoregulatory threshold which widens to plus or minus 2.5°C of 37°C, therefore widening the inter-threshold range over which regulatory responses are absent. This type of patient will therefore only have vasoconstriction and non-shivering thermogenesis available for heat production. Furthermore, non-shivering thermogenesis is only minimally available and total body oxygen consumption hardly increases.

Q. Can you describe the mechanisms of heat loss?

A. First of all, 60% of heat is dissipated to cooler surroundings; this is called *radiation* and is dependent on skin perfusion and the exposed surface area. Secondly *evaporation*, which accounts for 20% of heat loss under anaesthesia, is due to the latent heat of vaporization or the energy required to vaporize liquid from serosal or mucosal surfaces. It is dependent upon exposure and the ambient humidity. Thirdly, *convection*, which accounts for 15% of heat loss, is dependent on air flow over the exposed surface. Fourthly, *conduction*, which accounts for about 5% of heat loss and is dependent on transfer between adjacent surfaces.

Q. What happens to the core temperature when a person is feverish?

A. When a person is feverish, circulating pyrogens interfere with thermoregulation within the hypothalamus. The body's internal 'thermostat' is increased and therefore, as the fever develops, the patient experiences chills and shivering. Similarly, as the fever returns to normal, the patient feels extremely warm and so sweating and vasodilation occur.

BILE

Q. Where is bile produced?

A. In the liver.

Q. What is the function of bile?

A. Bile facilitates the absorption and digestion of fats.

Q. How does it do this?

A. Bile first acts as a detergent on fat that is digested. This way, fat is broken down into smaller pieces. Then, bile forms complexes with the lipids known as micelles. Micelles are more soluble and hence more readily absorbed via the intestinal mucosa.

Q. What would happen if a person had no bile?

A. The person would be unable to absorb lipids such as free fatty acids, mono-glycerides and cholesterol. They would pass through the intestine and present as steatorrhoea. In the long term, the person would suffer from nutritional deficiencies, especially of fat-soluble vitamins.

Q. What is bile made up from?

A. Bile is made up of:

- Bile salts
- Bilirubin
- Cholesterol
- Lecithin
- Water and plasma electrolytes i.e. Na^+, K^+, HCO_3^-.

Q. What is the role of the gallbladder in bile secretion?

A. Bile is secreted continuously by the liver. It travels from the liver to the gallbladder where it is stored until needed in the intestine to digest fat. The gallbladder also concentrates the bile by continuously absorbing water through its mucosa. The concentration of bile salts, cholesterol and bilirubin therefore increases.

Free fatty acids in the duodenum stimulate the release of cholecystokinin. This results in the contraction of the gallbladder and the simultaneous release of the Sphincter of Oddi. Bile is then released into the duodenum and fat absorption can then occur.

Q. Tell me about the enterohepatic circulation of bile.

A. The enterohepatic circulation of bile is the process by which bile is recycled in the body. Approximately 95% of the bile is reabsorbed through the wall of the small bowel. It then travels back to the liver via the portal system to be reused.

Q. How is bilirubin excreted?

A. Free bilirubin is formed from the breakdown of haemoglobin. It is extremely water insoluble and rapidly binds to albumin. It travels to the liver where it is conjugated and so becomes more water soluble (bilirubin glucuronide). It is then excreted into bile to the intestine where conjugated bilirubin is converted into urobilinogen. It is the oxidation of stercobilinogen and urobilinogen that gives stool and urine their characteristic colours.

Q. If a patient had extremely pale stools and dark urine, what would be your diagnosis?

A. My diagnosis would be obstructive jaundice.

FUNCTION OF THE PANCREAS

Q. Can you tell me what the pancreas secretes?

A. The pancreas functions as an exocrine and an endocrine gland.

Exocrine secretions (from the acini):

• Digestive enzymes – trypsin, chymotrypsin and carboxypolypeptidase
• Sodium bicarbonate.

Endocrine secretions (from the Islets of Langerhans):

• Insulin
• Glucagon.

Q. What is the main function of the pancreatic digestive enzymes?

A. The function of the pancreatic enzymes is to aid the digestion of protein, carbohydrates and fats.

Q. What causes the pancreatic enzymes to be released?

A. The secretion is stimulated by:

• Vagus nerve – acetylcholine, in the enteric nervous system
• Secretin – secreted by the intestinal (duodenum and jejunum) mucosa when acid food enters
• Cholecystokinin – secreted by the intestinal mucosa.

Q. Are these enzymes in their active or inactive form whilst in the pancreas?

A. They are in the inactive form whilst in the pancreas and become activated when they come in contact with intestinal mucosa.

Q. Why is this?

A. This is because they may digest the pancreas if they were stored in the active form.

Q. Can you think of any scenarios in which this may occur?

A. Yes, this may occur when the pancreas is blocked by a tumour or gallstones or is damaged (eg. by alcoholism). Acute pancreatitis then develops as pancreatic secretions accumulate and the usual inhibitor of the secretions, trypsin inhibitor, is unable to cope. The result is a widespread necrosis of the pancreas that can result in circulatory shock and is life threatening.

CALCIUM METABOLISM

Q. What is the normal range of serum calcium?

A. 2.3–2.7 mmol/l.

Q. What is the function of calcium?

A. Calcium is important for many physiological processes in the body. These include:

- Transmission of nerve impulses
- Blood clotting
- Contraction of smooth, skeletal and cardiac muscle.

99% of the body's calcium is stored in bones.

Q. How is the remaining 1% stored?

A. The remaining 1% is stored extracellularly (0.1%) and intracellularly (0.9%).

Q. Why is the metabolism of calcium in the body so tightly controlled?

A. The metabolism of calcium is tightly controlled as the nervous system is very sensitive to changes in serum concentrations. For example, hypercalcaemia can lead to depression of the nervous system and, similarly, hypocalcaemia can cause excitation of the nervous system.

Q. How does the body control serum calcium levels?

A. Calcium balance is maintained by dietary intake (milk, cheese, eggs) and urinary/ faecal losses. Calcium is absorbed in the intestines, aided by vitamin D. A small proportion of ingested calcium is absorbed and the rest is excreted in faeces. Some of the ingested calcium is also excreted in the urine. The body also derives calcium from gastrointestinal secretions.

Q. What hormones influence the balance of calcium in the body?

A. Hormones involved in the regulation of calcium include:

- Parathyroid hormone
- Calcitonin
- Vitamin D (1,25-dihydroxycholecalciferol).

Parathyroid hormone (PTH)

This hormone is produced by the parathyroid glands and is controlled by serum levels of ionized calcium. For example, hypocalcaemia results in the stimulation of parathyroid hormone production and hypercalcaemia causes the opposite effect. It has three main sites of action:

- Bones – PTH stimulates bone resorption and calcium release
- Intestine – PTH stimulates kidney production of active vitamin D which increases intestinal absorption of calcium
- Kidneys – PTH increases reabsorption of calcium in the kidneys and also increases phosphate excretion.

Calcitonin

Calcitonin is produced in the C cells of the thyroid gland. Its main action is to lower hypercalcaemia which it does by increasing calcium deposition into bones.

Vitamin D

Vitamin D is formed in the skin by UV radiation. In order to become active it is first stored in the liver and then converted to its active form in the kidney. Its main action is to increase serum calcium by increasing intestinal absorption. It also increases absorption of phosphate in the intestines. Its other actions include:

- Kidneys – reduces excretion of calcium and phosphate
- Bone – increases calcification.

Q. How is phosphate related to calcium metabolism?

A. Phosphate is closely linked with calcium metabolism in the body. It is readily absorbed from the intestine and excreted mostly in urine. Fluctuations in its serum concentrations, however, do not cause such dramatic physiological effects as occur with calcium.

High serum levels of phosphate result in hypocalcaemia as calcium phosphate precipitates out of solution and is deposited in the bones. Similarly, a low serum phosphate causes hypercalcaemia as calcium is released from the bones.

Q. What are the symptoms of hypercalcaemia?

A. Generally, hypercalcaemia is asymptomatic. However, if calcium is dramatically raised, the patient may develop:

- Thirst/polyuria

- Electrolyte imbalances – hyponatraemia and hypokalaemia
- Anorexia/constipation/nausea/vomiting
- Weakness/anxiety/depression/confusion/drowsiness/coma (if severe)
- Ectopic calcification – renal stones, calcification of blood vessels (if longstanding)
- Pancreatitis
- Hypertension.

If severe, hypercalcaemia may become a medical emergency.

IRON METABOLISM

Q. How is iron stored in the body?

A. Two thirds of the body's iron is in the form of haemoglobin. The rest is stored mostly as ferritin, a small proportion is stored as myoglobin and the remainder is within haem compounds.

Q. How is iron absorbed after it has been ingested?

A. Dietary iron is ingested in the form of meat. A small proportion may be absorbed from anywhere along the small intestine and generally according to body needs. For example, iron absorption may rise to as much as 25% of that ingested when a woman is menstruating or is pregnant.

The liver also secretes apotransferrin via bile into the duodenum. Apotransferrin is an iron-transporting protein which binds free iron and also iron compounds such as haemoglobin/myoglobin. Apotransferrin then becomes known as transferrin and binds to receptors within the intestinal epithelium. Any excess of iron within the intestine may also be absorbed into the mucosa where it remains available for absorption for a few days until it is released back into the lumen of the intestine.

Transferrin is then absorbed into the intestinal epithelium and then into the blood plasma.

Q. What regulates the absorption of iron?

A. Iron absorption is regulated by the body's need for it. This is obviously increased in women during pregnancy, childbirth and menstruation.

When apoferritin, the body's iron-transporting protein, is fully saturated with iron the resulting excess of iron in the intestinal mucosa results in a decrease in iron absorption. Also, as the body's iron stores become fully saturated, the liver decreases its production of available apoferritin, thereby reducing the amount of iron absorbed from the intestine.

Q. What is haemosiderin?

A. A small proportion of iron is stored as an insoluble form known as haemosiderin. When iron is in excess, haemosiderin may form large deposits in cells which can be viewed readily in histological slides.

In cases of iron poisoning, dangerous amounts of haemosiderin may be deposited around the body resulting in clotting abnormalities/haemorrhage and shock.

Q. What are the symptoms of iron deficiency anaemia?

A. Iron deficiency anaemia is the commonest type of anaemia. It is associated with tiredness, dizziness and occasionally palpitations on exertion. It may also cause spoon shaped nails (koilonychia) and in severe cases, cerebral oedema may occur.

Q. What is it generally caused by?

A. It can be diet related and tends to affect people in underdeveloped countries with poor diets. It can also be due to chronic blood loss.

Q. How is it diagnosed?

A. The diagnosis may be suspected on history and clinical examination. However, it is usually confirmed by a blood film. This demonstrates a microcytic, hypochromic anaemia as the absorption of iron from the intestine is not able to keep up with the amount of red blood cells (RBC) required and so the RBCs produced are small and lacking in haemoglobin. Blood tests also confirm the diagnosis by demonstrating a low serum iron, high/normal total iron-binding capacity and low serum ferritin.

SMALL INTESTINE

Q. What are the functions of the small intestine?

A. The small intestine is approximately 4 m long and is the major site of digestion and absorption in the body. This includes carbohydrates, fat, amino acids, ions, vitamin B_{12}, bile salts and water.

It is also a rich source of immunoglobulins and is responsible for the production of peptide hormones, such as gastric inhibitory peptide, which regulate the absorption and motor activity of the bowel.

Q. Why is the small intestine efficient at digestion?

A. The small bowel is efficient at digestion due to its widespread absorptive area:

- Mucosal folds ('*valvulae conniventes*')
- Villi – protrude from the mucosa into the lumen of the bowel
- Brush border present on each epithelial cell on every villus (microvilli).

(It is said that the absorptive area of the small bowel is approximately the size of a tennis court.)

The small bowel is also aided in digestion by the highly vascular nature of the villi and by the fact that they are continuously moving in order to absorb more fluid.

Q. How is water absorbed across the bowel wall?

A. Water is absorbed by osmosis, driven by gradients set up by the active transport of sodium, glucose and amino acids.

Q. Is this the same for digestion of fats?

A. Most ingested fat is digested in the small intestine; in order for it to be efficiently digested, it first has to be broken down into smaller globules. This emulsification occurs when it comes into contact with bile in the duodenum. Bile acts as a detergent in that it breaks it up into much smaller globules and makes it more water soluble.

Lipase is essential in the absorption of fats. It is produced in:

- Lingual gland (small amounts)
- Pancreatic fluid (large amounts)
- Enterocytes (small amounts).

The most abundant dietary fat is triglyceride. The pancreatic lipases split triglycerides into free fatty acids and 2-monoglycerides. These are both relatively insoluble, and so they form *micelles* with bile salts, which makes them more water soluble. They are then absorbed across the bowel mucosa.

Q. Why might someone need a small bowel resection?

A. The commonest causes for a small bowel resection include:

- Congenital abnormalities eg. Meckel's diverticulum
- Inflammatory conditions eg. Crohn's disease
- Trauma – blunt or open
- Idiopathic – during other surgical procedures such as hysterectomy
- Infarction/thrombosis of mesenteric vessels
- Bleeding e.g. angiodysplasia or Peutz–Jeghers syndrome
- Tumours e.g. carcinoid, lymphoma.

Q. What are the possible consequences of a small bowel resection?

A. Resection of a small amount of bowel should not affect the patient. However, resection of larger amounts may result in 'short bowel syndrome', where there is weight loss and malabsorption. Malabsorption of vitamin B_{12} and bile salts results if the terminal ileum is removed and so the patient may become anaemic and unable to absorb fat and fat-soluble vitamins.

With increasing removal of the small bowel, the patient develops diarrhoea due to having a short small bowel. Eventually, they may also develop steatorrhoea.

Q. Why are bacteria useful in digestion?

A. Bacteria are present in abundance in the bowel. They aid digestion by breaking down molecules such as gastrin and glycocholic acid. They also release folate which may then be absorbed

Q. What is the 'blind loop syndrome?'

A. The 'blind loop syndrome' is where a blind loop of bowel develops overgrowth of bacteria which then interferes with absorption. The blind loop may occur as a result of surgery but may also occur where multiple diverticuloses are present.

STEROID HORMONES

Q. Where are corticosteroids produced in the body?

A. Corticosteroids are produced by the adrenal cortex, situated within the adrenal gland at the superior poles of both kidneys.

Q. What are steroids made from?

A. Cholesterol, provided by circulating low density lipoproteins (LDL).

Q. What types of steroid hormones are produced by the adrenal cortex?

A. There are two main types – mineralocorticoids and glucocorticoids. A small amount of androgenic sex hormone is also produced.

Q. What is the essential difference between the two types?

A. Mineralocorticoids are mainly involved in the regulation of electrolytes such as sodium and potassium. Glucocorticoids are involved with carbohydrate metabolism and the stress response.

Q. How is cortisol involved in the stress response?

A. The stress response may be precipitated by:

- Fear/pain/mental stress
- Heat/cold
- Trauma/surgery
- Infection.

All of the above are associated with an increase in adrenocorticotrophic hormone (ACTH) from the anterior pituitary followed by an increase in cortisol in the circulation. The result is a quick mobilization of fatty acids and amino acids to provide glucose and energy.

Q. What effects does cortisol have?

A. These include:

- Stimulation of gluconeogenesis
- Decreases utilization of glucose by cells
- Increase in blood glucose concentration
- Reduces protein stores in the cells other than the liver
- Increases plasma proteins (to increase amino acid transport to the liver)

- Increases mobilization of fatty acids from adipose tissue and amino acids from muscle
- Depression of immune system (lymphopenia/eosinopenia)
- Anti-inflammatory effects (either by preventing it from occurring or speeding up resolution).

Q. How do steroid hormones exert their effects?

A. Steroid hormones travel in the circulation and are fat soluble. This means that they are able to pass through the cell membrane and then bind to their specific receptor protein. This hormone–receptor complex then travels to the cell's nucleus, where it binds to another receptor and stimulates the production of mRNA. The mRNA then leaves the cell nucleus, travels to the ribosome where translocation occurs and protein is produced. An increase in protein production then results in a physiological response.

Glucocorticoids result in a physiological response by increasing or decreasing transcription of genes and thereby altering synthesis of mRNA.

Q. What is Cushing's disease?

A. Cushing's disease is the hypersecretion of cortisol as a result of excessive amounts of ACTH from the anterior pituitary. It is the commonest cause of Cushing's syndrome. There is an increase in plasma ACTH and cortisol.

It is associated with the following:

- 'Lemon on a stick' appearance (central obesity, mobilization of fat from the lower body and deposited on the abdomen)
- Moon face (oedematous)
- Acne and hirsutism (androgenic effects)
- Increased blood glucose (due to increased gluconeogenesis)
- Weakness due to loss of muscle protein
- Suppressed immune system and increased risk of infection
- Thin skin and purple striae due to loss of skin collagen
- Osteoporosis due to loss of protein within bones.

Q. What specific concerns would you have regarding a patient undergoing surgery who has been on oral steroids for 3 years?

A. I would be worried about:

- Risk of infection
- Poor wound healing
- Impaired stress response
- Masking of symptoms of postoperative complications.

Patients who have been on long-term steroid therapy will have a depressed endogenous cortisol production, and will therefore require steroid cover. If they are taking more than 10 mg prednisolone per day, steroid cover is recommended for major surgery. This will involve 25 mg hydrocortisone at induction plus 25 mg 6 hourly for 48–72 hours.

TRANSECTION OF THE SPINAL CORD

Q. Describe the types of spinal cord injury that you know of.

A. **Primary neurological injury**

This is as a direct consequence of the initial injury, for example blunt trauma/ vertebral fracture/ligamentous rupture. This results in impingement of the spinal cord by bone or soft tissue. Also, penetrating injuries to the spinal cord result in primary neurological injury; however, these are rarely seen.

Secondary neurological injury

This is spinal cord injury as a result of a primary insult, for example hypoxia, mechanical abnormalities of the back, reduced spinal perfusion. Other examples include poor immobilization of the cord, oedema of a damaged cord, haemorrhage into/around the cord, electrolyte abnormalities such as hyper/hypoglycaemia, hypercalcaemia.

Q. What clinical features may lead you to suspect spinal cord injury in a trauma patient?

A. I would suspect a spinal cord injury in the following circumstances:

- History of multiple injuries/head injury
- Abnormal respiratory pattern due to diaphragmatic breathing
- Priaprism
- Abnormal reflexes – abdominal, anal and bulbocavernosus.

Q. At what level may a spinal cord injury cause respiratory difficulties?

A. A spinal injury occurring at C5 will result in paralysis of the diaphragm and at T12 will affect the intercostal muscles and interfere with breathing. Also, patients with spinal cord injuries have difficulties expectorating and have a tendency to V/Q mismatches. They may also have associated chest injuries e.g. rib fractures adding to the respiratory difficulties.

Q. What is spinal shock?

A. Spinal shock is characterized by:

- Flaccid paralysis
- Priaprism
- Diaphragmatic breathing
- Autonomic dysfunction
- Gastric dilatation.

It lasts for an indefinite period of time, although it usually lasts for approximately 4 weeks. As this state resolves, some areas of the spinal cord may recover; however, the permanently damaged areas become spastic.

Q. Apart from a complete spinal cord transection, describe the main injury patterns that you know of.

Brown–Sequard syndrome

Hemisection of the cord, often following direct trauma. Includes ipsilateral paralysis and loss of vibration and joint sense. Loss of pain and temperature sense contralaterally.

Central cord syndrome

More selective damage to the central grey matter leading to paralysis with variable sensory loss, which is greater in upper limbs due to fibre position within the cord. Urinary retention is common.

Anterior cord syndrome

Anterior spinal artery damage from aortic trauma or cross-clamping leads to cord ischaemia. Results in paralysis with abnormal light touch, pain and temperature sensation (cortico-spinal and spino-thalamic tracts). Posterior columns are preserved with normal vibration and joint position sensation.

Cauda Equina syndrome

GIT and GUT dysfunction associated with lower motor neurone signs in lower limbs. Sensory changes are variable. Associated with lumbar fractures.

Children/SCIWORA

Due to the high mobility of the bony spine, fractures are less common in children than in adults. There is Spinal Cord Injury WithOut Radiological Abnormality in 55% of children with a complete cord injury. The cervical region of the under 8-year-olds is most commonly damaged in this pattern. It should, however, be suspected in all age groups with all mechanisms of injury to the cord until excluded.

Q. Describe the physiological and autonomic changes seen in early spinal cord injury.

A. The pattern of injury depends upon the level and nature of the injury but the following should be considered.

The injury causes massive sympathetic discharge, causing a sudden profound rise in blood pressure and systemic vascular resistance. Direct sequelae of this include myocardial infarction, strokes and severe arrhythmias.

A

Airway loss, vomiting and aspiration risk. Impaired reflexes and gastric stasis.

B

Fractures above C4 result in no diaphragmatic action. Fractures affecting T2–12 allow intercostal-aided breathing; however, above this level they affect the diaphragm only. Breathing is also affected by a poor ability to cough and reduced tidal volumes. Poor muscle power and impaired cough may also result in sputum retention. Other effects on breathing include pulmonary emboli, neurogenic pulmonary oedema and ARDS.

C

Loss of sympathetic tone results in neurogenic vasodilatory shock. With damage above T1 affecting cardiac innervation, unopposed vagal tone may result in severe bradycardia/asystole.

D (neurology)

Muscle flaccidity and areflexia may last for weeks. Over 50% of T7 or higher lesions are associated with autonomic dysreflexia. Stimulation below the lesion allows a spinal reflex that has lost higher inhibition. Hypertension, bradycardia, sweating and flushing occur above the lesion. This can be fatal. Triggers are usually GIT or GUT in origin.

Other

Hypothermia from peripheral vasodilation; paralytic ileus; urinary retention; SIADH – water retention and hyponatraemia; glucose intolerance; DVT and PEs; stress ulceration of the gut; pressure sore and depression are common.

BRAINSTEM DEATH

Q. How do you certify/confirm death?

A. • Fixed dilated pupils
  • No response to pain
  • No central pulses
  • No respiratory effort.

Q. When did the concept of brainstem death materialize?

A. The development of ITU meant that patients who had sustained what would previously have been fatal cerebral insults were being maintained with cardiorespiratory support. This was first reported in 1959.

In 1968 (Harvard), 1971 (Minnesota) and the 1976 and 1977 conferences of the medical Royal Colleges and faculties in the UK, criteria governing the diagnosis were developed. It became increasingly clear that all the tests looked at brainstem function.

Q. Why is brainstem function important for life?

A. It determines:

- Wakefulness via the reticular activating system
- Cardiovascular control
- The ability to breathe independently
- All nerve fibres between the periphery and central nervous system pass through it.

Q. What are the common causes of brainstem death?

A.
- Head injury (> 50%)
- Subarachnoid haemorrhage (30%)
- Other intracranial causes (19%) – encephalitis, meningitis, abscess, tumour
- Extracranial causes – e.g. cardiac arrest (rare).

Q. Who should conduct the tests and when?

A. Two doctors each with more than 5 years' GMC registration, preferably consultants, and not members of any transplant team, on two separate occasions.

More than 6 hours after the onset of coma, or more than 24 hours following cardiac arrest.

Death is pronounced after the first set of tests – the second set is confirmatory and timing is discretionary.

Q. Is permission from relatives then required to discontinue ventilation?

A. No.

Q. Name the preconditions.

A.
- Coma dependent on ventilation
- Proven irremediable structural brain damage.

Q. Are there any exclusions?

A. Yes:

- Drug intoxication e.g. muscle relaxants/hypnotics (NB allow > $3\frac{1}{2}$ lives)
- Metabolic/endocrine disorders e.g. diabetic coma
- Hypothermia (< 35°C).

Q. What are the crucial brainstem reflexes that are tested, and that must be absent?

A.
- Pupillary response to light
- Corneal reflex
- Vestibulo-ocular reflex – iced water in external auditory meatus
- Gag/cough
- Facial response to painful facial stimuli
- Apnoea test.

Apnoea test

The patient must be pre-oxygenated with 100% O_2 for 10 minutes. The $Paco_2$ must be first recorded in the normal range (i.e. 4.5 – 6 kPa). The ventilator is then disconnected whilst insufflating 6 l/min O_2 via the endotracheal tube; and then observe. The patient must show no sign of respiratory effort and a repeat arterial blood gas must show a $Paco_2$ of > 6.65 kPa.

Q. If brainstem reflexes are not absent, when can you consider the persistent vegetative state (PVS)?

A. When sufficient recovery from the cerebral insult has been allowed, for example 3 months to 1 year.

Patients with PVS generally are still able to breathe, but make no purposeful voluntary movement and no meaningful response to the surrounding environment. The eyes may be open at times, but unable to follow movement consistently.

Q. What are the criteria for organ donation?

A. The donation of human organs is controlled by the Human Tissue Act (1961). Any donated organ comes from a patient who has given prior consent to do so. It is possible to donate individual organs: heart, lungs, kidney, liver, pancreas, bowel, bone, cornea, skin and more controversially face (skin and muscle).

Inclusion criteria include:

- Prior written consent
- Confirmed diagnosis of brainstem death (as discussed previously)
- No history of cancer (except brain tumours), HIV, hepatitis B
- Patient must be stabilized on a ventilator with no signs of sepsis.

Exclusion criteria (these vary according to the unit):

- Drug addicts
- Alcoholics
- Presence of diabetes or cardiac disease is a relative contraindication depending on the organ to be donated.

CRITICAL CARE

PRINCIPLES OF ANAESTHESIA

Q. What is anaesthesia?

A. Anaesthesia is derived from the Greek word anaisthesis, meaning without feeling. The word has been used for centuries to describe a lack of feeling, but was suggested by Holmes in 1846 to describe the state of sleep produced by ether. It is accepted that anaesthesia occurs at a particular, yet undefined, point along a continuum from awake to asleep. It is either present or absent therefore.

The classic description of anaesthetic stages was given by Guedel in 1937 in patients breathing ether in air.

Stage 1 (analgesia)

Normal reflexes remain intact and the stage ends with loss of the eyelash reflex and unconsciousness.

Stage 2 (excitement)

The pupils dilate and the eyes become divergent in gaze. Breathing becomes irregular and the patient may struggle. Laryngospasm may occur along with coughing or vomiting. The stage ends with the onset of automatic breathing and loss of the eyelid reflex.

Stage 3 (surgical anaesthesia)

This is divided into four planes:

- Plane 1. Pupils are now normal or small, lacrimation may be increased, and swallowing and vomiting are depressed. Gaze returns to the central position and the conjunctival reflex is lost.
- Plane 2 is until the onset of intercostal paralysis. The corneal reflex is lost, and the pupils enlarge. Lacrimation is increased and regular deep breathing begins.
- Plane 3 (ideal surgical anaesthesia). This is the onset of sole diaphragmatic breathing with complete intercostal paralysis. There is depression of the light reflex and laryngeal reflexes as well as lacrimation.
- Plane 4 includes diaphragmatic paralysis and depression of cranial reflexes.

Stage 4 (overdose)

This is seen with dilation of the pupils and apnoea.

The techniques used today disguise these stages, with plane 3 being reached very quickly.

Q. What are the essential principles of anaesthesia?

A. Anaesthesia involves hypnosis, analgesia and muscle relaxation.

Hypnosis

This occurs at induction. Propofol is a popular anaesthetic induction agent. It has a short half-life, quick onset of action and short recovery time. It can cause marked hypotension. Fentanyl, a strong opioid, may also be used with it, reducing the amount of propofol needed and it also has less of a hypotensive effect.

Inhalational agents are used to maintain hypnosis throughout the operation. Popular agents include isoflurane and desflurane.

Muscle relaxation

This is achieved using neuromuscular junction blocking drugs, and gives profound muscle relaxation. Other non-neuromuscular blocking anaesthetic agents may also give a limited degree of muscle relaxation.

This facilitates endotracheal intubation and intraoperatively aids the surgeon in intra-abdominal and thoracic surgery. Muscle relaxants used may be classified into depolarizing and non-depolarizing; non-depolarizing agents are more commonly used. Atracurium and vecuronium are popular agents due to their quick onset of action. Their effects last for approximately 30 min and may be reversed by the anticholinesterase neostigmine. The only depolarizing neuromuscular blocking agent in common use is suxamethonium, whose effects cannot be reversed.

Analgesia

Analgesia may be administered via the premedication and during the procedure. The choice of agent here depends on the required duration, ranging from the very short-acting alfentinil to fentanyl and to long-acting morphine. Other analgesics used during maintenance of anaesthesia include NSAIDs and paracetamol.

Q. Can you explain the principles of a 'crash induction?'

A. This describes what is normally called a rapid sequence induction which is used when a patient is not adequately starved prior to surgery. The stomach is assumed to be full due to the non-fasted state and so cricoid pressure is applied as the anaesthetic is being given to prevent regurgitation and therefore aspiration until the airway is protected. Propofol is generally avoided because of its hypotensive effects and thiopentone is often used instead. Cricoid pressure is only released when the endotracheal tube is correctly positioned and the cuff inflated.

MONITORING OF THE CRITICALLY ILL PATIENT

Q. What are the basic steps involved in monitoring the critically ill patient?

A. Even with critically ill patients, it is still essential to monitor simple and easily measured parameters. The pulse, blood pressure and respiratory rate should all be continuously recorded. Temperature should also be regularly measured. Pulse oximetry will help to assess oxygenation.

The majority of critically ill patients will have central venous access or a Swan–Ganz catheter helping to accurately measure cardiac and respiratory status. It is also routine to insert an arterial line for accurate blood pressure monitoring and blood gas sampling. A urinary catheter to measure urine output correctly is also required.

Blood tests are needed. Their type and frequency will depend on the exact nature of the underlying illness. The following blood tests would be considered routine in most critically ill patients. Full blood count to assess the presence of infection, anaemia and platelet count. Urea and electrolytes will monitor renal function and minimize the chances of electrolyte imbalance. Liver function and clotting status also need regular assessment in the critically ill, due to the possibility of multiorgan failure or coagulopathies.

ECG and chest radiograph are also essential baseline monitoring tools. They may need regularly repeating if clinically indicated.

Q. Could you tell me about the limitations of pulse oximetry?

A. Because of the shape of the oxygen-haemoglobin dissociation curve, a small drop in the oxygen saturation from say 99% to 94% is related to a large drop in the partial pressure of oxygen in the blood.

Pulse oximetry does not measure carbon dioxide levels in the blood. It is possible for critically ill patients to have unacceptably high levels of carbon dioxide, while maintaining good oxygen saturations.

Other factors that limit pulse oximetry include poor peripheral perfusion, anaemia, dirty skin and frequent movements, such as shivering.

When dealing with critically ill patients, regular arterial blood gas measurements are an important adjunct to pulse oximetry.

Q. What are the advantages of arterial cannulation?

A. Using a transducer it is possible to continuously measure arterial blood pressure. Arterial cannulation allows for simple and regular access to arterial blood for use in blood gas measurements.

Q. When would you consider the insertion of a central venous catheter?

A. When managing hypovolaemia and fluid replacement a central line is particularly helpful. They are used for the infusion of vasoactive drugs, irritant drugs and long-term intravenous therapies. Central venous pressure may also guide therapy in cardiac failure.

Q. Are there any drawbacks in the use of central venous catheterization?

A. Central venous catheterization is an invasive and non-trivial procedure. The insertion requires skill and experience. Complications include damage to local structures, pneumo- or haemothoraxes, damage to nerves, blood vessels, lymphatics and local tissue, or the loss of instrumentation within the body.

Central venous catheterization also predisposes to sepsis. The insertion of a foreign body can lead to either generalized sepsis or sepsis at the insertion site, if microbes are introduced during the procedure. The catheter is usually left in situ for several days, and acts as a focus for further potential sepsis.

Q. Can you tell me which parameters can be measured using a Swan–Ganz catheter?

A. When a Swan–Ganz or pulmonary artery (PA) catheter is correctly inserted the balloon at the tip is 'wedged' in the pulmonary artery. This will allow measurement of the pulmonary artery wedge pressure; other measurements are made with the balloon deflated. Physiological values can be calculated from the measured parameters.

When the tip of the catheter is wedged in the pulmonary artery, it connects a column of fluid from the transducer to the left atrium. Logically, it is then possible to gauge the left ventricular end diastolic pressure and in turn the left ventricular end diastolic volume, the true pre-load.

Cardiac output can be measured either by injecting a known volume of cold saline and measuring thermodilution or more commonly by cooling of an electrical element in the catheter by the blood flow round it.

Systemic vascular resistance, pulmonary vascular resistance, stroke volume and oxygen delivery and uptake can also be derived from the basic measurements made with a Swan–Ganz catheter.

Q. Could you draw the various waveforms generated by the different vessels and chambers that are seen when inserting a Swan–Ganz catheter into the pulmonary artery?

A. Yes. As you can see from the diagram (Fig. 11) the four wave types seen are derived from the position of the tip of the catheter. They change as the tip advances through the right atrium, the right ventricle, the pulmonary artery until it finally comes to rest in the pulmonary artery.

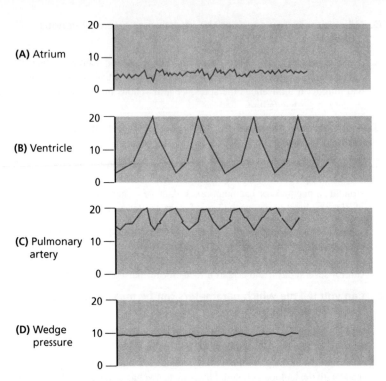

Fig. 11 Pressures (mmHg) and waveforms encountered during the insertion of a Swan–Ganz catheter.

Q. You have mentioned the use of transducers several times in your answers, could you give me some more information about them?

A. Transducers are devices that convert mechanical energy into an electrical output. Each of them varies in design and function depending on what is being measured. For example, a transducer is used to produce a display on a monitor next to the patient that shows the pressures measured while inserting a Swan–Ganz catheter.

It is important to be aware of the role of transducers because incorrect calibration can lead to spurious results being displayed.

LOCAL ANAESTHETICS

Q. What are local anaesthetics?

A. They are drugs that reversibly inhibit impulse transmission to nerve fibres. They may be classified structurally into amides or esters. Amides are hepatically metabolized and esters by cholinesterases.

Q. How do they act?

A. By blocking sodium channels. They are weak bases, stored as the hydrochloride salt in an acidic solution (predominantly ionized and water soluble):

$$BH \longleftrightarrow B + H^+$$
$$\text{Ionized} \qquad \text{Free base}$$

As the pH in physiological tissues is relatively more alkaline, the drug dissociates releasing the free base (more lipid soluble). It is the uncharged free base that readily diffuses intra-axonally, where it reionizes by combining with hydrogen ions at the lower pH. It is when the drug is in the ionized state that the sodium channels are blocked, preventing depolarization.

Q. What is the major determinant of the onset of conduction blockade?

A. pKa

Q. Do you understand the term pKa?

A. Yes, it is the pH at which the drug is 50% ionized/unionized.

Q. What is its significance?

A. The higher the pKa (i.e. the further from physiological pH) the more *ionized* the drug is, and thus the less lipid soluble it is. Conversely, when the pKa is closer to 7.4, there is more unionized drug, which is more lipid soluble. (The pKa of most local anaesthetics is above physiological pH.)

Q. Tell me about potency and what is the major determinant?

A. The more potent a drug is, less is required for the same effect. The main determinant is *lipid solubility*. The more lipid soluble the drug, the more readily it will cross membranes and it therefore has increased potency (bupivacaine is more lipid soluble than lignocaine).

Q. What main factor affects the duration of action of local anaesthetics?

A. Protein binding. Increased protein binding equates to an increased duration of action.

Q. Give me the maximum safe doses of three commonly used local anaesthetics.

A. Lignocaine 3 mg/kg
Bupivacaine 2 mg/kg
Prilocaine 6 mg/kg.

✔ **TIP**

For % to mg/ml conversion simply shift the decimal place one to the right:
Lignocaine   2% = 20 mg/ml
Bupivacaine 0.5% = 5 mg/ml
Bupivacaine 0.25% = 2.5 mg/ml.

Toxic doses can therefore be easily calculated. 20 ml of 0.5% bupivacaine = 100 mg; safe in anyone over 50 kg.

Q. What effect do local anaesthetics have on blood vessels?

A. Most local anaesthetics, with the exception of cocaine, cause a degree of vasodilation.

Q. What effect does the addition of adrenaline have?

A. This causes an increased duration of action – there is vasoconstriction and thus reduced systemic absorption, in addition to alpha effects enhancing blockade.

When added to lignocaine in a concentration of 1 in 200 000, it increases the safe dose from 3 mg/ml to 7 mg/ml (it has no effect on bupivacaine). Onset time is reduced.

Q. What are the symptoms and signs of local anaesthetic toxicity?

A. • Light headedness, perioral tingling and tinnitus
• Visual disturbance
• Muscular twitching
• Convulsions
• Coma
• Respiratory arrest
• Resistant cardiac arrhythmias and cardiac arrest.

Q. How would you treat these?

A. Treatment is supportive. I would give cardiorespiratory support consisting of ABC, oxygen and senior assistance (CPR may be considerably prolonged due to the refractory nature of the disrhythmias).

Convulsions require treatment with phenytoin or barbiturates. Cardiopulmonary bypass has been used in exceptional circumstances.

FLUID MANAGEMENT

Q. What percentage of the body is water?

A. Approximately 60% in the average male and 55% in females due to higher levels of fat.

Q. How is this divided up within the body?

A. Over 50–60% (30 l) of this water is intracellular, the rest is extracellular and may be divided up as follows:

- Interstitial – 10 l
- Intravascular – 5 l
- Transcellular (water in GIT, CSF, synovium, pleural and pericardial) – 1 l.

Q. What do you know about the distribution of electrolytes within these compartments?

A. Water readily crosses the cell membrane and equilibrates according to osmolality. Sodium and chloride ions are mostly extracellular and potassium is predominantly intracellular. They require an active pump to transport them across the cell membrane.

Q. What are the basal 24 hour fluid requirements of a normal adult?

A. Fluid requirements are dependent on size, age and temperature. Normally, this is around 2500 ml of water which the body obtains from food, water and as a result of the metabolic oxidation of CO_2. The bodily requirements of sodium and potassium are approximately 1 mmol/kg/day.

Water losses through urine, faeces, skin and through respiration amount to approximately 2500 ml.

Q. What is normal saline?

A. Normal saline is a crystalloid fluid that may be given intravenously and is composed of:

- Water
- 150 mmol/l sodium
- 150 mmol/l chloride.

Q. What would happen to water distribution in the body if you administered 1 l of 0.9% normal saline (NaCl)?

A. 0.9% sodium chloride is isotonic with plasma. An infusion would result in an expansion of the extracellular space. Some fluid would shift into the vascular space as the osmolality would increase by a small amount. Approximately 15% of it would remain in the intravascular compartment.

Q. Is this the same for 5% dextrose solution?

A. Generally dextrose solutions are distributed across all compartments and as a result only very small amounts remain in the intravascular compartments.

Q. What fluid regime would you prescribe for a healthy patient who was nil by mouth?

A. I would work out their basal requirements and losses and try to match this as closely as possible.

Q. Why is potassium so important?

A. Potassium is lost continuously through urine and faeces. A normal patient will become hypokalaemic if it is not replaced.

Q. What routes are available to you for administering fluids?

A. There are several possibilities:

- Intravenous
- Oral
- Subcutaneous
- Interosseous (in children).

Q. What would happen if you gave a patient too much potassium?

A. Hyperkalaemia can cause ventricular fibrillation. Care should be taken to give bags of fluid to which potassium has already been added. Bolus injection should never be done.

Q. What factors are important to consider preoperatively?

A. • Dehydration must be avoided
- Starvation alone often accounts for a 1–2 l fluid deficit (e.g. starved from midnight for late morning or afternoon surgery)
- For every degree increase in temperature, there is an approximate 10% increase in fluid requirement
- Excess bowel losses in emergency patients or those receiving bowel preparation.

Q. What happens to the distribution of water across the compartments as dehydration worsens?

A. Initially, water is lost from all body compartments. As the water losses become severe, hypovolaemia within the intravascular compartment stimulates the release of aldosterone. This stimulates the kidney to retain sodium which causes the plasma sodium to increase. Water then diffuses out of the cells and the following clinical features occur:

- Loss of skin turgor/dry mucous membranes
- Weakness and confusion
- Peripheral vasoconstriction
- Oliguria
- Concentrated urine.

Q. What is the essential difference between crystalloid and colloid solutions?

A. Colloid solutions are plasma substitutes and exert an oncotic pressure. An infusion of colloid, therefore, would result in an increase in the intravascular compartment as it is unable to cross through the capillary membrane. Crystalloids are a similar composition to plasma and so rapidly distribute throughout the extracellular compartments.

Q. Can you give me any examples of commercially available colloids?

A. Colloids may be given in the form of human plasma derivatives (from donor blood) or as synthetic plasma substitute.

Human plasma

Fresh frozen plasma, human albumin and purified protein fraction may be prepared from donated blood. Several donors are required to produce one unit. The process carries all the risks associated with blood transfusion and is also costly. Human albumin has an extremely long half-life of 10 days.

Synthetic plasma substitutes

- Gelatins – i.e. haemaccel, gelofusin. Produced from bovine collagen and remain in the intravascular compartment for approximately 30 min (half-life 2–4 hours). Low incidence of allergic reactions.
- Dextrans – i.e. dextran 40 and 70. Glucose polymer. Has been reported to cause allergies, coagulation abnormalities and interferes with the cross-matching process. Plasma half-life is approximately 12 hours.
- Hetastarch – i.e. hespan. Stays in the intravascular compartment the longest. Associated with coagulopathy if large volumes are infused. Plasma half-life approximately 24 hours.

Q. When would you consider using colloids instead of crystalloids?

A. The use of colloids over crystalloids in an emergency is controversial. Both types of fluids are able to expand the plasma volume; however more crystalloid is required to produce the same effect as a colloid.

Q. Can you give me any potential risks of colloid infusions?

A. The previously mentioned allergy/anaphylaxis, coagulation abnormalities and interaction with blood transfusion (high calcium content). Colloid infusion must be administered with caution as it can worsen oedema due to increased capillary permeability.

VENOUS ACCESS

Q. Under what circumstances would you consider performing a central venous cannulation?

A. Central venous cannulation can be performed for short-, medium- and long-term administration of irritant or potent drugs such as chemotherapy and antibiotics, total parenteral nutrition and dialysis. Central venous catheters are also useful for central venous pressure monitoring and administration of large volumes of intravenous fluid during resuscitation. Central venous cannulation may also be performed for procedures such as pulmonary artery catheterization and cardiac pacing.

Q. What is your preferred site of central venous catheterization?

A. Depending on the requirement, my preferred site of central venous cannulation is via the internal jugular vein. For central venous pressure monitoring, slow fluid administration, blood sampling and drug administration, I would use a triple lumen CVP line.

Q. Why the internal jugular approach?

A. It is, first of all, the approach with which I am most comfortable. Under most circumstances it is easier to perform and is reliable for short-term usage (up to 1 week). If the carotid artery is accidentally punctured, pressure may easily be applied and the bleeding controlled. This is not easily done in the subclavian approach. It is however possible to damage structures including the brachial plexus, phrenic nerve, thoracic duct (left-hand side) or sympathetic chain. It is also possible to damage the dome of the pleura causing pneumothorax. However, the risk of this complication occurring is far more likely with the subclavian versus the high internal jugular approach.

The subclavian vein approach, although having a higher incidence of pneumothorax and haemothorax and being more difficult to perform, is preferable for longer-term placement as it is more comfortable for the patient; it is also less likely to become infected as there is reduced movement in and out of the catheter at the site of insertion.

The femoral vein approach is often easier than the aforementioned approaches, especially in obese patients. Complications include a traditionally higher incidence of infection, thromboembolism and femoral arterial puncture. The pleura and lungs are also completely avoided.

Q. What other complications can you think of?

A. Apart from damage to the structures surrounding the area of insertion, the introduction of a central venous catheter into the heart may cause arrhythmias or cardiac perforation. Embolism is a very real risk in all techniques, particularly when the insertion site is above the level of the heart. As previously mentioned, catheter-related sepsis can be avoided by using a fastidious aseptic technique.

Q. What is the Seldinger technique?

A. The Seldinger technique is used for the insertion of cannulae. It involves the use of a guide wire and is thought to be safer and less traumatic than other techniques. The needle comes with a guide wire within it. The vessel is punctured using the needle, the guide wire is then advanced through it and into the vessel. The needle can then be removed and the guide wire remains within the vessel. A dilator is then advanced over the guide wire and removed. The cannula may then be easily advanced over the guide wire, safely into the vessel. The wire can then be removed and the cannula secured in place.

Q. When would you consider central venous pressure monitoring?

A. CVP monitoring is indicated in shock states, hypovolaemia, acute cardiovascular disease, major surgery and in the intensive care unit. It is useful in indicating right ventricular pre-load and cardiac function. In the normal heart, right ventricular and left ventricular functions are mirrored. It is only then that the CVP may be taken as a reflection of left ventricular pre-load. It is possible for the CVP to be normal in the presence of left ventricular failure and pulmonary oedema, or raised in right-sided failure, but with normal left-sided function. That said, CVP is a good starting point in the assessment of cardiac failure, cardiac tamponade, circulatory overload, vasoconstriction and superior vena caval obstruction (where the normal venous waveform may be lost).

Q. What does a CVP of 10 cm of water tell you?

A. Nothing in isolation. The normal range is between 0 and 8 cm of water. It should be used as a dynamic measurement. In other words, hourly measurements should be taken and change noted in response to fluid bolus administration. For example, a volume challenge of 250 ml of gelofusin leading to a persistent rise in central venous pressure of 5 cm or more of water is an indication of right ventricular failure; whereas the same rise followed by a reduction in CVP to the pre-existing level may either be normal or an indicator of ongoing haemorrhage. In haemorrhage, fluid resuscitation may not increase the CVP.

Other problems that lead to misrepresentation of central venous pressure monitoring include:

• Varying patient position whilst using manometer
• Different operators
• Lack of knowledge about how to operate the manometer
• A blocked catheter
• Incorrect three-way tap alignment.

It must therefore be stressed that CVP measurement should be conducted by somebody who is familiar with the technique, aware of the physiology expected, and is able to conduct serial measurements themselves. It should also not be used in isolation for determining fluid and inotropic resuscitation requirements. Other physiological parameters must be taken into consideration such as pulse, blood pressure and peripheral perfusion.

Q. In the initial resuscitation of haemorrhagic shock, which would you consider more useful, a CVP line or peripheral intravenous access?

A. During initial resuscitation of haemorrhagic shock, I would use two large 14-gauge venflons, sited in large arm veins.

Q. What are the flow characteristics of a 14-gauge venflon?

A. 240 ml per minute can be infused through a 14-gauge venflon. Thus two will enable a litre of fluid to be infused every 2 minutes. This is much faster than through central venous lines, which are longer and of smaller bore.

Poiseuille's law

This states that the rate of blood flow is proportional to the fourth power of a vessel's radius. Therefore diameter plays a large part in determining flow through a vessel.

$$Q = \frac{\pi.\,P.\,r^4}{8.\eta.\,l}$$

where Q = rate of flow, P = pressure difference between two ends of a vessel, r = radius of vessel, l = length of vessel, η = viscosity.

I would leave the insertion of large rapid-infusion lines such as the Swann–Ganz introducers to a competent anaesthetist.

PAIN CONTROL

Q. What are the benefits of good pain control postoperatively?

A. The World Health Organization has stated that 'it is a basic human right to have adequate pain control postoperatively'.

Besides the psychological impact of poor pain control, all physiological systems of the body will be affected. The physiological impact is best considered by system:

Respiratory

Pain causes poor intercostal muscle function, and diaphragmatic splinting; this leads to a drop in alveolar minute ventilation and functional residual capacity, leading to decreased Pao_2 and increased $Paco_2$. Poor cough, atelectasis and sputum retention predispose a patient to respiratory infection and thus increased morbidity and mortality.

Cardiovascular

Increased sympathetic tone causes tachycardia and hypertension, which combined with raised total peripheral resistance and increased myocardial oxygen demand predisposes a patient to myocardial ischaemia. This is more common in the elderly and those with pre-existing ischaemic heart disease.

Gastrointestinal

Pain causes gastric stasis and increases postoperative vomiting.

Genitourinary

Urinary retention is common.

Endocrine

The stress response to surgery is increased by pain. The hormones cortisol, anti-diuretic hormone and catecholamines lead to sodium and water retention, and poor diabetic control.

Central nervous system

Restlessness, confusion, agitation and poor sleep habit are all associated with poor pain control.

Psychological

Pain causes fear, anxiety, poor compliance and a reluctance to describe symptoms.

General

Immobility predisposes a patient to deep vein thrombosis and therefore pulmonary embolism.

Physiotherapy/rehabilitation are delayed or less effective.

Q. **What do you understand by the term multimodal approach to pain control?**

A. A multimodal approach to postoperative pain control involves not only drugs. It also includes specific techniques such as epidurals, patient-controlled delivery systems and psychological support of the patient. This approach allows the doses of opioids to be reduced, thus reducing the side effects of respiratory depression and sedation.

Pain is rarely completely removed, except by a few nerve-blocking techniques, but is made acceptable to the patient and kept at a level whereby recovery is not delayed.

Each patient defines pain as what they say hurts, not necessarily what the medical staff think. Simple traditional intramuscular opioid techniques have been shown to fail to work effectively in up to 70% of patients.

Analgesic drugs should be given in a stepwise 'analgesic ladder' approach, with a review after each step to check for effect and side effect, effectively titrating to the individual patient and their response. At any point, nerve blockade and non-steroidal anti-inflammatories (NSAIDs) can be considered. For example:

- Simple analgesics – paracetamol or NSAID unless contraindicated on request
- Regular prescription
- Combinations – paracetamol and weak oral opioid e.g. codeine or dihydrocodeine
- Oral opioid/equivalent – morphine, tramadol
- Intravenous opioids
- Specific nerve-blocking techniques.

The patient should have their pain assessed before and after each step, preferably by a scoring system such as a visual analogue score e.g. a pain ruler, and should be reassured and supported until analgesia is achieved. This dramatically increases success and satisfaction.

Successful pain control is best delivered by specially trained nurses backed by a pain control team, to whom difficult cases can be referred and from whom advice sought. This also allows training of ward staff and is an approach now being favoured by those Trusts that can staff such a team.

Q. What are the side effects of opioids?

A. Opioids can cause:

- Respiratory depression, can also predispose to atelectasis and chest infection
- Sedation
- Nausea/vomiting
- Dependence
- Tolerance
- Constipation – may be severe and require laxatives/purgatives
- Euphoria
- Pruritus.

Q. What non-opioid drugs or techniques do you know of? How do they work?

A. Non-opioid drugs can be classified into two groups, paracetamol and non-steroidal anti-inflammatory drugs (NSAIDs).

Paracetamol works as an analgesic and antipyretic by acting on the central nervous system prostaglandin synthesis but has little or no peripheral anti-inflammatory actions. It is useful as a background analgesic and is synergistic with simple oral opioids.

NSAIDs, e.g. ibuprofen and diclofenac, have anti-inflammatory, antipyretic and analgesic actions and are widely used for postoperative analgesia. In children they can have a similar effectiveness to opioids; in adults they are opioid sparing and are synergistic with opioids. They have a common mechanism of action of inhibition of cyclo-oxygenase, resulting in reduced prostaglandins, and pain mediator molecules at the sites of tissue damage.

The side effects of prostaglandin inhibition elsewhere include gastric ulceration, renal impairment, and altered platelet function, and this has led to the creation of cyclo-oxygenase 2 inhibitors like rofecoxib, which are believed to have more selective actions on pain over side effects.

Local anaesthetic blocks

Lignocaine and bupivacaine are commonly used in the UK and produce analgesia lasting for 2 – 4 hours depending upon the site used; occasionally it can last for much longer when directly applied to a major nerve or plexus. The powerful analgesic effect is caused by nerve action potential blockade, but the overall quantity and frequency are limited by the toxic side effects of the local anaesthetic.

Spinal/epidural local anaesthetic blocks

Applying these drugs into or around the central nerves allows for profound analgesia at minimal dosages, but is complicated by effects upon the sympathetic tone distally causing hypotension and motor blockade. These effects are minimized by low-dose techniques and infusions. They act synergistically with opioids applied via the same route. They require specific nursing care and insertion by skilled anaesthetists.

Q. **Are there any other possible routes of administering analgesia?**

A. Other routes include:

- Intra-nasal – mainly used in children
- Sublingual i.e. buprenorphine
- Inhalation i.e. nitrous oxide
- Transcutaneous i.e. fentanyl patches.

Q. **What are the side effects of NSAIDs?**

A. The side effects include:

- Gastric – reflux, gastritis, peptic ulcers
- Respiratory – bronchospasm may be induced, particularly in asthmatics
- Renal – acute renal failure
- Clotting – irreversible inhibition of thromboxane A_2 reduces the efficacy of platelet function and so bleeding occurs.

SHOCK

Q. Define and classify shock

A. Shock can be defined as inadequate tissue or organ perfusion as a consequence of acute circulatory failure, resulting in generalized tissue hypoxia. It usually occurs from inadequate cardiac output or misdistribution of blood flow. Traditionally, it has been divided into:

- Hypovolaemic including haemorrhagic, but also burns and dehydration etc.
- Cardiogenic i.e. pump failure, following MI, for example
- Obstructive i.e. impedance to ventricular outflow, e.g. PE or cardiac tamponade
- Septic.

Others causes of shock include anaphylaxis and high spinal cord injury (neurogenic).

Q. What clinical features are common as shock progresses?

A. The body responds to the cause of shock through the sympathetic nervous system, which causes tachycardia and usually vasoconstriction in an attempt to maintain cardiac output and 'reverse' the hypotension. Oliguria (<0.5 ml/kg) occurs as the body actively retains fluid, and metabolic acidosis as a result of inadequate oxygen delivery to the tissues. As shock progresses, there is increasing organ failure shown by the lungs (dyspnoea), brain (e.g. confusion) and heart (myocardial depression); hepatic and gastrointestinal failure may also occur.

Q. How much blood can a fit young adult lose before there is a marked change in blood pressure?

A. Young healthy individuals can vasoconstrict intensely, maintaining relatively normal systolic blood pressure, even after a blood loss of 1500 – 2000 ml, i.e. 30–40% blood volume. Only then might you see a fall in their systolic blood pressure. Initially, their diastolic pressure is raised, resulting in a narrower pulse pressure (SBP — DBP), associated with a tachycardia to maintain cardiac output (HR × SV). Other more subtle signs may include tachypnoea (air hunger), and decreased capillary refill (>2 seconds), as well as pale extremities and complexion. Young adults often become anxious or aggressive with ongoing large blood loss.

Q. How might the elderly differ in response to acute blood loss?

A. The elderly often differ as a result of coexisting pathology or medications they are on. They may not develop an appropriate tachycardia if they are on beta blockers for angina or blood pressure. Often they have very little reserve and may become hypotensive after minimal blood loss, or as a result of autonomic neuropathy, where they cannot vasoconstrict appropriately. Alternatively, an apparently normal blood pressure may not be normal in someone with marked pre-existing hypertension, and may in fact be a significant hypotension for that individual.

Q. What if a patient fails to respond to resuscitation?

A. Clinical improvement will occur and be sustained if you have replaced the correct amount of blood and other fluids, and ongoing losses have decreased or stopped. If a patient does fail to respond, you have to consider other sources of occult haemorrhage, e.g. chest, abdomen and pelvis, especially in the trauma patient. It is also important to rule out the causes of non-haemorrhagic shock in the trauma patient, such as pericardial tamponade, tension pneumothorax and cardiac contusion.

AIRWAY CONTROL

Q. What are the clinical features of upper airway obstruction?

A. These include:

- Dyspnoea/stridor
- Hoarseness
- Dysphonia
- Use of accessory muscles including abdominal musculature
- Tracheal tug
- Intercostal recession
- Cyanosis.

Q. What simple manoeuvres can you use to try to clear the airway?

A. Firstly, I would open the mouth taking care not to move the neck in a trauma case. Then I would look inside for any obvious obstruction; e.g. the patient may have food or teeth inside. I would sweep my finger inside to try to dislodge any foreign bodies. Then I would lift the chin and perform a jaw thrust in order to stop the tongue blocking the airway.

Q. What adjuncts are available for you to use in the emergency setting?

A. If a patient is maintaining their own airway but is hypoxic, I would administer 100% oxygen using a simple face mask or nasal cannula. If they were unconscious, I would use a Guedel or nasopharyngeal airway to help maintain the airway and administer 100% oxygen.

Q. Are there any problems associated with using a Guedel airway?

A. A Guedel airway will induce retching/vomiting in patients who are not deeply unconscious and also may induce a rise in intracranial pressure.

Q. Do you know what a Venturi mask is?

A. A Venturi mask is a mask used for administering oxygen and is used instead of a facial mask when an accurate assessment of inspired oxygen is needed. It is therefore known as a 'fixed performance' mask and can be used to give set amounts of oxygen i.e. 24%, 60%.

Q. When would you consider endotracheal intubation?

A. • I would consider endotracheal intubation in the following circumstances:
- Upper airway obstruction
- Apnoea/respiratory failure
- Prophylaxis – smoke inhalational injuries to the airway/protection against aspiration.

Q. If you had a patient with severe injuries to the larynx, nose or mouth making endotracheal intubation impossible, how would you secure the airway?

A. Under these circumstances, I would call for senior help and perform a needle cricothyroidotomy. This is a quick procedure that involves a small incision in the midline, over the cricothyroid membrane. A cannula is then inserted through the membrane and into the trachea and oxygen is attached using a Y connector. If this is not available, a hole in the side of the tubing may be used to periodically allow CO_2 to escape (intermittent insufflation).

Q. Is this an efficient form of ventilation?

A. No, it is only really a holding measure until a proper airway can be secured. It is not very effective at getting rid of the build-up of CO_2 and also requires considerable ventilatory effort if the patient is not paralysed.

Q. Would you perform a tracheostomy as an emergency?

A. No, I would use other techniques such as needle or surgical cricothyroidotomy in an emergency situation and a tracheostomy only as a last resort.

Q. You have an unconscious patient who you have just intubated and who appears to still be hypoxic. What is running through your mind?

A. I would be concerned about the possibility of one-sided intubation, a pneumothorax and lung collapse. I would quickly assess the patient, looking particularly for:

- Resonant percussion note
- Asymmetrical breathing/lack of breath sounds.

I would also check that my endotracheal tube was correctly positioned and that the tubing and ventilator were functioning normally.

Q. What action would you take if you suspected a pneumothorax?

A. If I suspected a tension pneumothorax, I would immediately place a large-bore cannula into the second intercostal space, mid-clavicular line on the affected side. There would be a 'hiss' of air as the tension is relieved. I would then insert a chest drain on the affected side, fifth intercostal space, mid-axillary line.

Q. What are the main indications for mechanical ventilation?

A. The indications for mechanical ventilation include:

- Respiratory failure
- Impending respiratory failure

- Coma with raised intracranial pressure
- Prophylactic in those at risk i.e. postoperatively in those with respiratory disease.

Q. Once ventilated, what are the aims of mechanical ventilation?

A. • Optimal gas exchange – improved arterial oxygenation and removal of carbon dioxide
- Reduced work of breathing.

Q. Can you think of any complications of mechanical ventilation?

A. These include:

- Problems associated with intubation
- Equipment failure – disconnection, power supply
- Cardiovascular – reduced cardiac output, reduced venous return, increased pulmonary vascular resistance
- Respiratory – alveolar collapse, V/Q mismatch, hypoventilation, reduced surfactant, damage to alveolar membrane, infection
- Barotrauma – pneumomediastinum, pneumothorax, emphysema
- Gastrointestinal – abdominal distension/ileus
- Liver impairment
- Water retention – mostly affecting the lungs, Reduced renal blood flow resulting in reduced urine output
- Psychiatric.

RESPIRATORY FAILURE

Q. Define 'respiratory failure'.

A. Respiratory failure is a syndrome in which the respiratory system fails in one or both of its gas exchange functions: oxygenation and carbon dioxide elimination. It is defined as a Pao_2 of <60 mmHg (8 kPa) while air breathing at rest, with or without a $Paco_2$ of >50 mmHg (6.5 kPa).

Q. How can it be classified? Give examples of the different types.

A. Respiratory failure can be divided into acute and chronic as well as type I and type II.

Type I failure is also known as hypoxaemic/hypoxic respiratory failure and primarily represents a failure of oxygenation (low Pao_2 with a normal Fio_2). It is characterized by a Pao_2 of <60 mmHg with a normal or low $Paco_2$ and can be associated with virtually all acute lung diseases (generally involving fluid filling or collapse of alveolar units). The pathology results in a mismatch between pulmonary ventilation and perfusion (V/Q mismatch). Typical examples are pneumonia, pulmonary oedema and lung contusion.

Type II failure is also known as hypercapnic respiratory failure and primarily represents a failure of ventilation (the ability to clear carbon dioxide). It is characterized by a Pao_2 <60 mmHg and a $Paco_2$ >50 mmHg due to alveolar hypoventilation for whatever reason. Asthma, acute exacerbations of COPD, excess opioid administration and coma are common causes, the former two causing alveolar hypoventilation by airflow limitation and the latter two by depressed central ventilatory drive.

Acute respiratory failure develops over minutes to hours. Acute type II failure results in a respiratory acidosis, whereas chronic type II failure develops over days, allowing renal compensatory mechanisms to near-normalize blood pH by bicarbonate retention. Arterial blood gases cannot readily be used to differentiate acute from chronic type I failure; however the presence of polycythaemia (increased red cell volume due to hypoxia-induced increased erythropoietin production) and cor pulmonale (right ventricular hypertrophy secondary to increased pulmonary vascular resistance resulting from chronic alveolar hypoxia) can be taken as clinical markers of chronic disease.

Q. What relevance does respiratory failure have to surgery? How is the type of surgery related to postoperative respiratory failure?

A. Postoperative morbidity and mortality are increased in patients with pre-existing chronic lung disease and those presenting preoperatively with acute respiratory failure. Death from pulmonary complications occurs in 7% of surgical patients with moderate to severe chronic pulmonary disease, and postoperative pulmonary morbidity occurs in 33% of patients with mild to moderate disease. This highlights the need for identification of such patients preoperatively (as well as those with additional known risk factors such as obesity and cigarette smoking) so that immediate treatment can be initiated in the acute cases, and appropriate pre-optimization of lung function in the chronic disease patients. Ensuring an adequate level of postoperative care and monitoring is available for such patients, such as in an ITU or HDU setting, should also form part of the preoperative planning.

Some of the persisting effects of general anaesthesia play a role in postoperative pulmonary complications (POPCs), such as alveolar collapse from reduced FRC and lung compliance; the effectiveness and choice of postoperative analgesia regimes are also important (e.g. opiate respiratory depression, evidence showing beneficial effects on respiratory function of epidural analgesia). The effect of surgery itself needs also to be taken into account. Postoperative respiratory failure is more common following emergency surgery and prolonged procedures (>4 hours). Thoracic and abdominal surgery increase the risk, both decreasing postoperative FEV1 and FVC by up to 50%. Some surgical procedures by their very nature cause a reduction in a patient's respiratory function and reserve (pulmonary resection), and in these an accurate assessment of preoperative severity of any chronic lung disease is essential as it impacts on patient selection.

Q. **Outline your preoperative assessment of a patient with longstanding COPD due for an elective laparotomy.**

A. Preoperative assessment should consist of history, examination and appropriate investigations, bearing in mind that a laparotomy will have potentially significant adverse effects on respiratory function in the postoperative period.

From the history it is important to ascertain the severity of the patient's respiratory disease and whether there is any evidence of an acute exacerbation of disease. Exercise tolerance, dyspnoea at rest or minimal exertion, the need for regular home bronchodilator nebulizers or home oxygen therapy are indicators of severity, as well as any previous HDU or ITU admissions for ventilatory support. A history of recent deterioration in exercise tolerance with escalation of nebulizer usage may point towards an acute element to their respiratory disease such as lower respiratory tract infection. The patient's cardiovascular status needs assessing (query orthopnoea/paroxysmal nocturnal dyspnoea/ peripheral oedema) for any contribution that it may be making to respiratory compromise, as well as additional risk factors (cigarette smoking).

On clinical examination, acute respiratory failure features to check for include patient confusion or drowsiness, asterixis, central cyanosis, tachycardia and tachypnoea with the use of the accessory muscles of respiration. Peripheral oedema and hepatomegaly may indicate cor pulmonale from longstanding disease.

Appropriate investigations would include (1) laboratory tests – FBC ?anaemia and polycythaemia, biochemistry – ?deranged LFTs due to cor pulmonale, ?magnesium/phosphate deficiency aggravating respiratory failure; (2) ECG – ?evidence of cor pulmonale or coexistent cardiac disease; (3) CXR – may reveal the cause of any acute element to respiratory failure as well as serving as a useful baseline study in a patient with chronic chest disease; (4) arterial blood gases – should be performed wherever respiratory failure, acute or chronic, is suspected to help confirm the diagnosis, assist in distinction between the types and severity, and guide therapy. Further tests may include echocardiography to assess LV and RV function and lung function tests to assess the severity of disease and any degree of reversibility.

Q. **Discuss your management of respiratory failure occurring in a patient 3 days post-laparotomy. What might be indications for ventilatory support for such a patient?**

A. Respiratory failure postoperatively can occur in a previously fit patient or as an acute exacerbation of an underlying chronic respiratory disease. The development of a lower respiratory tract infection, either hospital- or pre-hospital-acquired, combined with basal lung segment collapse is a reasonably common cause of such a postoperative scenario, especially where inadequate pain control is also a contributing factor.

Treatment is divided into supportive measures to improve oxygenation and hence tissue oxygen delivery immediately, as well as measures to treat the underlying causes and contributing factors. Such treatment is usually best managed in a HDU setting. Oxygen therapy is therefore the first-line treatment, but should be used cautiously in patients with a background history of chronic type II failure who are reliant on their hypoxic drive (but it must be remembered that the patient will die of hypoxia long before hypercapnia). Mechanical means of improving oxygenation in type I failure by alveolar recruitment include CPAP (continuous positive airway pressure) which might avoid the need for invasive ventilation if commenced early enough. Pharmacological treatments include the use of bronchodilators (ß2 agonists and theophyllines) to reduce airway resistance and the work of breathing, systemic corticosteroids if airway inflammation is an element (COPD exacerbation), antibiotics if there is evidence of pneumonia, and improved analgesia if pain is limiting ventilation. Chest physiotherapy including breathing and coughing exercises, ambulation and postural drainage should be performed by specialist personnel.

Mechanical ventilation (IPPV) is indicated in the presence of (1) gross hypoxia e.g. PaO_2 <8 kPa on 60% FiO_2; (2) worsening hypercarbia and respiratory or metabolic acidosis despite treatment; (3) patient exhaustion, restlessness, or an inability to clear sputum. IPPV is used to increase PaO_2, lower $PaCO_2$ and relieve respiratory muscle fatigue, whilst therapy directed at the underlying cause of the respiratory failure continues (IPPV in itself is not a curative treatment – it is supportive).

ARDS

Q. What do you understand by the term ARDS?

A. ARDS stands for acute respiratory distress syndrome. It is essentially non-cardiogenic pulmonary oedema with a normal pulmonary artery wedge pressure (PAWP), which is characterized by stiff lungs, refractory hypoxaemia and diffuse pulmonary infiltrates on chest radiography. It is associated with a mortality of approximately 50%.

Q. What causes it?

A. It is commonly caused by sepsis and aspiration. Other causes include trauma, pancreatitis, drug overdose, cardiopulmonary bypass and obstetric causes such as eclampsia.

Q. How does it present?

A. It can present up to 72 hours after a precipitating event. The patient becomes tachypnoeic with increasing hypoxia. Fine crepitations can be heard throughout the lung fields. The condition may be diagnosed by:

- Presence of precipitating cause
- Bilateral diffuse infiltrates on chest radiography
- PaO_2 > 8 kPa, FiO_2 <0.4
- PAOP <15 – 18 mmHg (normal).

Q. What is the underlying physiology of the condition?

A. The initial stimulus is inflammation, which causes an increase in vascular permeability and endothelial injury resulting in alveolar flooding. The affected areas become stiff and poorly oxygenated. This results in a decrease in functional residual capacity. The local blood vessels react by constricting and redirecting blood flow to better oxygenated areas. This creates a shunt and increases the pulmonary resistance. This results in high right-sided cardiac filling pressures and right ventricular dilation.

After 5–10 days, collagen is deposited in the interstitial spaces which may cause fibrosis, lung destruction and ultimately emphysema.

Q. How do we manage this condition?

A. Management of this condition is essentially supportive and aimed at treatment of the underlying cause. General measures include:

Respiratory	– mechanical ventilation
	– PEEP
	– permissive hypercapnia, to prevent barotrauma
	– inverse ratio ventilation, to help alveolar recruitment
Avoidance of pulmonary oedema	– restrict fluid
	– diuretics
Body position changes	– using gravity to redirect blood flow, to improve shunt
Physiotherapy	- not useful in the early stages
	– useful later in removal of secretions
Inhaled nitric oxide	– to improve ventilation–perfusion ratio with pulmonary artery vasodilation.

Other methods have been used such as aerosolized surfactant and prostacyclin but without much evidence of improvement. It is possible for patients to make a full recovery if treatment is effective.

INOTROPES

Q. What determines cardiac output?

A. Cardiac output = stroke volume × heart rate.

Q. What happens when the heart rate increases?

A. As heart rate increases, diastole is shortened and so less blood flows into the ventricle. Stroke volume therefore reduces.

Q. What do you understand by the term pre-load?

A. Pre-load is the amount the myocardium has been stretched at the end of diastole, just prior to ventricular contraction. It is mainly influenced by venous return.

Q. What does Starling's law of the heart state?

A. Starling's law states that 'the force of myocardial contraction is directly proportional to myocardial fibre length'. Stroke volume, therefore, increases as the end diastolic volume increases.

Q. Is this true at extreme levels of contraction?

A. No, when the myocardium is overstretched it is unable to contract efficiently and the stroke volume falls.

Q. How would you assess cardiac filling pressure?

A. Trends in the central venous pressure can be approximated to left-sided filling pressure in the normal heart, but central venous pressure measures the right-sided pressure so gives useful information on the volume status of a healthy patient.

Pulmonary artery catheterization allows for assessment of pulmonary artery pressures, which are more closely associated to left-sided filling.

Q. What would be your first-line therapy in the resuscitation process of somebody in septic shock?

A. My primary therapy would be initial fluid resuscitation using clinical end points. Initial fluid resuscitation is often under-performed for fear of pulmonary oedema as a complication, thus the need for invasive monitoring.

Q. What would you consider to be the optimal pulmonary artery occlusion pressure?

A. The optimal filling pressure is one that is associated with the greatest increase in cardiac output and stroke volume. For most patients this value is in the range 12 – 15 mm Hg.

Q. In terms of tissue perfusion, what would you consider to be the optimal haemoglobin concentration?

A. It is classically described that the optimal haemoglobin concentration taking into account plasma viscosity is 8 – 10 g/dl haemoglobin; this, however, may need to be altered in patients with low cardiac output or coronary artery disease. It must be stressed that in recent years, with the increased risk of blood transfusion and the increasing cost and availability of blood products, slightly lower levels of haemoglobin are becoming acceptable, but this refers more often to the uncomplicated perioperative state than to septic patients.

Q. When would you consider vasopressor therapy?

A. Vasopressors should only be considered in patients with:

- Refractory hypotension unresponsive to initial fluid resuscitation
- Tachycardia

- Low systemic vascular resistance
- Significant peripheral vasodilatation.

It is vital for improvement of organ perfusion that patients are not hypovolaemic prior to administration of vasopressors.

Q. What would be your first-line choice of inotrope?

A. Dopamine is often used as a first-line agent for increasing blood pressure. Adrenaline can be considered for refractory hypotension, although it is associated with adverse side effects.

Q. What are your feelings about dopamine for renal preservation?

A. Dopamine is a naturally occurring catecholamine and neurotransmitter in post-ganglionic sympathetic nerve endings and in the adrenal medulla. It is used as an inotropic drug in both septic and cardiogenic shock; however, uncertainty has arisen about its ability to confer any renal protection at low dose in the intensive care unit. There are also reports of reduction in gastric mucosal perfusion and gut hypoperfusion.

Q. Are there any other inotropes that you could use in these circumstances?

A. *Dobutamine* is another synthetic catecholamine that can be used as an inotrope in septic or cardiogenic shock. Predominantly it is a β-1 receptor agonist with β-2 and α effects. Dopamine receptors are not affected; an increase in myocardial contractility is seen with a reduction in the degree of induced tachycardia and myocardial oxygen consumption. It also has the effect of reducing left ventricular and diastolic pressure. The usual dosage is between 2.5 and 20 µg/kg /minute; high doses can cause ventricular arrhythmias. It is therefore best reserved for shock secondary to pump failure.

Dopexamine is another less commonly used inotropic drug, used more in cardiac failure and after cardiac surgery. It is predominantly a peripheral dopamine receptor agonist and a β-2 adrenergic agonist with indirect β-1 action. It is therefore a chronotrope, inotrope and a peripheral vasodilator. Doses between 0.5 and 6 µg/kg/minute are commonly used.

Noradrenaline is a catecholamine, and is the immediate precursor of adrenaline; it is a natural neurotransmitter and hormone predominantly stimulating the α-adrenal receptors non-selectively with some β-1 receptor activation. It is used as the inotrope of choice in sepsis with low systemic vascular resistance. It is an extremely potent vasopressor. Systolic and diastolic hypotension may indeed be corrected; however renal and mesenteric vasoconstriction are significant concerns for renal hepatic and gut blood flow.

Adrenaline is a catecholamine; it is both a hormone and neurotransmitter of the sympathetic nervous system and brainstem. It is released from the adrenal medulla and central adrenergic neurones. It stimulates both α and β receptors, displaying predominantly β effects of low dose and after effects at higher doses.

Adrenaline therefore has many clinical uses including treatment of anaphylaxis, cardiogenic shock, septic shock, as a bronchodilator and as a vasoconstricting agent with local anaesthetics. Adrenaline however may cause significant cardiac arrhythmias especially in the presence of hypercarbia, hypoxia and other drugs, in particular cocaine or halothane.

Q. When would you consider using an intra-aortic balloon pump?

A. I would consider using an intra-aortic balloon pump to support the circulation where the cardiac index was poor, particularly if this was secondary to myocardial ischaemia.

Q. How do they work?

A. They are inflatable balloons that are inserted via the femoral artery into the aorta. The correct position is just distal to the left subclavian artery. The balloon is inflated at the beginning of diastole in order to increase the pressure within the aortic root. This increases the amount of blood that flows into the coronary arteries. As the balloon rapidly deflates at the beginning of systole, after-load is reduced. The overall effect is to improve diastolic coronary blood flow, with a reduction in after-load, both of which improve cardiac output.

Q. Are there any contraindications?

A. These include:

Absolute

- Aortic aneurysm
- Aortic regurgitation
- Severe aortic disease.

Relative

- Cardiac arrhythmias.

STRESS RESPONSE TO SURGERY

Q. Tell me about the stress response to surgery.

A. The stress response is the metabolic and hormonal changes that follow surgery and which also occur following trauma, burns or haemorrhage. There is a release of polypeptides from damaged tissues. Whatever the mechanism, the neuroendocrine response is initiated.

Q. What hormones are involved in the neuroendocrine response you have just mentioned?

A. There is increased release of ACTH, endorphins, growth hormone, vasopressin and prolactin. There is also increasing catecholamine production from stimulation of the sympathetic nervous system. Increased cortisol levels occur and an increased aldosterone level which leads to a rise in renin and angiotensin.

Q. **What is the overall effect on the metabolic rate?**

A. The effect of the above is to lead to a marked increase in the metabolic rate, a rise in temperature, a rise in oxygen consumption, a rise in CO_2 production, salt and water retention and increased potassium loss from the kidneys. The intense catabolism that follows leads to mobilization of fatty acids. Amino acids are converted to carbohydrate and there can be quite a marked negative nitrogen balance. You will also see a rise in blood glucose and impaired production of insulin.

Q. **Is there a name given to the phases of this metabolic response?**

A. The phases are called *ebb* and *flow*. *Ebb* is the initial phase, occurring within the first 24 hours where a decrease in metabolic rate is seen. *Flow* is the next phase which is associated with an increase in metabolic rate. This may be associated with glucose intolerance and a catabolic state.

Q. **What are the clinical effects of the metabolic response to surgery/trauma?**

A. This response results in an increase in cardiac output, an increase in respiratory rate leading to alkalosis, hypoalbuminaemia and an activation of the clotting cascade which may result in DIC.

Q. **Can you tell me anything about the anaesthetic effects on the stress response to surgery?**

A. A lot of work has been done to try to attenuate the stress response to surgery; it appears that inhalation agents have little effect. The high-dose opioid techniques have been shown to attenuate a stress response; the use of etomidate by infusion does prevent excess cortisol production, but little else. Spinal and epidural use reduces the stress response to lower-half surgery but they tend to cause more suppression of glucose than cortisol. Spinal opioids have been shown not to ablate, but do show some modification of the stress response to surgery.

SEPSIS

Q. **What is the difference between sepsis and systemic inflammatory response syndrome (SIRS)?**

A. SIRS is a generalized inflammatory response by the body which may be caused by sepsis. Sepsis refers to infection only. SIRS is the response seen to a variety of clinical insults, manifest by two or more of the following:

- Temperature $>38°C$ or $< 36°C$
- Heart rate > 90
- Respiratory rate > 20 or $Pa_{CO_2} < 4.3$
- WCC $> 12 \times 10^9$ /l or $< 4 \times 10^9$ /l

Sepsis is defined as SIRS with documented infection, i.e. the immune response to an infection of some kind. Otherwise, SIRS can occur from a number of aetiological triggers including infection (bacterial, viral, fungal), but also hypovolaemic shock, trauma, burns, pancreatitis, tissue ischaemia etc.

Septic shock is SIRS with documented infection, but also including hypotension despite adequate fluid resuscitation, and abnormal or inadequate organ perfusion/hypoperfusion.

Q. What causes SIRS?

A. SIRS may be caused by:

- Sepsis
- Trauma
- Acute pancreatitis
- Burns.

Q. What is the role of cytokines in sepsis?

A. Cytokines are low molecular weight proteins. They are very potent, have a short half-life and are the local factors involved in the inflammatory and immune responses. They act via complex and interactive pathways, with positive feedback and amplification, not unlike the complement cascade. The important ones that appear to be implicated in sepsis and the body's response to infection are TNF-α (tumour necrosis factor-alpha), IL-1 (interleukin 1) and IL-6 (interleukin 6). They have a whole host of local and systemic effects, including vasodilatation, increased capillary permeability, impaired oxygen utilization and myocardial depression.

Q. What part do cytokines play in the pathophysiology of SIRS?

A. Cytokines are involved in SIRS since they make up the inflammatory response. Initially, a local inflammatory response is triggered whereby neutrophils and macrophages are induced and inflammatory mediators, like cytokines, are released. The inflammatory response then becomes progressively more systemic, leading to an overwhelming response involving IL-6, IL-8, IL-1 and TNF-α.

Q. What is the commonest cause of sepsis?

A. Bacterial infection is the commonest cause. Traditionally gram negative bacteria were the major cause of sepsis, but nowadays gram positive bacteria cause about the same percentage of cases as gram negative bacteria. Together, they account for more than 95% of cases of sepsis.

Q. What are some of the clinical features seen in the septic patient?

A. Initially hyperthermia is usually seen, along with tachycardia, hypotension, tachypnoea and warm bounding peripheries as a result of peripheral vasodilatation. This is the hyperdynamic circulation that results from decreased SVR (systemic vascular resistance) and increased cardiac output, and in this manner, septic shock differs initially from the other types of shock (where there is decreased cardiac output along with peripheral vasoconstriction).

Again, signs may differ in the extremes of age and those with pre-existing pathology.

In the later stages, hypotension with vasoconstriction may occur, especially if the patient is hypovolaemic or if there is poor myocardial function. Occasionally, you may also see more subtle signs by themselves such as oliguria, mild hypoxia, drowsiness or confusion.

Q. How might laboratory investigations help with the initial diagnosis?

A. Typically an FBC will show a high WCC, with neutrophilia, although the WCC may be low in overwhelming sepsis. Also, the platelet count may be decreased (consumption).

A coagulation screen usually reveals an increased INR, due to septic coagulopathy and DIC, although in the very late stages of septic shock any derangement may be due to hepatic dysfunction.

Urea and electrolyte results may show a degree of renal impairment, or indicate an element of dehydration if the urea (and sodium) is raised disproportionately compared to the creatinine.

Arterial blood gases may show a metabolic acidosis with a compensatory respiratory alkalosis (due to hyperventilation or 'air hunger' driving down the P_{CO_2}).

Lactate levels are often high as a result of tissue hypoxia.

Q. What are the treatment aims in sepsis?

A. Clearly, this depends on the nature of the initial insult and may be straightforward in some cases, e.g. oxygen, antibiotics and chest physiotherapy for lobar pneumonia. Generally, therefore, treatment is aimed at the underlying condition (i.e. find and treat the source of infection) whilst supporting vital organ functions. This essentially involves haemodynamic support with the main goal of maintaining oxygen delivery to the tissues and organs. Thus treatment will vary according to clinical state, and may well involve the support of failing organs with appropriate therapy – ventilation, dialysis, replacing platelets and clotting products, inotropic support, nutrition, etc.

Q. Are steroids useful in sepsis?

A. Some animal studies in the past have shown improved survival with steroid treatment in sepsis. Several large multicentre randomized human trials have shown no overall benefit. Corticosteroids do not improve outcome and may increase the mortality rate in a subset of patients with renal insufficiency, and also increase the incidence of secondary infection.

Q. What is the definition of multiorgan dysfunction (MOD)?

A. MOD is the presence of organ dysfunction in a critically ill patient, usually in two or more organs. It may be due to the direct effect of a triggering illness i.e. trauma, or it may be secondary to the development of SIRS.

Q. What is its mortality?

A. It generally has a grave prognosis, 70–90% if two or more organs are involved.

GASTROINTESTINAL BLEEDS

Q. A 45-year-old man who has had an external fixator applied to his right leg following trauma has an episode of haematemesis; what would your management be?

A. I would begin urgent resuscitation with intravenous fluid or blood products. I would also check that the patient had adequate venous access, with at least two large-bore cannulae.

I would check a full blood count, urea and electrolytes, liver function tests and clotting screen. I would make sure that at least four units of blood were cross-matched. Finally, I would arrange for an erect chest X-ray and abdominal X-ray if I had elicited some abdominal pain in the history or examination.

Q. What might your investigation show?

A. The full blood count will check the haemoglobin level, the haematocrit and the platelet function. The haemoglobin level and the haematocrit may be a guide as to the level of the bleeding. A normal level should however be regarded with respect to the timing of the bleeding. It takes several hours for the levels to drop to an accurate level. This is because immediately after an acute episode of bleeding, patients have a decreased circulating volume; as this normalizes, haemodilution occurs and the accurate levels become apparent.

Another clue as to the timing of the bleeding can be gained from the urea. If this is raised disproportionately when compared to the creatinine, it indicates that some form of bleeding has been occurring for at least 24 hours. The rise in urea results from the breakdown of blood within the gastrointestinal tract. Increased liver function tests may indicate advanced liver disease with the possibility of oesophageal varices. Any abnormalities in clotting will need to be corrected if found. An erect chest X-ray may show free gas under the diaphragm and the possibility of a perforated peptic ulcer as the underlying cause.

Q. Assuming that your patient has been stabilized, what would you do next?

A. I would arrange for urgent endoscopy.

Q. What would be the most likely cause for this patient's haematemesis?

A. Patients in hospital have haematemesis for two broad groups of reasons. The first is the unmasking of pre-existing disease such as a peptic ulcer (aggravated by ulcer-causing drugs such as NSAIDs) or bleeding from longstanding oesophageal varices. The second is due to stress ulceration, leading to widespread gastric and duodenal erosions.

Q. Do you know any mechanisms that cause stress ulceration?

A. Any patient who has sustained a major insult such as trauma, sepsis or burns is at risk of stress ulceration. It is caused by mucosal ischaemia. Approximately 90% of patients admitted to ITU will have some degree of mucosal ischaemia. Fortunately both H_2 receptor blockage and sucrulfate have been shown to significantly decrease morbidity.

Q. What is the place of surgery in managing acute haematemesis?

A. All patients should first undergo emergency endoscopy to try to identify the cause of the bleeding. Surgical intervention is rarely required due to the success of modern endoscopy. Therapeutic manoeuvres can be undertaken such as sclerotherapy to actively bleeding peptic ulceration or injection of oesophageal varices. Surgery is required where bleeding cannot be controlled. For gastric ulcers a Bilroth I is traditionally performed. This involves resection of the affected area, followed by anastomosis of the remaining stomach to the duodenum. For duodenal ulcers the most commonly performed procedure involves a pyloroplasty with under-running of the bleeding ulcer. Other options such as a Bilroth II (gastro-jejunostomy) are no longer performed.

Recurrence of ulcers is a known complication after surgery. There is usually a good response to medical therapy and no need for further surgical intervention. If this fails, it is possible that some antrum may have been left behind post-gastrectomy or the patient may have Zollinger–Ellison syndrome.

✱ TEACHING NOTE

In a viva situation you should never underplay the importance of basic resuscitation. While the occasional examiner may be irritated, they will never fail a candidate for mentioning it. However, failure to mention it may be considered by some examiners to be a pass/fail point.

SURGERY IN THE IMMUNOCOMPROMISED

Q. What groups of patients might you suspect to be immunocompromised?

A. The most likely causes of immunosuppression are:

- Drug-induced i.e. cytotoxics/steroids
- Malignancy
- AIDS (acquired immunodeficiency syndrome).

More rarely, the patient may have a congenitally acquired immunodeficiency such as Di George syndrome or Bruton's disease.

Q. Why are hospitalized patients at risk of immunosuppression?

A. Hospitalized patients may be immunosuppressed as a result of an underlying disease. They may also be at risk of immunosuppression as a result of critical illness. Critical illness can result in a widespread immune dysfunction affecting:

- T/B cells
- Macrophages
- Neutrophil function (impaired chemotaxis and intracellular killing).

Q. What would concern you about potentially performing an operation on an immunosuppressed patient?

A. I would have several concerns:

- Risk of infection – patients who are immunosuppressed are at risk of overwhelming sepsis from opportunistic pathogens
- Multiple infection
- Associated bone marrow suppression – thrombocytopenia and leucopenia
- Associated medical conditions – diabetes, Cushing's syndrome, pancreatitis, hepatotoxicity.

Q. What is an opportunistic infection?

A. An opportunistic infection is one that is usually non-pathogenic but can cause overwhelming sepsis in the immunocompromised, sometimes ending in death.

Q. Can you give me any examples?

A.
- Bacterial – *Salmonella, Listeria monocytogenes, Mycobacterium avium-intracellulare, Mycobacterium tuberculosis*
- Viral – *Herpes simplex, Herpes zoster, Cytomegalovirus*
- Fungal – *Candida albicans, Cryptococcus neoformans, Histoplasma*
- Protozoal – *Pneumocystis carinii* (PCP), *Cryptosporidium, Toxoplasmosis gondii.*

The commonest organisms that result in infection are bacteria, mostly gram negative bacilli e.g. *E. coli, Klebsiella* or proteus.

Q. What are the commonest sites of infection in this group of patients?

A. The commonest site is the chest/lungs. Other sites include the oral mucosa, genitourinary tract and central nervous system.

Q. What measures can be taken to prevent infection?

A. Infection in hospitalized patients usually originates from hospital staff, other patients, visitors and contaminated equipment. There are various measures, usually enforced by an infection control team, to reduce the incidence of transmitted pathogens. These include:

- Hand washing in between each patient using antimicrobial wash i.e. chlorhexidine
- Clean gowns/overshoes to be worn by staff/visitors
- Ward/ITU design allowing adequate space between each bed, with adequate hand-washing facilities
- Single cubicles for barrier/reverse barrier nursing
- The provision of staff training in aseptic technique.

Q. Are there any other sources of infection to consider specific to ITU?

A. In ITU, other sources of infection include:

- Ventilator tubing – needs changing every 48 hours
- Humidified water
- Ventilators – filters should be used
- Tracheal suction – use aseptic technique at all times
- Urinary catheters – aseptic, use an obstructed, closed-drainage system
- Central lines – infection from skin or nearby thrombus, replace every 5–7 days, used closed system (avoid three-way taps), consider tunnelling for TPN
- Wounds – should be inspected regularly.

Q. What is the role of the infection control team?

A. The infection control team have a role in monitoring hospital infection rates, regulating antibiotic usage and advising clinicians on appropriate sensitivities of antibiotic use.

They also have a role in staff training:

- Disinfection and sterilization
- Isolation procedures
- Vaccinations
- Needlestick injuries.

Q. If you were treating a patient on ITU who had liver failure and you suspected may have hepatitis B or HIV, what precautions would you undertake?

A. I would take steps to ensure that care was taken when handling urine, faeces and blood. I would also take care over protecting any skin cuts/abrasions/contact with mucosal surfaces. I would also ensure that specimens were clearly labelled as high risk and that thorough hand washing was undertaken before and after handling the patient.

Q. How would you deal with a needlestick injury?

A. I would explain the situation clearly to the patient and implement the Trust's policy. I would ask permission to take a virology sample from the patient and send one from myself. I would then contact the infection control team immediately regarding the possibility of commencing a course of anti-retroviral.

Q. What steps could you take to minimize the needlestick injury occurring in the first place?

A. These include:

- Safe needle practice – never re-sheath the needle, and discard immediately
- Don't leave sharps unattended
- Don't overfill a sharps box.

OLIGURIA

Q. How do you define oliguria?

A. Oliguria is a urine output of less than 0.5 ml/kg/hour. In an average adult male, this is approximately 30 ml/hour.

Q. What determines the urine output?

A. Urine output is determined by:

- Renal perfusion pressure (arteriolar tone and cardiac output)
- Functioning renal tubules
- Functioning urinary tract.

Q. You are an on-call surgical SHO called to see a 62-year-old gentleman who is post-anterior resection. He has a urine output of 15 ml over the last hour. What are the possible causes?

A. This gentleman has oliguria. The causes of this include:

- Pre-renal – as a result of reduced blood flow to the kidneys, for example, dehydration, haemorrhage, sepsis, major burns and conditions associated with a reduced cardiac output such as cardiac failure.
- Renal – i.e. underlying kidney disease which may be drug induced (NSAIDs, gentamicin), glomerulonephritis etc.
- Post-renal – obstruction secondary to renal stones or tumours.

The most likely cause in this gentleman is probably a combination of two or three of the above. For example, he may be hypotensive (pre-renal) as a result of the surgery with a background of underlying kidney disease (renal) possibly as a result of long-term NSAID use.

Q. **What are the commonest causes of oliguria postoperatively?**

A. The commonest causes include:

- The stress response to surgery (stimulation of ADH, circulating mineralocorticoids and glucocorticoids)
- Dehydration/blood loss
- Sepsis/vasodilation
- Acute tubular necrosis
- Urinary tract obstruction i.e. blocked catheter
- Intra-abdominal hypertension i.e. peritonitis.

Q. **What is acute tubular necrosis (ATN)?**

A. Acute tubular necrosis is acute renal failure due to injury to renal tubular epithelial cells. It usually occurs as a result of the hypoperfusion associated with shock. Renal perfusion is reduced and ischaemia develops.

Q. **How would you make a diagnosis of acute renal failure?**

A. I would make a diagnosis of renal failure by:

- Persistent oliguria (<0.5 ml/kg/hour)
- U+E – elevated urea and creatinine
- Urine osmolality increases/urinary sodium increases
- Other metabolic abnormalities – decreased Na^+, increased K^+, decreased Ca^+.

Q. **Describe the methods and management of impending renal failure in the surgical/critically ill patient.**

A. It is believed that early appropriate management of pre-renal failure may avoid the onset of renal failure, and thus the need for renal replacement therapy, and the increase in mortality and morbidity associated with renal failure.

Basic principles guide initial therapeutic strategies, before pharmacological interventions.

Optimize the circulating volume in order to reverse the actions of ADH and aldosterone. Accepted practice involves assessing the dynamic response of the CVP, urine output and haemodynamic markers to a fluid challenge. Spontaneous peripheral rewarming indicates adequate circulating volume.

Optimization, or adequate fluid resuscitation, may not be enough. The autoregulation of renal perfusion pressure versus renal blood flow is often lost, and so a mean arterial pressure (MAP) of 70 mmHg is thought to be acceptable. The patient's pre-morbid MAP, however, is more ideal (the lowest to maintain organ perfusion). Norepinephrine can be titrated to raise MAP and hence renal afferent arteriolar pressure, once volume status is corrected.

Abdominal compartment syndrome or intra-abdominal hypertension (>20–25 mmHg) can occur and should be excluded. Global reduction of renal blood flow or direct renal pressure may be the cause.

Avoidance of nephrotoxins is essential:

- Aminoglycosides i.e. gentamicin, NSAIDs (which inhibit renal prostaglandins)
- ACE inhibitors, cautiously used
- Iodinated radiocontrast agents.

Pharmacological manipulations are common but there is little if no good evidence to support their use.

Frusemide

Frusemide, a loop diuretic, is thought to reduce the oxygen requirements of the loop of Henle, and may increase renal blood flow via prostaglandins. It may induce a diuresis to aid fluid management, but has an influence on outcome. Intensivists favour low doses (10 mg) and infusions, unlike historical renal failure doses (4 mg/kg), as at high doses it is nephrotoxic.

Dopamine

Recent evidence from an Australian randomized control trial (RCT) has shown no benefit from the use of low-dose regimes, with higher-dose regimes relying upon the inotropic effects of the drug. It has many side effects, and even in surgical prophylaxis, the evidence is not substantial.

Mannitol

Mannitol is also nephrotoxic in high doses and there is no evidence for its use in acute renal failure.

SCORING SYSTEMS IN ITU

Q. **What is the aim of a scoring system in ITU?**

A. The aim of a scoring system is to use past experience to predict future outcomes. A 'prognostic estimate' is therefore obtained.

Q. **Can you name a few?**

A. I can think of APACHE 2, APACHE 3, SAPS, MPM, SOFA, GCS and TISS.

Q. **Could you define APACHE 2 for me?**

A. APACHE 2 is the acute physiology and chronic health evaluation. It has 34 variables in the original consensus, refined to 12 by statistical techniques and additional weighting for previous health, age and urgency of admission. The sum provides a score and this is converted to risk of death using probability theory with additional weighting to account for the primary diagnosis.

Q. Can you give me any idea of the problems associated with the APACHE 2 scoring system?

A. Yes – data collection is a problem because some of the parameters are only measured once in the initial stay and may be subject to variation. The GCS is heavily weighted and subjective and also the diagnostic labelling is not well established. Where resuscitation occurs prior to ITU admission the score is lowered by what is referred to as lead-time bias. There can also be 'selection bias', where prediction errors occur between the patient being evaluated and those patients used to create the reference database.

Simplified acute physiology score (SAPS), the Riyadh intensive care programme (RIP) and the sickness severity score (SSS) are all based on APACHE. None use diagnostic weights.

SAPS has been updated to SAPS II, now using 12 physiological variables with additional weights for age, weight and three underlying diseases (AIDS, metastatic disease and haematological malignancy). Urine output has also been shown to be a better predictor of outcome than serum creatinine.

MPM (mortality prediction model), with multicentre revision, is now seen as MPM II. It generates a direct risk of death at admission (MPM0) and at 24 hours (MPM24) using 15 binary variables, with 'yes/no' answers. Included are emergency admission, CPR, mechanical ventilation, renal failure, cirrhosis, cancer, coma, heart rate and systolic blood pressure.

SOFas (organ system failures) is seemingly simpler and easier to apply, but difficulty lies in defining varying degrees of system failure without being over laborious about physiological variables.

TISS (therapeutic intensity scoring system) is probably more useful for cost calculation by comparing ITU days to ordinary hospital bed days.

TRISS (trauma-related injury severity system), combines ISS and TS.

The ISS is the sum of the squared values in each of the six anatomical areas of AIS (abbreviated injury system), giving a linear relationship between score and outcome.

TURP SYNDROME

Q. What is TURP syndrome?

A. This is a syndrome following transurethral resection of the prostate. It occurs in about 10% of patients. In 1 – 2% it is severe and in around 8% mild. It follows the absorption of excess irrigation fluid, most commonly glycine. The syndrome is characterized by an increase in intravascular volume, dilutional hyponatraemia, intracellular oedema and the metabolism of glycine to ammonia.

Q. What physiological signs or symptoms might you expect to see?

A. Signs include a reduced pulse rate and blood pressure, the potential for symptomatic angina, dyspnoea, visual disturbance, mental irritation leading to a reduced level of consciousness and seizures.

Q. What measures can be taken to try to prevent TURP syndrome?

A. The incidence of problems related to the duration of surgery, the height of the irrigation fluid and thus the volume used. Also to be considered is the amount of hypotonic crystalloid infused perioperatively.

Q. How might you aid detection?

A. The use of regional anaesthesia allows for early detection of altered cerebral function. Central venous pressure monitoring should be used in at-risk patients. Measurement of plasma sodium can be useful as a fall of greater than 10 mmol/l signifies absorption of more than 2 l of irrigation fluid. Also, it may be diagnosed by adding alcohol to the irrigation fluid and measuring plasma alcohol.

Q. What are your management aims?

A. Treatment involves slow correction of low sodium with frusemide (or judicious use of hypertonic saline). In rare cases, rapid correction may lead to central pontine bleed (a rough guide to speed of correction is 1–2 mmol per hour). Further supportive therapy, including inotropes, is occasionally needed.

FAT EMBOLUS

Q. What are the causes or risk factors for fat embolism?

A. The fat embolism syndrome (FES) is most commonly associated with major trauma i.e. fractures of the long bones or pelvis. It has also been reported in:

- Acute haemorrhagic pancreatitis
- Diabetes
- Decompression illness
- Prosthetic joint replacement
- Liposuction
- Bone marrow transplantation
- Major burns
- Cardiopulmonary bypass
- TPN.

It is defined as the presence of fat globules within the lung parenchyma or peripheral microcirculation and has a mortality of 10–15%.

Q. What is the pathophysiology?

A. The fat emboli are thought to originate from exposed bone marrow, and as these globules enter the circulation, they impact in capillaries in the microcirculation, resulting in local tissue damage and ischaemia. There is also a biochemical theory as well as a mechanical explanation, whereby free fatty acids (FFA) are released as a result of lipase activation by stress hormones. These FFAs are thought to cause a local inflammatory response.

Typically, FES occurs 1–5 days after long-bone fractures, in about 5% of major trauma patients.

Q. Which systems are typically involved?

A. Respiratory insufficiency (tachypnoea and cyanosis) results from emboli entering and lodging within the pulmonary circulation. The intravascular deposition of globules into the arterial circulation, either via the pulmonary arterial capillaries or via pulmonary shunts, also leads to neurological dysfunction i.e. hemiparesis or encephalopathy. There are also cutaneous manifestations in which a petechial rash completes the classic triad.

Q. What features may be seen to aid diagnosis?

A. Cardiovascular, respiratory and nervous system signs are similar to those seen with air embolism.

Respiratory distress occurs as is evident by dyspnoea, tachypnoea and hypoxaemia. The patient may have a cough or haemoptysis, and pulmonary hypertension may occur, leading to pulmonary oedema.

Cerebral features include restlessness, confusion, coma and convulsions, and exist in up to 80% of patients.

The petechial rash typically occurs on the chest, neck and axillae, but can also be found on the oral mucosa and conjunctivae.

Other features include pyrexia (>38°C), tachycardia, hypotension and retinal haemorrhages/exudates.

Q. What other investigations might be performed?

A. As well as blood gases to confirm hypoxaemia, a chest X-ray may show bilateral fluffy shadowing ('snowstorm' appearance), but is usually normal at presentation.

An ECG may show evidence of right heart strain, and laboratory results may indicate coagulation abnormalities, anaemia and thrombocytopenia.

Fat droplets are often seen in cells recovered from bronchopulmonary lavage in trauma patients with FES, but the appearance of fat globules in the urine is neither sensitive nor specific for FES. Lipid emboli may be visualized in the retinal vessels on fundoscopy. Fat droplets may also be stained for histologically, using Sudan black stain.

Other investigations include:

- FBC – low Hb (as a result of trauma), high ESR
- Clotting – high FDPs (associated with DIC)
- U+Es – query abnormal renal function, low calcium (chelated by circulating lipids).

Q. What is the management for these patients?

A. Supportive therapy is the mainstay of treatment in these cases. Adequate oxygenation is imperative and mechanical ventilation with PEEP may be required in severe cases.

Specific treatment of dehydration, sepsis, DVT prophylaxis and nutrition should also be addressed.

Q. Is it possible to prevent FES?

A. Early immobilization of fractures is necessary, and early fixation is thought to reduce the incidence of FES. A number of specific therapies, including corticosteroids, albumin, heparin, aprotinin and alcohol infusions, have all been tried and suggested, but there is no firm evidence to support their use in the treatment of FES.

COMMUNICATION SKILLS

INTRODUCTION

Communication skills are an essential part of any clinician's skills, from which surgeons are not exempt. Good communication allows for greater patient and staff satisfaction. Patients' knowledge and compliance are increased. Good communication has been shown to positively influence health and will prevent many dangerous, libellous and time-consuming situations. Most complaints can be dealt with and anticipated by appropriate communication. Awkward and threatening situations can usually be dealt with immediately and amicably, when doctors communicate effectively with their patients.

Communication *can* be done well. It is extremely satisfying to communicate successfully. When patients go away happy with their consultations, you will know it. Improvements in your skills are also easy to recognize and enjoyable to experience. Knowing that you did something better than the last time is a self-fulfilling exercise and will spur you on to further improvement.

Good communication can be learnt and improved. It is better to be a bad communicator who has taken steps to improve, than a bad communicator who has not. The suggestions below are designed to be included in your daily routine. They can and should become second nature to you. Hopefully you will absorb these skills for the rest of your working life.

Communication is about more than the words that come out of your mouth. It is about your whole manner. Through non-verbal techniques you convey messages that are just as important as the actual words. The way you are perceived, during a consultation, will colour the judgement of anyone you speak to, ultimately affecting the way in which they rate your ability.

The advice incorporated into this chapter is exactly that, advice. It is based on personal experience and the current evidence about communication skills training. By far the best method for developing communication is from personal improvement, reflecting positively on aspects of communication that you do well. Practice is vital if you want to improve. This chapter will hopefully be a small part of that lifelong process of improving and changing the way you communicate.

The initial section of this chapter outlines the structure of the exam, which contains three different components: information giving, information gathering and a written exercise. Areas which interest the examiners and for which they award marks are highlighted. This book is primarily designed to help you pass the surgical membership exam and an exam setting is not a normal environment. However 'normal' the scenario is, it can never be perfect. Therefore we have included relevant advice, tips and techniques for the exam situation.

The next section describes techniques to improve your communication skills. By working through these techniques and absorbing them into your practice, you will be able to deal with any scenario that the exam should throw at you.

We then provide an outline for a typical consultation. This gives a framework around which discussions can be based and breaks up the consultation into four areas that follow naturally from each other and will cover all the aspects needed in a comprehensive discussion.

Some specific scenarios are then given. These are scenarios that have been used previously in the exam and are all common situations that any SHO who has completed the prerequisite 20 months of basic surgical training should have encountered.

Practice scenarios, for each part of the exam, are then given at the end of the chapter. These will allow you to practise the skills highlighted in this chapter and prepare for the exam in a structured way.

Communication skills are just like any other part of medicine; they are learnt. Nobody is born with knowledge; it has to be acquired in whatever way you choose. Usually communication skills are acquired from personal experience. Once you become confident with these skills, you will notice an improved level of patient and self-satisfaction. Improved feedback will start almost as soon as you attempt to apply these skills to your everyday practice. Your patients and their families will leave your room happy and you will be aware of this.

This chapter is designed both as a guide to passing the Royal College exam and to try to give surgeons advice on how to communicate properly for the rest of their professional careers. The scenarios presented in the exam are also designed to familiarize junior doctors with management situations, which are likely to occur as they progress in their careers, and how they should deal with them. A consultant surgeon is not only responsible for patient care but is also in charge of a large team of people and so must possess more than just technical ability.

FORMAT OF THE COMMUNICATION SKILLS SECTION OF THE EXAM

It is important to be totally familiar with the current examination format. Full details can be found on all the college websites or by writing directly to the Colleges. The communication skills section is initially taken together with the viva section. Candidates who pass the viva section but fail the communications section can proceed to the clinical section, but not vice versa. They will have to reapply separately for the communications section as many times as required within the specified time limit from first sitting the viva (currently 2 years). The communication skills section must be passed before the MRCS is awarded.

Under the new intercollegiate examination the communication skills section has three parts, as follows:

Part 1 Information giving

This is a role-play section using an actor. You will be given 5 minutes to read through a scenario, usually a history. The candidate is then taken to the test room where the examiners will introduce themselves, but not the actor who will be playing the part of a patient or relative. The candidate has 10 minutes to provide the required information to the actor. The examiners will not interrupt the interview but will be present while it is conducted. It is not necessary to take up all of the allotted time and you will not be penalized for using less time.

The structure of this section revolves around an individual scenario, which you are given. It is unlikely to be simply a surgical clerking, but more likely a discussion guided by you.

Part 2 Information gathering

This is another role-play section using an actor and lasts a total of 15 minutes. Candidates receive a broad outline of the case and are allowed 5 minutes for preparation. The candidate then has 10 minutes with the actor, who may be playing the part of a patient or a relative, to communicate the required information. Again, a discussion lasting less than 10 minutes is not necessarily seen as a sign of poor performance.

The examiners will introduce themselves to the candidate but will not introduce the candidate to the actor. A copy of the scenario will be available in the room should it be required. Notes cannot be made during the preparation but paper will be available in the test room if the candidate wishes to draw a diagram to facilitate the discussion. At the end of the discussion with the actor you should present the information you have gathered to the examiners, who will be playing the part of your consultant.

This is the most straightforward of the communications skills sections, it is primarily a surgical clerking. History taking is something that happens each day that you practice and you should already be familiar with doing it. The emphasis that you put on the different parts of the clerking depends on the exact scenario that you are given.

Part 3 Written section

In this section, you will be presented with an anonymous set of patient notes for review. An internal or external referral letter, will then need to be written using the information supplied. This may be a letter to a GP, a hospital colleague or a written request for a test.

SPECIFIC MRCS EXAM TECHNIQUE

The emphasis of this section is obviously your ability to communicate with others. Theoretical knowledge is being tested in the other parts of the examination and the scenarios that you will be given are unlikely to involve highly specialized areas of surgery. That means that you will be expected to be factually correct about what you do say, as the surgical topics discussed are considered routine. You can fail this section of the exam, even if you communicate well, if you get basic surgical facts wrong.

Specific areas that are of interest to the college are:

1. The greeting between the candidate and the actor
2. The style of the questioning, with open not closed questions
3. An appropriate pace with good facilitation
4. Focused on the primary topic
5. Allowing time for questions
6. Being empathic without making incorrect assumptions about how the patient feels
7. Body language and eye contact
8. Summarizing.

All of these areas and ways to improve in each of them are discussed in this chapter.

Marking scheme

Each test has a separate marking sheet for the examiners to indicate the candidate's performance on various points, some of which will be specific to each scenario. This sheet is an aide-memoire for the examiners.

The examiners will score each section on a scale of 1 to 4, with '1' as the lowest and '4' as the highest score. There are four marks altogether, with information gathering having two separate marks, one for the interview and one for the presentation. The overall mark is the sum of the four individual scores. Any candidate who passes but scores a '1' in any section, and borderline candidates, will be discussed by the examiners. The actor's opinion will be taken into account for these candidates.

Personal presentation

Your dress is also extremely important. It is not the place of this book to tell you how to dress on an everyday basis, although it is the place of this book to tell you how to dress to pass the MRCS exam.

Men should wear a suit. Make it dark and simple, with a tie. Women should also dress simply, with a degree of restraint.

For the exam, arrive without smelling of cigarettes, alcohol or strong food. Each one of these could annoy the actor or your examiners.

If you are carrying a mobile phone ensure that it is switched off.

Mental preparation

Mentally prepare for the discussion before it starts. In the information giving and gathering sections you have 5 minutes' preparation time; make sure that you use it.

What is the main point of the scenario? For example, informed consent – are there any other clues given about what I might encounter or issues which need to be addressed? For example, previous adverse reaction to anaesthetic – something which should be addressed during consenting.

You should think about what you are going to need to say and how you are going to say it. Imagine what questions you could be asked and try to formulate good answers. For example, if you had to tell someone that they were suffering from bowel cancer, they might reasonably ask you how long they have got to live or what the treatment options are. Both are questions that a surgical senior house officer (SHO) should be expected to answer.

The environment

The examination guidelines may state that furniture can be rearranged as appropriate. You should not be afraid to do this if you do not like the setup provided.

Try to sit in a position either level with or below the person you are talking to. This enables the doctor to appear less overbearing and authoritative, establishing trust and rapport. Towering over patients and relatives is intimidating and can be a particular problem for large doctors. If there is a desk in a consultation room, try not to sit behind it in such a way that you are looking across it, as this can alienate some people. Pull the actor's chair to the side so you are not facing each other across the desk.

A normal performance

Try to treat the discussion with the actor like any other consultation. Pretend that it is a real hospital setting not an exam setting. It will still be stressful, all exams are, but you will perform much better. You will come across as more normal, allowing your communication skills to come through. Try to make the artificial environment of the examination into a real-life situation.

If the person you are talking to starts to cry, do what you would do in real life: 'Here, let me give you a tissue' and offer a non-existent packet. The actor is likely to react normally and pretend to take one. This shows the examiners your presence of mind and calmness. You are making the artificial environment of the exam into a real situation. Your efforts at play acting will be rewarded with good marks.

The actor

The first two sections of the exam involve the use of an actor. Actors are a commonly used part of medical training and should be familiar to many candidates.

Actors are a fantastic learning tool, who improve the quality of training. Difficult and sensitive issues can be discussed in a safe atmosphere, allowing individuals to build up their own skills. They are very realistic, most are 'too good', almost the perfect model. When questioned appropriately they will give you all the information that you need. Real patients are rarely as accommodating or straightforward.

Practice

This is essential if you are going to improve. You can do this by yourself, rehearsing answers to set questions, so that on the day they flow beautifully. Or, you could pretend to be in an exam situation answering questions spontaneously and thinking afterwards what your answers were like.

Practise with colleagues who have either done the exam or are doing it with you. It is helpful to take turns at the different roles within the group, rotating between examiner, candidate and actor. It is amazing how different and revealing it can be to play and watch the different roles. Organize a mock examination or arrange to practise with an actor before the examination. This will provide excellent constructive criticism and perfect practice for the examination.

Many people feel self-conscious practising with people they know. Positive feedback, particularly when you are just starting to revise or immediately before the exam, will help to increase your confidence.

Timing is also important. The various sections of the examination have specific time limits. You should wear a watch to the examination, to time yourself. While you are practising, make a habit of timing yourself. This helps to pace the consultation appropriately and ensure that you don't overrun. Asking questions at the end of the discussion, which may result in a long and detailed answer, can then be avoided.

Specific questions

If you are asked detailed surgical questions which you do not know the answer to, say so. Apologize and tell the person that you will find out and let them know.

The anxious patient, 'Exactly what number of bowel operations does Mr Smith do each year?'

Candidate, 'Sorry, I do not know the exact figure. He has done about two every week while I have been working for him. Would you like me to find out the exact number for you?'

Pictures

Pictures and sketches are an excellent way of communicating in surgery. They are good at helping patients to understand and remember what is going on. The examination makes specific allowance for pictures, providing paper in the test room. The use of pictures is mentioned in the Colleges' advice to candidates. We would encourage their use whenever possible in the examination.

Use of 'allied' health professionals

Throughout surgery, many other health-care professionals, such as surgical specialist nurses, physiotherapists, occupational therapists and social workers, are encountered. They are a common and essential part of normal work. During the exam it is important to refer to other health-care professionals whenever possible. It helps with the flow of consultation in the exam setting, making it feel like a normal consultation. It also demonstrates a level of experience to the examiners; it shows that you've 'put your time in' on the wards and are ready to become a registrar.

The letter

This part of the examination is not a formal test of the English language and perfect English is not required. Put an address in the top right-hand corner, the date, a simple greeting, a farewell, your name written legibly and a signature. If you are filling out a test form, the patient information should be completed thoroughly, as this is a common reason for tests to be declined.

This letter is just like any other professional letter that you would write as an SHO. When you write any letter or complete a request form, think 'is this professional, complete and written in a reasonable space of time?' Very quickly, you will have prepared for this section of the exam without having had to worry about it too much.

Royal College of Surgeons,
Edinburgh,
31.12.03

Dear Dr/Miss/Colleague

I am writing to you....

Yours sincerely,
A. Butcher

GENERAL TECHNIQUES FOR IMPROVING COMMUNICATION SKILLS

There are a lot of general skills which are helpful in improving communication. They are methods of viewing and improving your performance as a whole. These are simple techniques that can be learnt and remembered so that they become a routine part of your consultation skills. In the months leading up to the MRCS examination, try to include these general skills in as many of your clinical encounters as possible. This will help to make these skills routine. When the examination comes, you will be in a position where these skills are second nature and have become part of your normal approach to patients and their relatives. You will be in a strong position to answer whatever scenarios you are given in the exam.

Many of the subjects included in this list are issues which have been identified as particular problems in surgical consultations; they are generally simple things that should not be too difficult to master.

Introductions

Unbelievably, doctors do not always introduce themselves or explain their role. This is usually due to oversight; nevertheless it comes across as arrogant and rude.

An oversight such as this cannot be allowed to happen in the exam setting. This is an area of specific concern to the examiners in the MRCS. If you do not introduce yourself appropriately at the start of your consultation, it alerts the examiners to a candidate who is a poor communicator and you will be playing 'catch up' for the rest of this section.

'Hello my name is... and I work for...'. This phrase is an extremely simple way of establishing rapport with a patient. If this is something that you do not do, or forget to do, then it must be learnt. By the time of the examination there is no excuse for not introducing yourself in a polite and simple manner each time you encounter a patient or relative.

It is also important to define your role. The medical system is complicated and hierarchical. Most people will not be aware of the way that the system works and it is important to explain 'where you fit in'. Some people will think you are the consultant and some will think that you do not look old enough to make the tea. By explaining who you are and what you do, you will remove any doubts as to your role. Some people will only want to see the consultant but most will be happy to see a doctor who is part of the team caring for that individual.

The scenario that you are given in the examination will dictate the exact nature of your greeting. If you have never met a patient before then a thorough introduction is needed. 'Hello, I'm Doctor Smith and I work for Mr Jarvis, the consultant. I will be helping to look after you while you are in hospital'.

If you are meeting relatives or patients who you are supposed to know already then a shorter introduction should still be made. 'Hello, I'm Doctor Smith, we met before your operation'.

While introducing yourself you may wish to shake hands and ask the patient to sit down.

How would you like to be communicated with yourself?

It can be helpful to consider how you would like to be communicated with yourself.

Reflection on what you consider to be important helps you to assess and improve your own deficiencies. Research has shown that appearing to be interested in your patients is extremely important. People like to be spoken to by someone who appears concerned. For the individual this is not just another hernia repair, it is their hernia repair.

Reflect on previous good consultations

This is a vitally important technique for self-improvement. We would strongly recommend, at least once, thinking about a specific consultation that went well. It does not matter about the exact circumstances, just what was good about it. Most people find this a rewarding exercise. It emphasizes good communication. It shows you that you can communicate well, at least for that moment. Any positive lessons should be absorbed and taken forward into future consultations.

Look at others

Another method that some people find useful for improving their own communication skills is to look at colleagues. They assess what were the good points of the consultation and what were the bad.

A good way to start using this technique is to think of an incident when a colleague said something grossly inappropriate. It would be rare for such an event not to have occurred at some point in your medical training. Without being judgemental, make a mental note not to use the same words or mannerisms if you are ever in the same situation.

Once you are comfortable with this technique, concentrate on the positive aspects of other peoples' consultations. If they use mannerisms, phrases or tone of voice that you like, try to adapt them and incorporate them into your own practice.

Body language

In communication, the use of non-verbal skills is as important as the use of verbal skills. The manner you convey is extremely important in determining how you are perceived by that person. It affects the way people react to you and what they say to you.

If possible try to sit in an open position, facing the person you are speaking to. Do not lean too far back or forward. Become familiar and comfortable with a neutral sitting position, with your hands held comfortably. Some people prefer to sit with their legs crossed. This is acceptable, if you can avoid looking like a chat-show host. We would not recommend crossing your arms. This is a particularly negative piece of body language and best avoided.

Positive movements, such as nodding your head in agreement or encouraging hand gestures, are forms of body language that we use all the time. These things help to build up good relationships with people that you are speaking to. They create a natural pace and aid good facilitation.

The other person's body language will affect the way you lead the consultation. The information that you learn from them is huge. Are they responding to you in an open and receptive way? Does their non-verbal communication indicate that they are happy with the course that the interview is taking? Or are they turned away from you, with their arms tightly crossed and frowning?

Listening skills

The way in which you listen to other people is important and an extension of your body language. If you appear to be listening with real interest, then the chances are that the posture you have adopted will be a good one. The person that you are communicating with will feel listened to by a caring and competent surgeon.

Nodding, smiling, sometimes echoing important words are all methods of showing that you are listening. Ultimately, they all help to encourage people to talk.

Use silence

This is a very underrated tool in communication. It allows difficult issues to be absorbed. It allows people to frame questions in their minds before asking them and to express their emotions without interruption.

In the exam setting do not leave too long without speaking, as the flow of the consultation will be interrupted. Pauses of a few seconds are acceptable.

The candidate breaking bad news "I'm very sorry to tell you that the operation did show that you have cancer"

The actor bows their head and sobs, without responding.

The candidate "I know this is difficult, take your time", pause for a few seconds then continue "I'm sorry but there are some other things that we need to talk about today"

Eye contact

Eye contact is important in establishing trust and rapport. Assessing the eye contact that you receive also helps to guide your verbal responses. Is the person you are talking to shy and nervous; are they angry or sad? All of these are feelings and emotions conveyed with eye contact. It is not necessary to stare directly at someone or gaze longingly into their eyes. It is, though, important to catch a person's eye during the consultation. Sometimes it is necessary to hold another person's eye contact, particularly at important points in a consultation, helping to emphasize specific comments.

If you find eye contact a difficult skill then begin by building up the number of times you catch a person's eye during a consultation. As you become more comfortable with eye contact, try to increase the length of time that you hold a person's gaze. You will quickly become familiar and confident with the appropriate use of eye contact.

Physical contact

The degree of physical contact that you have with your patients will depend on the situation and the personalities of those involved. The level of contact ranges from nothing to a kiss and a hug.

Generally, some degree of contact is appreciated and thoughtful. In the MRC3 exam, the appropriate use of physical contact will impress and add to the overall impression of a caring, competent communicator.

If you are not used to any form of contact whatsoever it can be daunting to start to try. An easy first step to build physical contact into your communications skills base is to touch the other person on the arm while you are sitting on the edge of their bed. Be confident but gentle with your movement. As you feel yourself becoming more confident, holding a patient's hand is the next step. The manner and timing of how and when to use physical contact will develop as you try to use it more.

Apologize

This really is one of the most useful things to learn. If a mistake or misunderstanding has occurred, say so and apologize. The vast majority of people that you will ever deal with are decent normal people, who respect and listen to the medical profession; they are not out to cause trouble or complain. If something has gone wrong, most simply want an apology and recognition of the fact that something is not right. If you were not present, it is important not to attribute blame; your apology is to simply acknowledge that the person has concerns. An apology is often unexpected but usually welcomed. It helps dispel the air of arrogance which often accompanies doctors.

Here are two different responses to the same situation. Try to imagine yourself in the position of the relative in the scenario and it is obvious that the second response is much better than the first.

You are the daughter of an elderly lady with a hip fracture who has booked an appointment to see you at 2 p.m. You have been delayed in theatre and it is now 3.40 p.m. The orthopaedic SHO has had no lunch and there are three patients in accident and emergency who have been referred to them. As the relative of the patient, you would be completely unaware of these facts. You are only concerned with the wait and the health of your mother.

First response, while eating a sandwich, 'I am in a real hurry. I can talk to you for 5 minutes and then I have to go'.

Second response, 'I am so sorry to have kept you waiting. An emergency came up in the operating theatre that we did not expect. I also have emergency patients waiting to see me in accident and emergency. I am afraid that I can only stop for a short while. Would you mind if I eat this while we talk, as I have missed lunch?'

This second response acknowledges that you have kept someone waiting for 1 hour and 40 minutes. It explains why you were late and why you cannot stay for long. The overall impression is of a busy but caring, competent doctor. The first response implies that you could not care less.

Expectations and concerns

Patients' expectations are an important issue in most consultations. The person who you are communicating with will have specific expectations of the consultation. They have come to you in your professional capacity, for particular questions to be answered. What do they expect to have achieved from this consultation? Did they expect an operation and not get one or vice versa?

Alongside the expectations, establish exactly what the concerns are of your patient or their relatives. Ask the patient how you can help and what their concerns are. The college examiners are looking out for you to elicit any expectations or concerns during the examination.

Patient "How do you know that I won't get a thrombosis or bleeding after my operation. I had a relative who had complications in this hospital"

Doctor "You seem particularly concerned about the side effects of the operation. We could go through them again if you'd like? Are the complications that your relative suffered worrying you?"

Start with open questions

Any questioning should begin by being very broad; try not to focus too early on particular issues. It is very easy to start asking closed questions, which may not elicit the information that is required.

Initial questions should be broad, 'How can I help?' or 'Do you know what this meeting is about?' All these first enquiries will allow the person to express what is of particular concern to them, rather than what you think is the matter.

As the conversation moves to more detailed discussions, to try to remain as open as possible in your questions. This will allow the consultation to develop in ways that answer the patient's most relevant questions.

Here is an example of the different use of open and closed questions and the subsequent outcome.

Closed questioning "You seem worried about the operation, is it the pain afterwards?"

"Yes, that's right"

Open questioning "You seem worried about the operation, which bit is most troubling you?"
"Well, it is a bit embarrassing, but I'm worried about the bag that I will have after the operation"
The second, more open, question allows the patient to express the problem that is really worrying them.

Show understanding and empathy

The ability to show understanding and empathy is another area for which marks are awarded in the MRCS examination. For example, phrases like 'that must have been hard' or 'Is money a bit of a problem?' are simple and add empathy to the discussion.

It is easy to jump to the wrong conclusions and a note of caution should be made not to make assumptions about how the other person is feeling. People react to situations in many different ways, with different reactions resulting from historical events which are out of your control as a doctor. The death of a relative is not always unwelcome to other family members. Major surgery, however hazardous, may be greeted with joy by some, who feel that it is worth it whatever the risks.

Use the other person's language

Use the other person's language and avoid the use of jargon. Getting the right level of communication with a patient is difficult. To show empathy and compassion, ensuring a patient understands what you are talking about without being patronizing, is hard.

Calibration is the process of establishing the level of intelligence and specific medical knowledge of the person that you are talking to.

One approach is to start at a low level of language and work upwards. Try to find a level of understanding that you think the other person is comfortable with. Start with basic facts and build upwards. As the conversation develops, introduce more complex facts and concentrate on areas that seem to be of concern.

Here are two different examples of this technique, both using the same scenario. The scenario is that you have to tell a mother her 7-year-old son needs an appendicectomy; it is midnight.

First scenario

Doctor "Your son needs an operation to remove his appendix, we will do this in the morning"
Mother "What is the appendix?"
Doctor "A small piece of tissue in the tummy, that can go rotten and needs to come out"
Most mothers would know what the appendix is and that it often becomes inflamed in children. This lady did not and so that is where the explanation should start and then work upwards.

Second scenario

Doctor "Your son needs an operation to remove his appendix, we will do this in the morning"

Mother "I thought that was what was wrong by the way he was holding his tummy. It will be like his sister's operation 2 years ago. Why are you not doing this now though?"

Doctor "It is important to stabilize children before operations with fluids and antibiotics. We also know that most operations, including this one, are best done the following morning, when senior staff are easily available and people are less tired".

The mother is familiar with the operation from her daughter's experience. Her concerns are different and need to be answered appropriately. Her level of understanding of the condition is much greater, and the level and complexity of the language which can be used are also higher.

Medical jargon such as 'lap chole', or abbreviations like I & D should be avoided. The time spent in medical training and practice has meant that these terms are part of your everyday language. Patients and their relatives do not have this level of knowledge. The use of medical terms which are not understood diminishes the quality of any discussion.

Allow time for questions

You should allow questions to be asked at any time during a consultation. If, during a specific consultation, someone is constantly asking questions that are disrupting the conversation, then politely tell them that you will make time for questions at the end. Often you will have answered most of their questions already.

At the end of every consultation it is very important to allow time for questions. Ask if there are any questions. This gives the opportunity of clarifying any remaining worries and concerns. It also empowers the other person and is known to improve patient satisfaction with the consultation.

The understanding

As little as 30% of what is said in a consultation is remembered and understood. It is important to reinforce points that you think are important. You should try to establish exactly what your patient or relative has understood. It may not be possible to make a person understand everything that has occurred at a single occasion. You may need to schedule further interviews, to repeat certain points or introduce further information, which it was not appropriate to deal with at a previous interview.

Summary

Summarizing is one of the most crucial parts of any consultation, which you need to incorporate into every consultation.

It can be done as short summaries scattered throughout the discussion, usually with a final summary at the end. Sometimes a single summary at the end is sufficient if you feel that the information you are giving is brief or the person has a good understanding of what has been said.

After a summary, it is usually a good idea to ask the person what they have understood about what you have just said.

Reflect on each consultation/personal debriefing

After each consultation you should try to think about it. Telling people difficult truths is hard. It is difficult and uncomfortable, particularly at first. With practice it does become satisfying to do it well. Seeing your skills develop is one of the most rewarding ways of watching your communications skills base grow.

When you are ready, try to think through communication difficulties, positives and negatives. Try to concentrate on what went well. Ask yourself some simple questions, to help break down the consultation into manageable areas. What were the good things about it? How did you feel about it overall? Good or bad? Were there parts of it that you did not like? What would you do differently if you were faced with the same situation? How can you improve the next time?

A 'NORMAL' CONSULTATION

In order to conduct a focused and well-paced consultation, it can be helpful to divide it into sections. By going through these sections in order you will ensure that you do not forget anything and will have a framework with which to conduct the discussion.

The chances are that the majority of your consultations follow a similar pattern, but if you have particular problems with this section of the exam then it may be worth learning to follow this framework.

The following framework has been divided into five sections. The examples given at the end of the chapter are all based around this framework. The sections are:

1. **Preparation**
   Before any consultation try to think through what is about to happen. You are given designated time in the exam to prepare, and you would be stupid not to use it. What is the scenario about? What information do I need to elicit or cover? What questions could I expect to be asked?

2. **Connecting**
   The first part of any discussion involves establishing trust and rapport. You should introduce yourself and begin to converse with the person. This might include preliminary questions about the person's age or where they live or possibly some small talk to help put the person at their ease.

3. **Consulting**
   This is the part of the discussion when you try to gather the information that you require. This is when open and thoughtful questioning will help. Your rapport with your patient should continue to increase, while you carefully guide the conversation to points relevant to the discussion. Your body language and empathic manner will all help to smooth the passage of the consultation.

4. **Summarizing**

As we have said, the summary is an essential part of all discussions. Using a summary helps to clarify what has been said and to establish what the patient has actually understood.

5. **Housekeeping**

In the same way that a person starts any consultation with certain expectations, they will finish the consultation with further expectations. This final section of a consultation is used to deal with those expectations. What are the plans for follow-up? What is the person expecting you to do now? For example, writing to the GP or arranging an ultrasound? This final section also allows you to deal with any issues that you may have forgotten and to tie up any loose ends.

SPECIFIC SCENARIOS

The following are specific situations that have been frequently encountered in the exam. We have outlined general templates around which to base a consultation, including some of the general points discussed above.

Breaking bad news

This is one of the most commonly asked scenarios. You must be familiar with how to answer it. It can be disguised in a variety of forms; the death of a patient, an operation that has gone wrong or a serious diagnosis. It does not matter what form it is presented in, you must be able to give a good answer.

Bad news cannot be broken gently, but it can be given in a sensitive manner and at an individual's own pace. Receiving bad news is often accompanied by denial. This may be reflected in the responses that you get from the actor. Denial is rarely total though. As diseases progress, denial generally subsides. In the exam, if you are faced with a situation in which the actor is in a state of denial, try to challenge this in a sensitive manner, remembering that patients need time to adjust to bad news.

You may also be faced with difficult questions such as 'How long have I got?' Often there are particular reasons for such questions, such as a family wedding or birth. In general, specific estimations of prognosis are best avoided.

Anger is another common reaction. It is important not to take this personally. It is not aimed at you. There are often personal and family issues which are beyond your control and role as a surgeon. Keeping calm and professional is usually enough to defuse these situations.

When breaking bad news, either in the exam or on the wards, the first thing to do is to prepare. Are you ready? Do you have all the information that you need? Have you made enough time available to deliver the bad news? Are you the best person to deliver the news? Is the environment right? Have you remembered to inform the nursing staff about what you are doing? In the exam setting, all these questions are irrelevant but they are extremely important in real life.

Introduce yourself and establish your position within the team.

A good starting point is to establish what the patient/relative already knows. 'What do you know about what has happened while your mother has been in hospital?' This lays the groundwork for approaching the real problem. The individual may be expecting the worst and have a large degree of insight into the situation. Alternatively, this may be the first time that any hint of bad news has arisen, and so a more circumspect approach is required.

Here is the same clinical situation, viewed through the eyes of two different relatives. A previously frail 90-year-old woman has deteriorated acutely after an emergency total hip replacement. She has been seen by the consultant geriatrician, who feels that she should be kept comfortable and allowed to die peacefully.

The first relative is an eldest daughter, who has cared for her mother for the last 5 years. She was with her when she was admitted this morning.

Doctor "What do you understand about what has happened so far?"

Daughter "Mother has had an operation on her hip. She was very poorly before she had the operation, she's not been right for the last 9 months or so. The doctor in casualty said that an operation would be difficult and was very dangerous"

Doctor "That is right, your mother was very poorly before the operation"

This woman appreciates the reality of the situation. She knows her mother was in generally poor health. She has been warned already that things could go wrong by the doctor in accident and emergency. The impending bad news is not unexpected and can be tackled directly. She is likely to be upset rather than shocked.

The second scenario involves an eldest son, who has not seen his mother since his annual visit on Boxing Day, 9 months previously.

Doctor "What do you understand about what has happened so far?"

Son "My mother has had an operation on her hip, when will I be able to see her? I can't believe she is in here, she was very well when I last saw her"

This man does not have an appreciation of the situation. He needs to have the background to the admission explained before breaking the bad news. The bad news will be a shock to him as well as upsetting.

Next, it is important to establish if the person is ready to hear the bad news. In the exam, they almost certainly will be. In reality, they may not. You should respect their wishes and offer the possibility of a future discussion. The majority of people do eventually want to know their diagnosis, the treatment options and the prognosis, even when the outlook is bleak.

You are now ready to break the news, fire a warning shot, 'I've got some bad news'. Once this has had a moment to sink in, continue. Break the news in stages, using brief simple language, avoiding jargon and using an appropriate level of language.

The specific scenario will dictate what language you use, but it must be clear and honest.

Cancer is a very specific situation. The word cancer must be used if this is the diagnosis. Phrases such as 'lump', 'growth' or 'lesion' are misleading and confusing to many people. Often, the person does not register the significance of these words. In the exam if you have to break bad news regarding cancer, the examiners will be listening for the word cancer. If you do not use it, you are likely to be marked down.

It is important at this stage to check for understanding. It may be necessary to go over the bad news again.

Once you are certain that the patient has understood, you should allow silence, show empathy and acknowledge the upset and distress that has occurred.

As with any consultation, allow time for questions. Now is the time to arrange follow-up and it is extremely important that the patient or relative has a point of future contact. This is an excellent opportunity to involve other health professionals such as palliative care nurses and to show your breadth of clinical experience.

After any consultation, or relaxing at home after the exam, it is important to take time to debrief. Reflect on the good and bad points. Consider how you could improve for the next time.

Collusion

This is a common scenario, occurring between relatives and patients. It is the situation where relatives do not wish their loved ones to be told bad news. 'Please don't tell Mum she has cancer, she won't be able to take it'.

It is generally an act of love. In many cases the individual concerned suspects the diagnosis anyway. It is very important that this situation is not allowed to continue. It leads to far more problems than it solves. Patients resent their relatives for not telling them and secrecy surrounds the patient and family, making communication very hard between family members. Patients also have a right to medical knowledge, which their family cannot veto.

When this is explained to relatives they will usually accept it and allow their relative to be told the bad news. If they are still not happy, you should tell them that you are going to tell them anyway, explaining your reasons again. It is the patient you are treating, not their relatives.

Angry patient

This is a situation in which surgeons often find themselves. The angry patient can be extremely intimidating and confrontational. Dealing with angry people requires particular skills to help diffuse the situation.

Several factors are important when dealing with angry people. Firstly, an appropriate environment is essential when dealing with angry people. It is not acceptable to have a shouting match on the ward. In fact, a shouting match is the last thing that is needed. As a professional person, you must remain calm and collected throughout, whatever state the other person may get themselves into.

Next, it is important to listen to the person; a lot of anger can be released simply by listening without interruption to the other person. Try to convey a sense of understanding and empathy while doing this.

The final part of dealing with an angry person is to offer a solution to their problem, even if that is a further meeting or involvement of others to take matters further.

Dealing with complaints

This is another situation where early considerate management can result in a quick and satisfactory outcome for all sides. The modern NHS has systems in place for dealing with complaints and written complaints should be dealt with by your consultant and the hospital management.

If you are faced with a complaint in a one-to-one discussion, then the technique for managing the situation is very similar to that used when dealing with an angry patient. Remain calm and listen to the other person.

You should explain the complaints procedure in your hospital, which involves writing to the hospital's chief executive, who will acknowledge the complaint immediately. A full response will usually be issued within 28 days of receiving the complaint.

It may be appropriate to apologize, although you should avoid blaming individuals, particularly regarding events where you were not actually present.

Informed consent

The following comment was written on the consent form of a patient for an elective aortic aneurysm repair: '...repair of the big pipe in the middle of your body, which carries blood around the body. It is a very dangerous operation, you might die. Without the operation you are more likely to die'. Compare this with another example that we have all seen, 'AAA repair'.

Usually something between these two approaches is adopted. The first option is far more informative. It sums up what is going to happen and leaves little doubt that a patient is aware of the mortality that is involved in an operation of this severity. The second gives virtually no information to a patient that will be of any use to them.

After connecting with your patient it is important to say what informed consent is and why you are doing it.

If you are given this scenario you will be expected to discuss complications, both those that are general to all surgery and those specific to the operation. The potential mortality risks will also need to be discussed, if appropriate.

Summing up is important. The patient or relative should understand why the operation is taking place and what the outcome and main complications are likely to be. Make sure that you ask the person what they have understood about these two areas.

CONCLUSION

Hopefully some of what you have read here will be of use as you prepare for the MRCS examination. In addition, your skills as surgical communicators should be better for the rest of your career. This will improve not only patient satisfaction, but also your own satisfaction as well. Good communication will also improve your time management. A little extra time spent talking to people thoroughly will lead to fewer complaints and reduce the need for future additional discussions.

It is also essential to remember that communication skills can always be improved and that they are a learnt skill, not an inherited one. The key to that improvement is through self-directed learning, using the skills that you have learnt in life as well as those you have learnt from this book, and using them on a daily basis. If you take the trouble to do this, you will see how you have improved as a communicator and how much more your patients and their relatives think of you.

CASE SCENARIOS

Information giving

Case 1

You are asked to see a 76-year-old married man who has gone into urinary retention for the first time. Your examination revealed a smoothly enlarged prostate gland. He has just been catheterized. You are required to discuss the immediate and long-term treatment options, including potential surgery.

He is a type II diabetic, well controlled on diet alone.

Preparation. The information you are going to give needs to be split into two sections, the immediate management and the long-term management. To score full marks you are given other information which you need to work into your discussion. Does type II diabetes and an operation on the prostate have any connection? Why mention he is married? To really impress the examiners, your history should cover his sexual history in detail, as a TURP and type II diabetes are causes of impotence. It is important, therefore, to elicit his sexual function before any surgery. Remember not to use the phrase TURP without a full explanation of what it means.

Connecting. The fact that you have examined him implies you have already met and you are returning to tell him about his treatment options; therefore a brief 'Hello, again' should be sufficient.

Consulting. The consultation should begin broadly, while focusing on the issues that you are required to discuss. Inform him that the catheter was necessary to relieve the mechanical obstruction posed by the prostate and that it is likely to remain in position until surgery is performed. The leg bag should also be explained to him in detail. He should be told that he is likely to remain as an inpatient at least overnight.

Once the immediate situation has been dealt with, the scenario requires you to focus the discussion onto long-term treatment options. You should explain that he is likely to go into retention again without any definitive treatment. You should tell him you think that he will require surgery, probably within a few weeks. The type of surgery should now be discussed.

Now is also a good time to discuss the side effects of surgery. You should discuss those common to all surgery and those specifically associated with this procedure, such as incontinence or erectile dysfunction. This would also be an appropriate time to discuss his sexual history.

Summarizing. Sum up what you have said and what the likely course of events is going to be, for example, admission from the Emergency department to the ward or discharge home with a leg bag. Reiterate the fact that surgery is going to be the best long-term option, but that it will not be on this admission. Now is the time to ask if he has any questions.

Housekeeping. Is there anything that you might have left out? Let the patient know when they are likely to see you again, on the morning round for example. Say goodbye and finish the consultation.

Case 2

You are an orthopaedic SHO and have been asked to see the son of an 85-year-old man and discuss his father's condition. You have never met the son before; unfortunately his father has suffered postoperative complications. He has a wound haematoma with a secondary MRSA infection, which needs to be evacuated under anaesthetic.

Preparation. This scenario revolves around breaking bad news. The background that you are given implies that you will need to cover a lot of different ground. This includes why his father had the operation in the first place, the complications and the severity of the situation. Questions about why this has happened are almost certain to be asked and you should prepare for them.

Connecting. The scenario clearly says that you have not met this man before; a full introduction is therefore required. You are about to give bad news, your manner and tone should reflect that from the beginning of the consultation.

Consulting. As you have not met this man before, it is appropriate to ask him what he already knows about his father's condition. His response will give you a very good starting point. He may be fully aware that his father had an operation 3 days ago. Alternatively, he may have only found out about the hospital admission and surgery that morning.

Once the background knowledge regarding the original operation has been established, you should move on to the subject of postoperative complications. He will need a clear explanation about both MRSA and the wound haematoma. The need for surgery as the correct course of treatment should also be discussed.

The dangers of repeated surgery in a patient of this age group, including the additional morbidity of an MRSA infection, need to be highlighted.

Summarizing. Repeat the main points of the discussion again, in the order in which they occurred. Allow time for questions and make sure what you have said has really sunk in.

Housekeeping. Take a moment to think if you may have forgotten to say something. Assuming that you haven't, explain what is going to happen next, when his father's operation will take place and when you will be able to give him more information. Give the son the information he needs to contact you again, 'If you would like to speak to me, don't hesitate to ask the nurses to arrange a time'.

Case 3

You are the SHO in a busy, one-stop breast clinic. A 27-year-old woman who has not previously attended the clinic has told the nursing staff that she will only see the consultant. Radiology and cytology performed in the clinic have confirmed that the patient has a fibroadenoma. The consultant has had to leave the clinic early.

Preparation. This lady is likely to be angry, possibly aggressive towards you. It is important that you remain calm when talking to this person, whatever she may say to you. The prime objective of this scenario is to get this lady to talk to you. The secondary objective is to tell her that, as a lady under 30 years old, she has a benign lesion which can be removed if she wants.

Connecting. Introduce yourself and establish your place as an integral part of the consultant's team. Acknowledge that this lady wishes to see the consultant. Apologize that the consultant is not available and explain that you are capable of conducting this consultation. If she is still angry, politely explain that it is not always possible, or usual, to see the consultant in an NHS clinic. Let her know that the consultant is ultimately responsible for her care, and any queries or concerns that persist at the end of the consultation will be discussed with the consultant at a later date.

If this is still not satisfactory, it is the patient's right to see the consultant. She will then need to be told that she will have to be re-booked at a time when the consultant can see her. This may, however, be some time in the future. As this is not a diagnosis of cancer, it is not likely to be in the immediate future and the decision as to when it will occur rests with the consultant.

Consulting. Once it is established that you can lead the consultation, move to the subject of her fibroadenoma. It is now time to discuss the surgical management of a fibroadenoma in a young woman. It is important that you offer her the option of surgery, while emphasizing that this is a benign condition. The breast clinic will have breast-care specialist nurses available and you should offer the patient the opportunity to talk to one. You may also offer the option of leaving it alone and attending the clinic in 6 months' time for a follow-up ultrasound. This will determine whether or not the lump has grown in size and she can make a decision at this time about surgery. Emphasize to her that this is a benign lump and does not predispose her to breast cancer.

Summarizing. The summarizing should concentrate on the surgical aspects of the condition, what you have told her and what her options are.

Housekeeping. This will involve arranging appropriate follow-up regarding her breast lump. At this stage you could tactfully enquire into the quality of your services. Patients in this situation are excellent guides to how good you were. 'Thanks very much Doctor, I'm sorry about earlier, I was just worried' is the usual outcome. If they hurry away muttering under their breath, then you probably haven't done a great job.

Case 4

You are a neurosurgical SHO working on a neurology intensive care unit. A 42-year-old man who has been on the unit for the last 3 weeks has been pronounced brainstem dead by two consultants. His family, who you have got to know well, need to be told the bad news. Your consultant has asked you to talk to the family about switching off the life support and also the potential use of the patient's organs for transplantation. He was not carrying a donor card.

Preparation. This case is centred around breaking bad news, but with several subtle differences. The information that you are given says that you already know the family well; therefore your introduction should be tailored as such. You will then need to tell the family the bad news. It is likely that they will be aware that the patient is about to have his brainstem function assessed, with a poor outcome expected. The last section of the consultation then needs to be steered towards potential organ transplantation. It is also implicit that you will need to obtain their written consent.

Connecting. Although you know the family well, it is still important to say hello. The conversation should then be swiftly moved on to the bad news.

Consulting. With empathy and understanding, tell the family the result of the examination and the poor chances of recovery. Use clear language, explaining the implications of the diagnosis. Use pauses and silence to allow time for the implications to be absorbed.

Making it clear that you are moving on to a new and difficult topic, begin to discuss switching off the life support and the possibility of organ transplantation. If the family is receptive you should explain how the process will be carried out. You will need to mention which organs can be used, although exactly which ones are taken is at the family's discretion. Stress that they can take their time and will be allowed to spend some time with their relative before any decision is made.

As he was not carrying a donor card you should mention that you will need their formal written consent.

Summarizing. In this scenario, short brief summaries during the consultation, followed by periods of silence could be particularly effective. A long final summary about the brainstem death is likely to be somewhat redundant. Instead, it may be appropriate to concentrate on the positive aspects such as enabling another patient to have a chance of normal life.

Housekeeping. Any further questions which you have not already answered should be cleared up. Assuming that they are in agreement with organ donation, it is important to let them know what is now going to occur. Include an approximate time frame and arrange a time when you can obtain their consent for the procedure. If they do not wish to be left alone for a short while, a final act would be to offer to accompany them to see the patient, to spend some final time with their loved one.

Case 5

A 55-year-old woman with Graves' disease has been referred to your clinic by her GP for a total thyroidectomy. She is currently euthyroid and taking carbimazole. Last year a trial without carbimazole resulted in a rapid return of the thyrotoxicosis. The lady is expecting to have surgery and you need to tell her that radioactive iodine would be a more appropriate course of treatment.

Preparation. What are the important factors to consider before meeting this lady? She needs to be told that surgery is not the best option for a woman of her age. It is also important not to be overcritical of the GP. It is unprofessional and the management of thyroid disease has until recently been contentious. Early surgery without radioiodine was accepted treatment until relatively recently.

Connecting. A full introduction should be made, giving your name and position within the surgical team. You could begin by asking her what she already knows about her condition and what she thinks are the reasons for the consultation.

Consulting. It is important to tell this lady that she will be having radioiodine treatment. She will also need to be informed of the side effects and the precautions that will need to be taken immediately after receiving the treatment. The long-term likelihood that she may require replacement thyroxine, if she becomes hypothyroid, should also be mentioned. The procedure including the referral to a radiotherapist needs to be outlined.

You are likely to have to spend some time listening to her. She will almost certainly have some questions about the change in management, which she had not been expecting. The lack of surgery will not necessarily be seen as beneficial.

Summarizing. This will involve clarifying the treatment she is going to receive. Some of the more important side effects and precautions should also be re-emphasized.

Housekeeping. You need to tell her how her treatment will now proceed, who will contact her next and approximately when this will be. Most thyroid clinics will have access to literature on radioiodine and you could offer this to her.

Case 6

You are an SHO working for a cardiothoracic team. Your unit is involved in an established clinical trial comparing surgery with a new medical treatment. You are required to explain to a 64-year-old man, who fits the trial entry criteria, about his options.

Preparation. While preparing, consider what you know about clinical trials and what information you need to pass on to the patient. Let him know that he is not a 'guinea pig'. For a clinical trial to have reached this stage, there must be evidence that both treatments are at least equal and the new treatment may even be beneficial. You will also need to mention ethics committees and that every patient has the right to refuse entry into trials without detriment to their treatment.

Connecting. Introduce yourself in the usual manner and explain your position within the firm.

Consulting. Firstly, establish what he knows already and what he is expecting from the consultation. He may be aware that he has coronary artery disease needing treatment or he may not know the results of his angiogram. Once the need for treatment has been established, then the treatment options can be discussed. You need to clearly explain that the unit is involved in a trial and the reasons for this. The processes involved in the trial, such as randomization, should also be touched upon. The safeguards and its voluntary nature need to be discussed. He does not need to make up his mind right at that moment; most people will need a little time to consider what you have said.

Summarizing. You will need to emphasize the need for treatment, whether he decides to enter the trial or not. Outline the basics of the trial once again. It is his decision to enter and, whatever he decides, it will not affect his treatment in any way.

Housekeeping. Assuming that he has agreed to enter the trial, you will now need to get this organized. Usually this will involve contacting a coordinating centre for randomization. Let him know that he will get a decision either way very soon and he will be contacted in the near future. Do not forget to thank him; volunteers for trials are essential to medical progress.

Case 7

As an SHO in general surgery, you are required to speak to the mother of an 11-year-old boy who has been diagnosed with a probable acute torsion of his left testicle. He is due for immediate exploratory surgery and you need to obtain her consent for an operation.

Preparation. This is a relatively straightforward scenario. You need to explain about the diagnosis and the surgical treatment. You also need to obtain written consent. Due to the urgency of the clinical situation, you will need to inject urgency into the conversation. Finishing before the full time limit is highly likely, even desirable.

Connecting. Introduce yourself and begin the conversation immediately. 'I am afraid that I have some bad news about your son's testicle'.

Consulting. After a brief description of the surgical condition, the need for urgent exploratory surgery needs to be addressed. The operation should be explained in detail. It would also be reasonable to address the issue of fertility, a concern of any parent. Next, the issue of consent should be tackled. As he is a minor, she is required to sign the consent form for her son. Without great length, albeit thoroughly, discuss the process of consent and the associated risks of anaesthesia and surgery. She needs to be told that her son may lose a testicle even with surgery.

While time is a problem, this is still a great shock; therefore empathy and understanding need to be shown. It is appropriate to offer to come back after the surgery so that you can talk about things in greater depth and what your surgical findings were. Explain that due to the urgency of the situation you cannot talk about things as much as you would like to.

Summarizing. Give a very brief summary of what has happened and what is about to occur. Ask her if she has any questions left.

Housekeeping. Tell her that surgery is about to start and you will come back and speak to her again after the operation, when you will have more information available. Say goodbye and leave.

Case 8

You are a thoracic SHO. A previously fit 73-year-old smoker has undergone an 'open and close' thoracotomy today for a small cell carcinoma of his left lung. Thoracotomy showed extensive thoracic involvement and infiltration of the mediastinum. Curative surgery was not possible.

You are due to see him after he has recovered from the anaesthetic to tell him the bad news. On the morning ward round he was inappropriately cheerful.

The nursing staff have informed you that he has not even told his wife he is unwell. He has delayed coming into hospital for several weeks until his wife was due to go on holiday, so she would not know.

Preparation. This is going to be an extremely difficult few minutes. It is likely to be very emotionally draining and the outcome is uncertain. The crux of the situation is to break bad news to a man who appears to be in complete denial of his illness. This is the 'pass and fail' issue in the scenario.

Thinking through the information you have been given, you will need to deal with the patient's refusal to tell his wife about his illness. To gain full marks for the discussion, this needs to be adequately addressed.

Connecting. Say hello and sit down. He is likely to be tired and a bit drowsy so soon after surgery. Your manner should be restrained to set the tone for the rest of the conversation.

Consulting. Start immediately with the bad news, using simple and direct language. The degree of denial will dictate how you then respond. This patient has, after all, consented for surgery; therefore he has to be aware of a potentially poor outcome. He needs to know that he has cancer which cannot be cured. The potential options for palliative measures also need to be addressed. This would be a good time to talk about the use of the palliative care services.

Now is the time to address the issue of his wife. With sensitivity, explain that his wife cannot be informed without his consent, but in your experience withholding information is rarely the best long-term strategy. It is not necessary to really push this issue at this time. All the teams involved in his care from now on are likely to say the same things about his wife and, as his illness progresses, his views are likely to change.

Summarizing. This is a scenario where it is important to take your time. Emphasize all the important points once again. Use silence and allow a long time for questions.

Housekeeping. It is extremely important that this gentleman is not left feeling helpless. He needs to know when someone is going to see him next and what the next course of his treatment will be. Tell him you are going to tell the nurse in charge what has happened and they will look in on him in a few minutes.

Offer to see him again if he wants. Say goodbye and without rushing leave the room.

Information gathering

Case 1

A healthy 83-year-old man has been referred to your outpatients clinic regarding a troublesome right inguinal hernia. He had an inferior myocardial infarction 10 years ago.

Preparation. This is a relatively easy clerking. The two main areas needing to be covered are his hernia and his medical history.

You will be required to take a detailed history of the hernia. This should include:

- The length of history
- Predisposing causes – chronic cough, heavy lifting, constipation, symptoms of prostatism/difficulty passing urine
- The size
- Reducibility
- Elucidate any potential complications i.e. obstruction/strangulation (tender lump, abdominal pain, vomiting)
- How much it bothers him.

His medical clerking will also be relatively limited. A myocardial infarction 10 years ago without further complications should not prevent an operation occurring, if the patient is well. You should ask about chest pain and any limitation in function due to his infarct, such as shortness of breath on exertion. You do not need to pursue this too rigorously, providing he is symptom free.

If you are concerned about his fitness for anaesthesia, you could suggest an anaesthetic or cardiac opinion before his operation.

You also need to ask about his medications. If he is not taking any, it would be reasonable to ask him to see his GP to review this.

Ask about smoking and alcohol and, allowing for his age, a brief social history. You should pay particular attention to his plans for the immediate post-discharge period.

The consultation. Introduce yourself and begin to take a normal surgical history. Use the outline that you have formulated during your preparation time to guide your questions.

When you have all the information that you want, you need to summarize and allow time for questions in the normal way.

He should be given a point of contact and you should explain to him what will happen next. Let him know that he will need to give his written consent before he has the operation, and that he will see further doctors, such as an anaesthetist, before he has the operation.

End the discussion by saying goodbye, and indicate to the examiners that you have finished.

Case 2

A previously well 53-year-old business woman has been referred to the urology outpatients clinic having passed several episodes of frank blood in her urine. She is otherwise well, but does travel frequently to Africa.

The GP letter states that she was extremely reluctant to be referred to your clinic because she feels that there is nothing wrong with her.

Preparation. Your questions will revolve around her urinary symptoms; obviously it is important to gain as much information as possible about them. The scenario you are given also implies that you will need to ask her about her travel history. The African travel implies schistosomiasis is a potential diagnosis that the college would like you to cover.

The information given says that she was reluctant to attend the clinic. In reality, she is highly likely to be concerned about her symptoms. It is important to be understanding and to try to give her the opportunity to discuss those anxieties during your clerking.

The consultation. Say hello and introduce yourself. After gentle preliminary questions such as her name and age, begin to concentrate on her presenting complaint. When you have finished asking her about this, complete the history taking with questions about other symptoms and her general health. A social history is important, but likely to be brief.

Now is a good time to address her anxieties about her referral. Use open questions which allow her to express her concerns: 'Do you have any questions or concerns?' or 'Would you like to talk about possible diagnoses?' The remainder of the consultation will be dictated by her responses.

After summarizing the surgical aspects of her case, inform her of the likely investigations that you will instigate. Finally, politely end the consultation, indicating to the examiners that you have finished.

Case 3

A 17-year-old girl has been referred to you from the Emergency department. She is unwell with a 2-day history of colicky central abdominal pain which has now localized to her right iliac fossa. She has been obstructive with other members of staff and refused all examination and investigations.

The casualty SHO notices that she has a previous casualty card from an attendance at the department 6 weeks earlier. She was raped by a member of her family. She is currently living on her own in a woman's refuge.

Preparation. This is obviously a difficult situation. The clinical situation implies that she has appendicitis, possibly requiring surgery, and this needs to be clearly explained to her.

It is important to be sensitive and understanding. You should acknowledge her right not to be examined further but explain that it will be extremely helpful if you could do so. She must also be aware that by not complying fully with the examination, you cannot be sure what is wrong and she may be subjecting herself to a needless operation. You will need to mention other diagnoses, such as ectopic pregnancy and its implications. The possibility of an appendicectomy should also be discussed in detail.

Whether you talk directly about the incident 6 weeks before will depend on how the consultation is proceeding. Discussing the rape is the only way you will score full marks, but it is not essential to passing, as long as your manner is appropriate and you cover the surgical clerking well enough.

During the social history you should enquire whether or not she has a social worker assigned to her and offer to arrange for one if necessary.

The consultation. Introduce yourself as usual and begin to ask her some routine questions. Building rapport is very important here and it may be worth spending extra time chatting about things that you would not normally do; the weather or current affairs, for example.

Then move onto the detailed surgical history, concentrating on the relevant issues regarding her pain and medical history. You should tell her about the possible diagnoses and the potential impending operation.

After this, you can move on to more sensitive issues and ask her about her reluctance to be examined. If things are going well, now would be a good time to talk gently about the rape.

Summarizing will be focused on her surgical condition and it is not necessary to remind her of painful memories. Housekeeping will involve telling her of the immediate plan and that she will need to sign a consent form before any operation can take place.

Case 4

A 52-year-old woman with severe asthma is referred to the general surgical outpatients for removal of a longstanding sebaceous cyst. The GP's letter documents a previous anaphylactic reaction to local anaesthetic; however, the patient does not remember exactly which anaesthetic it was.

Preparation. The most important information that you need to elicit is her anaesthetic history and you should devote the majority of the clerking to this issue. Asthma is a major worry for a general anaesthetic and an anaphylactic reaction is also a major issue for a local anaesthetic.

It also changes the questions you ask her about her cyst. In addition to the usual questions regarding any lump, the degree of distress that it causes should be sought. You will need to tell the patient your concerns about anaesthesia and potentially advise the patient against surgery.

The consultation. After introductions and the relatively brief surgical history, concentrate on her anaesthetic and medical history.

After the history has been completed it is important to establish just how badly she wants to have her cyst removed, telling her that you will require an anaesthetic opinion before surgery is appropriate.

If she is still adamant that she wants an operation, then during your summary, re-emphasize the potential risk that she is taking; she must be informed that it is still not certain to go ahead. Your housekeeping will depend on the outcome of your conversation, but hopefully will be a discharge back to her GP!

WRITTEN SECTION

Here are three examples of scenarios that you may be given in the written section of the exam. They include the typical information that you should include when writing your letter or filling out a form in the exam. The key is to keep things brief, but comprehensive.

Example 1. Discharge letter to a GP. This covers the patient's details and the dates that he was in hospital. It includes his primary diagnosis and his surgical management. It covers the course of his illness and the additional treatment that he received. It ends with his current drug history and the plans for follow-up. Any changes in medications should also be highlighted. The results of major investigations should also be included, although each full blood count is probably over the top.

Royal College Hospital
London
08.01.04

Dear Doctor,

Re. Paul Smith
DOB 31.03.1970
Admitted 02.12.03
Discharged 12.12.03

This man was admitted as an emergency following a road traffic accident. He was knocked off his bicycle and suffered trauma, primarily to his right leg.

After initial assessment by the trauma team his only serious injury was an open fracture to his right tibia and fibula. This was operated on the evening of his admission. He had an external fixator applied and thorough wound debridement. There was a good surgical result.

Postoperatively, he suffered a superficial skin infection. Although he initially received intravenous antibiotics, there did not appear to be any deep-seated wound infection or osteomyelitis and therefore these were discontinued.

He is now taking no medication.

We will continue to review him in fracture clinic on a weekly basis. It is likely that the external fixator will be removed after 8 weeks.

Yours sincerely

A. Butcher, orthopaedic SHO to Mr A Carpenter

Example 2. An internal referral to a neurologist, following a postoperative cerebrovascular accident (CVA). According to the materials that you are given, this could be a letter to the consultant's secretary or an entry in the hospital notes. It will follow a similar pattern to the discharge summary above, although you should include more background information to enable the attending consultant to immediately get an idea of the clinical situation. You are not a specialist, hence the referral, but basic medical facts relating to the likely diagnosis should be listed.

The format given here would be equally applicable to an external referral letter too, although you would need to include some contact details for the patient as well.

Date 10.02.04

Dear consultant neurologist

My consultant would be extremely grateful if you would review this 63-year-old man. He was admitted for an elective reversal of a stoma following an anterior resection 12 months ago. There was no evidence of recurrence.

On the second postoperative day (yesterday) he suffered an acute left-sided weakness and slurring of his speech. Clinically, he has continued weakness in both his arm and leg, although his speech has recovered.

The on-call medical registrar felt that a CVA was the most likely diagnosis and suggested a CT scan. This was performed as an emergency. The results suggest a moderately sized infarction on the right side of his brain.

He has a history of hypertension, which has been well controlled, both before and during admission with atenolol 50 mg od only. He has no other past medical history of note and is taking no other medication. He does, however, continue to smoke.

We would value your opinion on future management and follow-up.

Yours sincerely

F. Spencer, SHO to consultant bowel surgeon

Example 3. Filling in a form. While this seems rather mundane, the college may give you a form to fill in as the written section of the exam. As long as you keep your wits about you, this section should be easy and present very little problem to anyone who has worked in a UK hospital.

The details you fill in will depend on which form you are given and which investigation is required. The points that you need to remember are twofold. Firstly, the clinical details need to be complete so the request cannot be declined on clinical grounds, and secondly, the patient information must be complete. Many requests for investigations are declined because the patient information is not completely filled in. You will fail this section of the exam if you simply put the patient's name and date of birth; all sections should be completed if the information is available to you.

APPENDICES

USEFUL NAMES

The following is a list of eponyms, Latin terms and names of famous surgeons/physicians that you may be expected to know:

Claudius Amyand – performed the first ever appendicectomy in 1736 in Westminster Hospital. The patient was an 11-year-old-boy who presented with a faecal fistula secondary to a right scrotal hernia. At the time of operation, Amyand found the appendix within the scrotum. The appendix had been perforated by a pin. The patient made a full postoperative recovery.

Arthur Sydney Blundell Bankart – 'Bankart's operation' was for recurrent dislocation of the shoulder. The joint capsule is sutured to the detached glenoid labrum without duplication of the subscapularis tendon. Otherwise known as 'Broca–Perthes–Bankart operation'.

Christiaan Barnard – South African cardiac surgeon. Performed the world's first human heart transplant in Groot Schuur Hospital in Cape Town, 1967. The patient was 53-year-old Louis Washkansky, a dentist with diabetes and incurable heart disease who faced almost certain death. He lived for 18 days after the operation before rejecting the heart. Barnard famously said, 'If a lion chases you to the bank of a river filled with crocodiles, you will leap into the water convinced you have a chance to swim to the other side. You would never accept such odds if there were no lion'. He was forced to give up surgery in 1983 due to rheumatoid arthritis and died in September 2001.

Sir Charles Bell (born 1774) – popular amongst Middlesex/UCLH surgeons. Charles Bell was a professor of surgery in Edinburgh and the Middlesex Hospital. He gallantly went to the grounds of the Battle of Waterloo and operated day and night on gunshot wounds. He named 'Bell's palsy,' paralysis of the facial nerve, and also extensively researched anterior and posterior nerve roots (Bell–Magendie rule).

August Bier (born 1898) – performed the first successful spinal anaesthetic. Later gave his name to 'Bier's block', intravenous regional limb anaesthesia.

Christian Albert Theodor Bilroth (born 1881) – trained in Berlin, professor of surgery in Zurich. Gave his name to the removal of the pylorus with end-to-end anastomosis of the stomach to the duodenum (Bilroth I). Bilroth II involved closing off the proximal duodenum and anastomosing the gastric stump to the jejunum. Also began the practice of audit and famously wrote: 'Statistics are like women. Mirrors of purest virtue and truth, or like whores, to use as one pleases'.

Sir John Bland-Sutton (born 1855) – born in Enfield, Middlesex, and trained at the Middlesex Hospital. One of the founders of gynaecological surgery and reported the first case of splenectomy for a 'wandering spleen'. He insisted on using silk for suturing and would buy balls that were 1 mile long. Apparently was very wealthy due to a large private practice and never quite lost his cockney accent. His ashes are kept in an urn in the Bland–Sutton Museum of Pathology, Middlesex Hospital.

Peter Camper – professor of medicine, surgery and anatomy in Holland. He named the superficial fatty layer of the fascia of the abdominal wall.

Charles Chassaignac – French surgeon who named the carotid tubercle of the sixth cervical vertebra.

Claudicare – to limp (Latin).

Colles' fracture – Abraham Colles, Irish professor of anatomy (Royal College of Surgeons of Ireland), named this fracture of the distal radius. Also named the superficial perineal fascia.

Sir Astley Paston Cooper – surgeon at Guy's and St Thomas' Hospital. Also President of the Royal College of Surgeons. Named the iliopectineal ligament and the fibrous ligaments in the breast. Also, in the treatment of aneurysms, was the first to ligate the carotid artery and the abdominal aorta. Said to be one of the hardest working surgeons in history and was also one of the wealthiest. He famously reported a straightforward haemorrhoidectomy resulting in mortality due to blood loss.

Harvey Cushing – trained at Yale and Harvard, Boston. Neurosurgeon who is known for describing the pituitary tumour that causes Cushing's syndrome. Also produced the first ever anaesthetic chart and introduced the practice of measuring blood pressure intraoperatively.

Fascia of Denonvilliers – fascia between the prostate and the rectum named after French anatomist Charles Denonvilliers.

Pouch of Douglas – The rectouterine pouch named after James Douglas (anatomist and obstetrician).

Baron Guillaume Dupuytren – French professor of surgery. Named contractures of the palmar and plantar fascia. Also pioneered lower jaw excision, excision of the cervix and lumbar colostomy. Spectacularly rose from poverty to extreme wealth; it has been said that he was forced to use cadavers' fat for the oil in his lamp whilst a student. Extremely hard working and enthusiastic, he was unable to take any criticism: 'First among surgeons, last among men'. The beast at the Seine, the brigand of the Hôtel-Dieu, the miser who would give the king one million francs, the Napoleon of surgery.

Sir Peter Freyer (1852–1921) – urologist from Belfast. Adept at crushing bladder stones using the lithotrite, was rewarded handsomely by the Rajah of Rampur for his work. Gave his name to the 'Freyer prostatectomy' involving a suprapubic approach with bladder drainage through a suprapubic tube. Caused much controversy when he announced that he was the first person to perform a total prostatectomy. This was not true and in response Freyer quoted Sidney Smith by saying, 'man is not the discoverer of any art who first says the thing, but he who says it so long and so loud and so clearly that he compels mankind to hear him'.

Sir Harold Gillies – plastic surgeon from St Bartholomew's Hospital. Famous for his reconstructive work during World War I and, of course, his forceps.

Robert James Graves (1797–1853) – Irish physician; besides his disease he also described angioneurotic oedema, scleroderma, erythromyalgia and the pin-hole pupil from pontine bleeding. Sometimes sarcastic; in dealing with a colleague's attack on the use of the stethoscope which he and Stokes advocated, he wrote, 'We suspect Dr Clutterbuck's sense of hearing must be injured: for him the 'ear trumpet' magnifies but distorts sound, rendering it less distinct than before'. Henry Clutterbuck 1770 – 1856.

William Stewart Halsted (born 1852) – American surgeon. Surgical career took a turn for the worse when he became a cocaine addict whilst experimenting its local anaesthetic use. Fortunately overcame this addiction at 35, although apparently was never quite the same again. Gave his name to the radical mastectomy: removal of breast, chest wall muscles (pectoralis major and minor) and all lymph nodes in axilla. Also introduced the use of rubber gloves.

John Hilton – surgeon from Guy's Hospital, born in Essex in 1807. Coined 'Hilton's law' which states that a nerve crossing a joint supplies the joint and the muscles surrounding it. Also named 'Hilton's line' which is a white line at the junction of the perineum and the anal mucosa which is meant to be palpable. Conducted a series of famous lectures known as 'Rest and pain' whereby he encouraged the use of rest in the healing of damaged tissues: 'a man received a blow on the chest from a fall upon the part…I could find no fracture of the ribs; but I observed that the patient had a most worrying wife…… I requested that his wife should not say a word to him. From that time, he got quickly well by local rest'.

Thomas Hodgkin (1798–1866) – Guy's Hospital, London, physician and most prominent British pathologist of his time; described his disease in 1832. Unpopular with the board at Guy's because of his liberal and stubborn views, he was denied professional advancement. Despite his reputation in London he made no success of practice – having sat up all night with a wealthy patient, he was given a blank cheque which he filled in for £10, saying the man did not look like he could afford more; the patient did not consult him again. Many friends would not consult him as he would not accept a fee. Published a paper on AR 20 years before Corrigan, described the biconcavity of the RBC, and the first case of appendicitis where perforation was noted to be the cause of death. The obelisk, erected by his friend Sir Moses Montefiore, in his now forgotten and overgrown grave in Jaffa bears the inscription 'Here rests the body of Thomas Hodgkin MD of Bedford Square, London. A man distinguished alike for scientific attainments, medical skills and self-sacrificing philanthropy'.

Johann Horner – Swiss professor of ophthalmology. Described 'Horner's syndrome', sympathetic chain damage leading to ptosis and pupil constriction.

Houston's valves – John Houston, Irish surgeon. Described mucosal folds within the rectum.

John Hunter – 'the father of modern surgery'. Born in East Kilbride, near Glasgow in 1728. Famous for describing testicular descent, naming the gubernaculum and several studies involving grafting. He is also famous for his extensive pathological specimen collection–plants, humans and animals. What is left of them after the bombings of 1941 are displayed in the Royal College of Surgeons. Perhaps the greatest anatomist of all time, founded experimental pathology, and put surgery on a scientific footing which laid the foundations for the 20th century's developments. 'Don't think, try the experiment', sums up his attitude, which inspired generations of modern surgeons. His marriage was delayed due to his experiments on venereal disease. He believed two diseases could not exist in the same organ at the same time; thus gonorrhoea and syphilis were thought to be different symptoms of the same disease. He lanced his own glans and prepuce to inoculate himself with some fluid from a lesion found on a prostitute. Unfortunately for Hunter, and medicine for years to come, she had both syphilis and gonorrhoea – which were, and thus continued to be thought of as the same disease. There is some doubt as to whether this actually occurred but the cure is said to have taken 3 years. He paid £500 for the body of an Irish giant who had wished to be buried at sea to form part of his massive comparative anatomical collection. Died after an argument with the board of St George's Hospital, and was buried initially in St Martin's in the Fields. Later moved, to be one of only three doctors buried in Westminster Abbey.

Jonathan Hutchinson – performed the first successful operation for paediatric intussusception. Treatment prior to this involved the use of enemas and rectal bougies. Trained at St Bartholomew's Hospital, London, and coined 'Hutchinson's triad' (Hutchinson's teeth, interstitial keratitis and labyrinthine deafness seen in congenital syphilis). Also gave his name to 'Hutchinson's pupil,' seen in extra-dural haemorrhage where the pupil on the same side dilates and becomes unresponsive to light. Was knighted in 1908 (aged 80) after much arm twisting from his friends.

Gustav Killian – German ENT surgeon. Named the weak area occurring between the thyropharyngeus and cricopharyngeus within the inferior constrictor. 'Killian's dehiscence' is where a pharyngeal pouch is likely to occur.

Emil Kocher – Swiss surgeon. Named 'Kocher's incision' which is a subcostal approach to the gallbladder and also described a method of mobilizing the duodenum by incision of the lateral peritoneal fold.

Carl Koller (born 1884) – Vienna. First doctor to develop regional anaesthesia using cocaine to anaesthetize the eye.

Joseph Lister (born 1827) – UCL trained, son of a Quaker, born in Upton Park (now a council block in East London). Pioneered the antiseptic use of carbolic acid in compound fractures. Knighted in 1883.

Antoine Louis (1723–1792) – French surgeon, physiologist and historian. Was at the forefront of the struggle to free Parisian surgeons from the grasp of the domineering physicians; submitted his MD dissertation in Latin demonstrating that surgeons were as liberally educated as their physician peers. Shortly before his death, he began construction of an executing machine with Joseph Ignace Guillotine (1738–1814) that bears his co-inventor's name.

Charles McBurney (born 1845) – surgeon from New York, named a muscle-splitting incision for appendicectomy and 'McBurney's point' which is the usual site of tenderness associated with acute appendicitis: "very exactly between an inch and a half and two inches from the anterior spinous process of the ilium on a straight line drawn from that process to the umbilicus".

Ephraim McDowell – performed the first elective laparotomy in 1809 in Danville, Kentucky. The operation was an ovariotomy for a large ovarian cyst misdiagnosed as a full-term pregnancy. McDowell transported the lady to his house on horseback and performed the laparotomy in his front room. The house is now a museum. McDowell had a preference for operating on Sundays. The inscription on his tombstone reads: 'Beneath this shaft rests Ephraim McDowell MD, the father of ovariotomy......'

Johannes Freiherr Von Mikulicz–Radecki (born 1898) – Heineke–Mikulicz pyloroplasty, a gastric pyloroplasty used to enlarge the gastric outlet and thereby render it non-functional. The pylorus is opened using a longitudinal incision and closed transversely. It is used in conjunction with a truncal vagotomy for the treatment of peptic ulcer disease.

W T G Morton – administered the first public general anaesthetic using ether in Massachusetts, 1846. The operation was to remove a jaw tumour.

Sir William Osler (1849–1919) – Canadian physician and Regius Chair of Medicine at the University of Oxford. Upon leaving Johns Hopkins in 1905, he gave a good-bye lecture in which he referred to the 'relative uselessness of men over 40 years of age'. Founder of clinical bedside medicine – 'To study medicine without books is like going to sea on uncharted waters; to study medicine without patients is like not going to sea at all'.

Sir James Paget – surgeon from St Bartholomew's Hospital. Named Paget's disease of the bone and the nipple.

Ambrose Paré – 16th century French military surgeon, discovered that the use of ligatures in gunshot wounds was more effective than boiling water or hot iron cauterization. 'I dressed the wound and God healed him'.

Patey (surgeon from the Middlesex Hospital) – modified mastectomy, sparing the pectoralis major.

Eugen Alexander Polya – Polya's gastrectomy, a modification of Bilroth II. A posterior gastro-enterostomy involving resection of two thirds of the stomach with closure of the duodenal stump and anastomosis of the stomach to the duodenum.

Poupart's ligament – Francois Poupart was a French surgeon. He gave his name to the inguinal ligament.

Pringle's manoeuvre – named after James Pringle, Glaswegian surgeon. Involves controlling bleeding from the hepatic artery by compressing the foramen of Winslow.

Benjamin Pugh (born 1846) – writer, traveller, obstetrician and surgeon. Born in Shropshire and worked in Chelmsford. The first to invent an obstetric forceps with a pelvic curve. More famously remembered by anaesthetists as the first person to use an 'air pipe'. It was used in breech deliveries where he inserted the pipe, trans-vaginally, into the baby's larynx and blew in air to expand the lungs, thereby preventing suffocation. He also used the practice of mouth-to-mouth resuscitation on neonates which wasn't taken up for a further 20–30 years.

Wilhelm Conrad Röntgen (1845–1923) – professor of physics in the University of Würzburg. Developed the first ever X-ray of his wife's hand showing the bones of her hand and her wedding ring. Some physicians at the time thought X-rays were intrusive to clinical practice. Awarded a Nobel prize in 1901.

Scarpa's fascia – named after Antonio Scarpa, Italian professor of surgery. The fibrous layer of the superficial fascia of the abdominal wall.

Sharpey's fibres – fibres of connective tissue between periosteum and bone. Named after William Sharpey, professor of anatomy, UCL.

Shenton's line – Edward Warren Hine Shenton – a curved line visible on X-ray formed by the top of the obturator foramen and the inner neck of the femur. It is used to diagnose fractures or congenital dislocation of the head of the femur.

John Snow – anaesthetist; in 1853 in London, he administered chloroform to Queen Victoria whilst she gave birth to her eighth child. He was particularly concerned for the safety and comfort of his patients. He kept copious records of all anaesthetics he administered and particularly described the five stages of anaesthesia. Was the greatest anaesthetist of his time, never accepted a fee from a patient and died suddenly from apoplexy. His death was not acknowledged by the *BMJ* or *The Lancet*.

Sir Henry Sessions Souttar (born 1875) – a general surgeon trained at the London Hospital Medical School, performed the first mitral valvotomy on a 15-year-old girl. 'To hear a murmur is a very different matter from feeling the blood itself pouring back over one's finger'.

Sir Frederick Treves – surgeon from the London Hospital. Named 'the bloodless fold of Treves' otherwise known as the iliocaecal fold. Famous for operating on the appendix of King Edward VII in 1902.

John Collins Warren (1778–1856) – professor of surgery at Harvard and performed the first operation under ether anaesthesia at Massachusetts General Hospital, Boston. The operation involved the removal of a lump from Gilbert Abbot's neck.

Ernst Wertheim (born 1900) – radical abdominal hysterectomy developed for the treatment of cervical cancer. Involves removal of the uterus and as much parametrial tissue as possible.

Wharton's duct – Thomas Wharton – a 5 cm long duct belonging to the submandibular salivary gland which opens in the mouth lateral to the frenulum.

Samuel Alexander Wilson (1877 – 1937) – neurologist, Queen's Square, London. Offered five points of advice based on his experience: (i) never show surprise, (ii) never say the same thing twice to a patient, (iii) never believe what the patient says the doctor said, (iv) be decisive in your indecision, (v) never take a meal with your patient.

Foramen of Winslow – named after Jacob Winslow, French professor of anatomy. The foramen is the opening to the lesser sac (epiploic foramen).

ABBREVIATIONS

A – airway
ACTH – adrenocorticotrophic hormone
ADH – antidiuretic hormone
AIDS – acquired immunodeficiency syndrome
AP – anterior–posterior
ASD – atrial septal defect
ATN – acute tubular necrosis
αFP – alphafetoprotein
B – breathing
BCC – basal cell carcinoma
BSE – bovine spongiform encephalopathy
C – circulation
CABG – coronary artery bypass graft
CDK – cyclin-dependent kinases
CEA – carcino-embryonic antigen
CIN – cervical intra-epithelial neoplasia
CNS – central nervous system
CPR – cardiopulmonary resuscitation
CRP – c reactive protein
CSF – cerebrospinal fluid
CT scan – computerized tomography scan
CXR – chest X-ray
DCIS – ductal carcinoma in situ
DIC – disseminated intravascular coagulation
DNA – deoxyribonucleic acid
DVT – deep vein thrombosis
EBV – Epstein Barr virus
ECF – extracellular fluid
ECG – electrocardiograph
EGF – epidermal growth factor
ERCP – endoscopic retrograde cholangiopancreatography
ESR – erythrocyte sedimentation rate
FBC – full blood count
FDP – fibrin degradation products
FEVI – forced expiratory volume
FFP – fresh frozen plasma
FNA – fine-needle aspiration cytology
FVC – forced vital capacity
GFR – glomerular filtration rate
GIT – gastrointestinal tract
G+S – group and save (blood grouping)
5-HIAA – 5-hydroxyindole-acetic acid
HIV – human immunodeficiency virus
HPV – human papilloma virus
HTLV 1 – human T lymphotrophic virus 1

IgE – immunoglobulin E
IGF – insulin-like growth factor (I and II)
IMS – industrial methylated spirit
LCIS – lobular carcinoma in situ
LFT – liver function tests
MEN syndrome – multiple endocrine neoplasia syndrome (I and II)
MRI – magnetic resonance imaging
NO – nitric oxide
nCJD – new variant Creutzfeld Jacob disease
PAOP – pulmonary artery occlusion pressure
PDGF – platelet-derived growth factor
PE – pulmonary embolus
PLAP – placental alkaline phosphatase
PR – per rectum
PVS – persistent vegetative state
RNA – ribonucleic acid
SCC – squamous cell carcinoma
SCID – severe combined immune deficiencies (T and B lymphocytes)
SHO – senior house officer
T4 – thyroxine
TB – tuberculosis
TED stocking – anti-embolism stocking
TGFβ – transforming growth factor β
TPA – tissue plasminogen activator
TPN – total parenteral nutrition
TSH – thyroid stimulating hormone
U+E – urea and electrolytes
UV – ultraviolet
VMA – vanillyl mandelic acid
VSD – ventricular septal defect
WCC – white cell count
X-match – cross-match of blood prior to transfusion

USEFUL DEFINITIONS

Abscess – pocket of pus surrounded by granulation tissue.

Aneurysm – an abnormal dilatation of a blood vessel/the heart.

Autopsy – post-mortem examination or 'necropsy'. Used to determine the cause of death.

Biopsy – an examination of tissues: needle/endoscopic/incisional.

Chemical pathology – the diagnosis of disease from chemical changes in body tissues or fluids.

Cyst – a fluid-filled space lined with epithelium.

Cytology – the examination of dispersed cells i.e. FNA from a breast lump.

Cytopathology – the investigation and diagnosis of disease from individual cells.

Disease – an abnormality that manifests itself with clinical symptoms and signs.

Endotoxins – lipopolysaccharides from the cell wall of gram negative bacteria i.e. *E. coli*.

Exotoxins – enzymes secreted from bacteria i.e. pseudomembranous colitis (*Clostridium difficile*).

Fistula – an abnormal connection between two epithelial surfaces, lined with granulation tissue.

Forensic pathology – 'legal pathology'. The investigation of death due to suspicious causes.

Genetic defects – abnormalities which may be inherited or acquired:
- Autosomal dominant – structural lesions affecting adults
- Autosomal recessive – biochemical lesions affecting children.

Genetic polymorphisms – genetic variations that determine eye, hair, skin colour etc. and may predispose to certain diseases.

Histopathology – the investigation and diagnosis of disease from the examination of tissues.

Infarction – necrosis secondary to obstruction of the circulation.

Sinus – an abnormal connection between a fluid-filled space/abscess and skin/mucosa, lined with granulation tissue.

venous blood oxygenation 239
venous cutdown 96, 97
ventilation 302
 in acute respiratory distress syndrome 307
ventilation—cont'd
 and brainstem death 281
 mechanical 302–3, 306
 complications 303
 mechanics of 247–8
 after respiratory failure 305–6
ventilation–perfusion mismatch 248, 249,
 250–1, 303
ventilation–perfusion ratio 94, 251
ventricular failure 262
ventricular filling, excessive 237
ventricular systole 262
Venturi mask 301
vertebrae
 cervical 69
 thoracic 68–9
 vertebra prominens 69
vertebral column 67–70
viral infection 316
viruses
 carcinogenic 166–7
 HIV 167
 testing donated blood 231
 see also specific viruses
vitamin D 272
vitellointestinal duct 11
vocal cords 41, 60
voice disorders 60–1, 114
vomiting
 in cervical spine injuries 136
 with small bowel obstruction 123–4

walking phases 32–3
warfarin 109
web space infections 22
'wedged' radiation fields 207
whiplash 135
Whipple's operation 88, 89
WHO guidelines for screening programs 212
wound closure 132–3
 abscesses 83
 delayed primary/secondary 133
 difficult/inappropriate 201
 emergency fasciotomy 135
 lymph node biopsy 79
 options to direct skin closure 202
 sternotomy 119
wound dehiscence 204–5
 abdominal, management of 205
 general/local risk factors 204
wound dressing 84
wound healing 153–4
 cell growth factors in 149
 factors affecting 133
 factors controlling/delaying 154
 by primary/secondary intention 154

X-rays in spinal injuries 135, 136

yolk sac 7

Ziehl–Neilson stain 159
zygomatic arch 70

Lightning Source UK Ltd.
Milton Keynes UK
31 March 2010

152162UK00001B/19/P